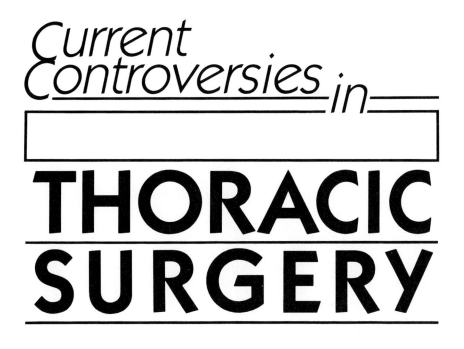

Current Controversies in THORACIC SURGERY

C. Frederick Kittle, M.D.

Professor of Surgery
Rush Medical College
Director, Section of Thoracic Surgery
Rush-Presbyterian-St. Luke's Medical Center
Chicago, Illinois

1986

W. B. Saunders Company

PHILADELPHIA □ LONDON □ TORONTO □ MEXICO CITY
RIO DE JANEIRO □ SYDNEY □ TOKYO □ HONG KONG

W. B. Saunders Company: West Washington Square
Philadelphia, PA 19105

Library of Congress Cataloging in Publication Data

Main entry under title:

Current controversies in thoracic surgery.

1. Chest—Surgery.   I. Kittle, C. Frederick.   II. Title: Thoracic surgery.   [DNLM: 1. Thoracic Surgery.   WF 980 C976]

RD536.C87   1985   617'.54059   85–2387

ISBN 0–7216–5461–4

Editor: Carroll Cann
Designer: Terri Siegel
Manuscript Editor: Elizabeth Galbraith
Production Manager: Bill Preston

Current Controversies in Thoracic Surgery   ISBN   0–7216–5461–4

Last digit is the print number: 9   8   7   6   5   4   3   2   1

Dedicated to
Ann, Candace, Bradley, Leslie, and Brian
for their understanding, love, and encouragement.

Contributors

AMJAD ALI, M.D.

Associate Professor, Rush Medical College, Chicago, Illinois; Associate Attending, Department of Diagnostic Radiology and Nuclear Medicine, Rush-Presbyterian–St. Luke's Medical Center, Chicago, Illinois

The Use of Radionuclide Scans in Lung Cancer: The Case for Routine Multiorgan Scans

KAREN H. ANTMAN, M.D.

Assistant Professor of Medicine, Harvard Medical School, Boston, Massachusetts; Assistant Physician, Dana-Farber Cancer Institute, and Associate Physician, Brigham & Women's Hospital, Boston, Massachusetts

Malignant Pleural Mesothelioma: A Combined Modality Approach

PHILIP G. ARNOLD, M.D.

Associate Professor of Surgery, Mayo Medical School, Rochester, Minnesota; Consultant in Plastic and Reconstructive Surgery, Department of Surgery, Mayo Clinic and Mayo Foundation, Rochester, Minnesota

Muscle Flaps and Thoracic Problems: Chest Wall Defects: Reconstruction with Autogenous Tissue

CHRISTOS A. ATHANASOULIS, M.D.

Professor of Radiology, Harvard Medical School, Boston, Massachusetts; Head, Section of Vascular Radiology, Massachusetts General Hospital, Boston, Massachusetts

The Management of Massive Hemoptysis: Control by Angiographic Methods

MANJIT S. BAINS, M.D.

Associate Professor, Cornell University Medical College, New York, New York; Associate Attending Surgeon (Thoracic), Memorial Sloan-Kettering Cancer Center, New York, New York

The Extent of Resection for Localized Lung Cancer: Lobectomy

ROBERT BOJAR, M.D.

Assistant Professor of Surgery (Cardiothoracic), Tufts University School of Medicine, Boston, Massachusetts; Assistant Surgeon, Department of Cardiothoracic Surgery, Tufts-New England Medical Center, Boston, Massachusetts

The Surgical Management of Recurrent or Persistent Pneumothorax: Pleurectomy Pneumothorax

JAY B. BRODSKY, M.D.

Associate Professor of Anesthesia, Stanford University School of Medicine, Stanford, California; Director of Anesthesia Services, Operating Rooms, Stanford University Medical Center, Stanford, California

Management of Postoperative Thoracotomy Pain: Lumbar Epidural Narcotics

JOEL D. COOPER, M.D.

Professor, Department of Surgery, Faculty of Medicine, University of Toronto, Toronto, Ontario; Head, Division of Thoracic Surgery, Toronto General Hospital, Toronto, Ontario

The Use of Mediastinoscopy in Lung Cancer: Preoperative Evaluation

JOSEPH M. CORSON, M.D.

Professor of Pathology, Harvard Medical School, Boston, Massachusetts; Chief, Surgical Pathology Division, Brigham & Women's Hospital, Boston, Massachusetts

Malignant Pleural Mesothelioma: A Combined Modality Approach

TOM R. DeMEESTER, M.D.

Professor of Thoracic and Cardiovascular Surgery, Creighton University School of Medicine, Omaha, Nebraska; Chief of Surgery, St. Joseph Hospital, Omaha, Nebraska

The Use of Radionuclide Scans in Lung Cancer: Gallum-67 Scanning for Preoperative Staging

JAMES DUCKETT, M.D.

Clinical Assistant Professor of Anesthesia, University of Pennsylvania School of Medicine, Philadelphia, Pennsylvania

The Use of Lasers for Tracheobronchial Lesions: Utilization of Nd:YAG Lasers for Endobronchial Lesions

TIMOTHY DUPONT, M.D.

Anesthesiologist, Mercy Hospital, San Diego, California

Management of Postoperative Thoracotomy Pain: Intermittent Epidural Infusion of Morphine

MARLENE R. ECKSTEIN, M.D.

Assistant Professor of Radiology, Harvard Medical School, Boston, Massachusetts; Assistant Radiologist, Massachusetts General Hospital, Boston, Massachusetts

The Management of Massive Hemoptysis: Control by Angiographic Methods

NABIL M. EL-BAZ, M.D.

Assistant Professor of Anesthesiology, Rush Medical College, Chicago, Illinois; Associate Attending Anesthesiologist, Rush-Presbyterian–St. Luke's Medical Center, Chicago, Illinois

Management of Postoperative Thoracotomy Pain: Continuous Epidural Infusion of Morphine; New Anesthetic Techniques for Intrathoracic Operations: One-Lung High-Frequency Ventilation for Thoracic Surgery

F. HENRY ELLIS, Jr., M.D., Ph.D.

Clinical Professor of Surgery, Harvard Medical School, Boston, Massachusetts; Chief of Section of Thoracic and Cardiovascular Surgery, Lahey Clinic Medical Center, Burlington, Massachusetts, and Division of Thoracic and Cardiovascular Surgery, New England Deaconess Hospital, Boston, Massachusetts

The Management of Zenker's Diverticulum: Cricopharyngeal Myotomy

L. PENFIELD FABER, M.D.

Professor of Surgery, Rush Medical College, Chicago, Illinois; Associate Dean, Surgical Sciences and Services, and Associate Vice President, Rush-Presbyterian–St. Luke's Medical Center, Chicago, Illinois

Malignant Pleural Mesothelioma: Operative Treatment by Extrapleural Pneumonectomy

ERNEST W. FORDHAM, M.D.

Professor of Diagnostic Radiology and Nuclear Medicine, Rush Medical College, Chicago, Illinois; Associate Chairman, Department of Diagnostic Radiology and Nuclear Medicine, and Director, Section of Nuclear Medicine, Rush-Presbyterian–St. Luke's Medical Center, Chicago, Illinois

The Use of Radionuclide Scans in Lung Cancer: The Case for Routine Multiorgan Scans

WILLARD A. FRY, M.D.

Associate Professor of Clinical Surgery, Northwestern University Medical School, Evanston, Illinois; Chief of Section of Thoracic Surgery, Evanston Hospital, Evanston, Illinois

Needle Biopsy for the Diagnosis of Intrathoracic Lesions: Transthoracic Needle Biopsy

ROBERT J. GINSBERG, M.D.

Associate Professor, University of Toronto, Toronto, Ontario; Surgeon-in-Chief and Head, Division of Thoracic Surgery, Mount Sinai Hospital, New York, New York

The Use of Mediastinoscopy in Lung Cancer: Preoperative Evaluation

JAIME O. HERRERA-HOYOS, M.D.

Critical Care Medicine, O'Horan University Hospital, Merida, Yucatan, Mexico

New Anesthetic Techniques for Intrathoracic Operations: High-Frequency Low-Compression Ventilation

LUCIUS D. HILL, M.D.

Head, Section of General, Thoracoesophageal, and Vascular Surgery, Virginia Mason Medical Center, and Clinical Professor of Surgery, University of Washington, School of Medicine, Seattle, Washington

The Management of Zenker's Diverticulum: The Utilization of Intraoperative Manometry

PAUL E. HOEKSEMA, M.D., Ph.D.

Professor of Otorhinolaryngology, State University, Groningen, the Netherlands; University Hospital, ENT-Department, Groningen, the Netherlands

The Management of Zenker's Diverticulum: Endoscopic Diverticulotomy

LAUREN D. HOLINGER, M.D.

Associate Professor, Rush Medical College, Chicago, Illinois, Instructor, Department of Otolaryngology–Head and Neck Surgery, Northwestern University Medical School, Chicago, Illinois, and Clinical Instructor, Department of Otolaryngology–Head and Neck Surgery, Abraham Lincoln School of Medicine, Chicago, Illinois; Associate Attending, Rush-Presbyterian–St. Luke's Medical Center, Chicago, Illinois, Active Attending Otolaryngologist, The Children's Memorial Hospital, Chicago, Illinois, and Section Head and Active Attending Bronchologist, University of Illinois Eye and Ear Infirmary, Chicago Illinois

The Management of Zenker's Diverticulum: Endoscopic (Dohlman) Diverticulotomy

ANTHONY D. IVANKOVICH, M.D.

Professor of Anesthesiology, Rush Medical College, Chicago, Illinois; Chairman of Anesthesiology and Senior Attending Anesthesiologist, Rush-Presbyterian–St. Luke's Medical Center, Chicago, Illinois

New Anesthetic Techniques for Intrathoracic Operations: One-Lung High-Frequency Ventilation; Continuous Epidural Infusion of Morphine

ROBERT J. JENSIK, M.D.

Professor of Surgery, Department of Cardiovascular-Thoracic Surgery, Rush Medical College, Chicago, Illinois, and Clinical Professor of Surgery, University of Illinois College of Medicine, Chicago, Illinois; Senior Attending, Cardiovascular-Thoracic Surgery, Rush-Presbyterian–St. Luke's Medical Center, Chicago, Illinois

The Extent of Resection for Localized Lung Cancer: Segmental Resection

C. FREDERICK KITTLE, M.D.

Professor of Surgery, Rush Medical College, Chicago, Illinois; Director, Section of Thoracic Surgery and Senior Attending, Rush-Presbyterian–St. Luke's Medical Center, Chicago, Illinois

The Surgical Management of Recurrent or Persistent Pneumothorax: Pleurectomy

RALPH J. LEWIS, M.D

Clinical Associate Professor of Surgery, University of Medicine and Dentistry of New Jersey, Piscataway, New Jersey; Chief of Thoracic and Cardiovascular Surgery, St. Peter's Medical Center, New Brunswick, New Jersey, and Somerset Medical Center, Somerville, New Jersey; Senior Attending, Thoracic and Cardiovascular Surgery, Middlesex General Hospital, New Brunswick, New Jersey, and Consultant, Thoracic and Cardiovascular Surgery, Hunterdon Medical Center, Flemington, New Jersey

Malignant Pleural Mesothelioma: A Nonsurgical Problem

ALEX G. LITTLE, M.D.

Associate Professor, University of Chicago Pritzker School of Medicine, Chicago, Illinois; Chief, Thoracic Surgery, University of Chicago Medical Center, Chicago, Illinois

The Use of Radionuclide Scans in Lung Cancer: Gallium-67 Scanning for Preoperative Staging; The Management of Zenker's Diverticulum: Cricopharyngeal Myotomy and Diverticulopexy

DONALD J. MAGILLIGAN, M.D.

Clinical Associate Professor of Surgery, University of Michigan Medical School, Ann Arbor, Michigan; Head, Division of Cardiac and Thoracic Surgery, Henry Ford Hospital, Detroit, Michigan

The Management of Massive Hemoptysis: Control by Bronchial Artery Embolization

JAMES B. D. MARK, M.D.

Johnson and Johnson Professor of Surgery, Stanford University School of Medicine, Stanford, California; Head, Division of Thoracic Surgery, Stanford Medical Center, Stanford, California

Thoracoscopy: Its Use for Diagnosis and Therapy; The Use of Radionuclide Scans in Lung Cancer: The Case Against Routine Multiorgan Scans

DAVID H. MARTIN, B.Sc., M.D., FRCP(C)

Respiratory Fellow, McMaster University, Hamilton, Ontario

Thoracoscopy: A Clinical Perspective

NAEL MARTINI, M.D.

Professor of Surgery, Cornell University Medical College, New York, New York; Chief, Thoracic Surgery, Memorial Sloan-Kettering Cancer Center, New York, New York

Malignant Pleural Mesothelioma: Operative Treatment by Pleurectomy; The Extent of Resection for Localized Lung Cancer: Lobectomy

STEPHEN J. MATHES, M.D.

Professor of Surgery, University of California, San Francisco, California; Head, Division of Plastic and Reconstructive Surgery, University of California Medical Center, San Francisco, California

Muscle Flaps and Thoracic Problems: Coverage of a Chronic and Infected Mediastinal Wound

BRIAN C. McCAUGHAN, M.B., B.S.

Royal Prince Alfred Hospital, Sydney, Australia

The Extent of Resection for Localized Lung Cancer: Lobectomy

PATRICIA M. McCORMACK, M.D.

Assistant Professor of Surgery, Cornell University Medical School, New York, New York; Assistant Attending Surgeon, Thoracic Service, Memorial Sloan-Kettering Cancer Center, New York, New York

Malignant Pleural Mesothelioma: Operative Treatment by Pleurectomy; The Extent of Resection for Localized Lung Cancer: Lobectomy

RICHARD McELVEIN, M.D.

Associate Professor of Surgery, University of Alabama at Birmingham, Birmingham, Alabama; Chief, Division of Thoracic Surgery, University of Alabama Hospitals and Veterans Administration Hospital, Birmingham, Alabama, and Assistant Chief of Staff, University of Alabama Hospitals, Birmingham, Alabama

The Use of Lasers for Tracheobronchial Lesions: Treatment of Obstructing Lesions by the Carbon Dioxide Laser

JOHN H. MEHNERT, M.D.

Active Teaching Service, Mercy Hospital, San Diego, California; Active Surgical Staff, Mercy, Sharp Memorial, Sharp Cabillo, Children's and Harbor View Hospitals, San Diego, California

Management of Postoperative Thoracotomy Pain: Intermittent Epidural Infusion of Morphine

C. DALE MERCER, M.D., FRCS(C)

Assistant Professor of Surgery, Queen's University, Kingston, Ontario, and Former Howard Wright Fellow, Virginia Mason Medical Center, Seattle, Washington; Attending Staff, Kingston General Hospital and Hotel Dieu Hospital, Kingston, Ontario

The Management of Zenker's Diverticulum: The Utilization of Intraoperative Manometry

JOSEPH I. MILLER, M.D.

Associate Professor of Cardiothoracic Surgery, Emory University School of Medicine, Atlanta, Georgia; Attending Cardiothoracic Surgeon, Emory University Hospital, Crawford W. Long Memorial Hospital, Piedmont Hospital, and Atlanta Veterans Administration Hospital, Atlanta, Georgia

Muscle Flaps and Thoracic Problems: Applicability and Utilization for Various Conditions

MICHAEL T. NEWHOUSE, M.D., M.Sc., FRCP(C), FACP

Clinical Professor of Medicine, McMaster University Medical School, Hamilton, Ontario; Chief, Service of Respirology and Head, Firestone Regional Chest and Allergy Unit, St. Joseph's Hospital, Hamilton, Ontario

Thoracoscopy: A Clinical Perspective

DAVID D. OAKES, M.D.

Associate Professor of Surgery, Stanford University School of Medicine, Stanford, California; Chief, General and Thoracic Surgery, Santa Clara Valley Medical Center, San Jose, California

Thoracoscopy: Its Use for Diagnosis and Therapy

PETER C. PAIROLERO, M.D.

Associate Professor of Surgery, Mayo Medical School, Rochester, Minnesota; Consultant in Sections of Thoracic and Cardiovascular Surgery and of Vascular Surgery, Mayo Clinic and Foundation, Rochester, Minnesota

The Management of Zenker's Diverticulum: Diverticulectomy; The Surgical Management of Recurrent or Persistent Pneumothorax: Abrasive Pleurodesis; Muscle Flaps and Thoracic Problems: Chest Wall Defects: Reconstruction with Autogenous Tissue

GRANT V. PARR, M.D.

Clinical Associate Professor of Surgery, University of Pennsylvania School of Medicine, Philadelphia, Pennsylvania; Chief, Division of Thoracic and Cardiovascular Surgery, Presbyterian-University of Pennsylvania Medical Center, Philadelphia, Pennsylvania

The Use of Lasers for Tracheobronchial Lesions: Utilization of Nd:YAG Lasers for Endobronchial Lesions

W. SPENCER PAYNE, M.D.

Professor of Surgery, Mayo Medical School, Rochester, Minnesota; Consultant in Section of Thoracic and Cardiovascular Surgery, Mayo Clinic and Mayo Foundation, Rochester, Minnesota and Consultant in Thoracic Surgery, St. Mary's Hospital and Rochester Methodist Hospital, Rochester, Minnesota

The Management of Zenker's Diverticulum: Diverticulectomy; The Surgical Management of Recurrent or Persistent Pneumothorax: Abrasive Pleurodesis

JEFFREY M. PIEHLER, M.D.

Assistant Professor of Surgery, Mayo Medical School, Rochester, Minnesota; Consultant in Section of Thoracic and Cardiovascular Surgery, Mayo Clinic and Mayo Foundation, Rochester, Minnesota

The Management of Zenker's Diverticulum: Diverticulectomy

JAMES E. REJOWSKI, M.D.

Instructor, Rush Medical College, Chicago, Illinois; Active Staff, Hinsdale Hospital, Hinsdale, Illinois, and Attending Staff, La Grange Memorial Hospital, La Grange, Illinois

The Management of Zenker's Diverticulum: Endoscopic (Dohlman) Diverticulotomy

JAMES W. RYAN, M.D.

Associate Professor, Department of Radiology (Nuclear Medicine), University of Chicago Medical School, Chicago, Illinois; Chief, Section of Nuclear Medicine, University of Chicago Medical Center, Chicago, Illinois

The Use of Radionuclide Scans in Lung Cancer: Gallium-67 Scanning for Preoperative Staging

SHUJI SEKI, M.D.

Associate Professor, Acute Medicine, Okayama University School of Medicine, Okayama, Japan; Department of Acute Medicine, Okayama University Hospital, Okayama, Japan

New Anesthetic Techniques for Intrathoracic Operations: High-Frequency Ventilation

RICHARD J. SHEMIN, M.D.

Assistant Professor of Surgery, Harvard Medical School, Boston, Massachusetts; Associate Cardiovascular Surgeon, Brigham & Women's Hospital, Consultant in Surgery, Dana-Farber Cancer Institute and West Roxbury VA Medical Center, Associate in Cardiac Surgery, Children's Hospital Medical Center, and Medical Director, Cardiac Surgical Intensive Care Unit, Brigham & Women's Hospital, Boston, Massachusetts

Malignant Pleural Mesothelioma: A Combined Modality Approach

JOHN P. SHERCK, M.D.

Clinical Assistant Professor of Surgery, Stanford University School of Medicine, Stanford, California; Associate Chief, General Surgery, Santa Clara Valley Medical Center, San Jose, California

Thoracoscopy: Its Use for Diagnosis and Therapy

P. C. SHETTY, M.D.

Senior Staff Radiologist, Henry Ford Hospital, Detroit, Michigan

The Management of Massive Hemoptysis: Control by Bronchial Artery Embolization

THOMAS W. SHIELDS, M.D.

Professor of Surgery, Northwestern University Medical School, Evanston, Illinois; Chief of Surgery, Veterans Administration Lakeside Medical Center, Chicago, Illinois, and Attending in Surgery, Northwestern Memorial Hospital, Evanston, Illinois

The Use of Mediastinoscopy in Lung Cancer: The Dilemma of Mediastinal Lymph Nodes

MARK S. SHULMAN, M.D.

Assistant Professor of Anesthesia, Stanford University School of Medicine, Stanford, California; Attending Anesthesiologist, Stanford University Medical Center, Stanford, California

Management of Postoperative Thoracotomy Pain: Lumbar Epidural Narcotics

ULF H. SJÖSTRAND, M.D., Ph.D.

Professor and Chairman of Anesthesiology, Örebro Medical Center Hospital, Örebro, Sweden; Clinical Professor of Anesthesiology, The University of Texas Health Science Center at San Antonio, San Antonio, Texas

New Anesthetic Techniques for Intrathoracic Operations: High-Frequency Low-Compression Ventilation

DAVID B. SKINNER, M.D.

Chairman and Dallas B. Phemister Professor, Department of Surgery, University of Chicago, Chicago, Illinois

The Management of Zenker's Diverticulum: Cricopharyngeal Myotomy and Diverticulopexy

R. BRIAN SMITH, M.D.

Professor and Chairman, Department of Anesthesiology, University of Texas Health Science Center at San Antonio, San Antonio, Texas; Anesthesiologist, Bexar County Hospital District, Consultant Anesthesiologist, Audie Murphy Veterans Hospital, and Consultant Anesthesiologist, State Chest Hospital, San Antonio, Texas

New Anesthetic Techniques for Intrathoracic Operations: One-Lung High-Frequency Ventilation

PAUL A. THOMAS, M.D.

Professor of Surgery, University of Illinois College of Medicine, Chicago, Illinois; Chief, Surgical Service, Veterans Administration West Side Medical Center, Attending Surgeon, University of Illinois Hospital, and Attending Surgeon, Cook County Hospital, Chicago, Illinois

Thoracoscopy: An Old Procedure Revisited

MICHAEL UNGER, M.D.

Assistant Professor of Clinical Medicine, University of Pennsylvania School of Medicine, Philadelphia, Pennsylvania; Associate Chief, Pulmonary Section, Presbyterian-University of Pennsylvania Medical Center, Philadelphia, Pennsylvania

The Use of Lasers for Tracheobronchial Lesions: Utilization of Nd:YAG Lasers for Endobronchial Lesions

JOSEPH J. M. VAN OVERBEEK, M.D., Ph.D.

Clinical Instructor and Staff Member, Department of Otolaryngology, State University, Groningen, the Netherlands; University Hospital Groningen and Deaconess Hospital Groningen, Groningen, the Netherlands

The Management of Zenker's Diverticulum: Endoscopic Diverticulotomy

ARTHUR C. WALTMAN, M.D.

Associate Professor of Radiology, Harvard Medical School, Boston, Massachusetts; Associate Radiologist, Massachusetts General Hospital, Boston, Massachusetts

The Management of Massive Hemoptysis: Control by Angiographic Methods

KO-PEN WANG, M.D.

Associate Professor of Medicine (Respiratory) and Otolaryngology, and Director of Panendoscopy Research and Training Program, Johns Hopkins Hospital, Baltimore, Maryland

Needle Biopsy for the Diagnosis of Intrathoracic Lesions: Transbronchial Needle Biopsy

DOV WEISSBERG, M.D., F.R.C.S.(C), F.A.C.S., F.C.C.P.

Visiting Assistant Professor of Surgery, Albert Einstein College of Medicine, New York, New York; Chief, Department of Thoracic and General Surgery, E. Wolfson Hospital, Holon, Israel

The Surgical Management of Recurrent or Persistent Pneumothorax: Pleuroscopy and Talc Poudrage

GEORGE L. ZORN, JR., M.D.

Associate Professor of Surgery, University of Alabama at Birmingham, Birmingham, Alabama; University of Alabama Hospitals, Birmingham, Alabama

The Use of Lasers for Tracheobronchial Lesions. Treatment of Obstructing Lesions by the Carbon Dioxide Laser

PREFACE

Controversy has existed since communication between people began; it is an inherent and basic intellectual characteristic. Whether we designate these conversations as Socratic, erotetic, Fabian, lively, or simply a weekly case conference, in the practice of medicine they serve the purpose of examining old and new concepts and of reviewing their assumptions, their purpose, their experiential data, and their justification. The strength and quality of our existence depend upon maintaining past beliefs as long as they are rational and logical, replacing them when they become incorrect or obsolete, and realizing that the dimension of time inevitably brings new diseases and new problems requiring new solutions.

This volume was planned to provide the reader with informative, logical, and cogent discussions about important controversies in the daily practice of thoracic surgery. The various viewpoints are presented without editorial bias; the reader must decide for himself and by his own rational judgment which opinion he can accept. Like the fable about the blind men describing an elephant, a final picture is best achieved by the logical integration of many viewpoints. Regardless of the eloquence of its presentation, any arbitrary authoritative imposition of conclusions without understanding and logic should be avoided. Obviously all the current unsettled issues in thoracic surgery cannot be listed and discussed here, since for some sufficient information is not available, and for others a definite opinion has not been formulated.

The introductory comments to each section provide perspective and additional information for the general topic. Often the historical aspects are given. History allows us to stand on the shoulders of our predecessors and reminds us that opinions once strongly enunciated have changed and that they may change again in the future.

The practice of surgery depends on the ability and ease with which we can answer for any problem the *what* (the pathology, the anatomy, the physiology, and so forth), the *how* (the technique, the preoperative and postoperative care), and the *why* (the results—immediate and late). This contrasts with the authoritarian approach, so prevalent and accepted in previous centuries.

I am grateful and bear a continuing debt of appreciation to my associates, L. Penfield Faber, Robert J. Jensik, Frank J. Milloy, and William H. Warren, who in their daily discussions and at frequent conferences constantly demonstrate the *what, how,* and *why* for general thoracic problems. They epitomize the general thoracic surgeon's approach to problem-solving and demand without hesitation a consideration of all alternatives before any acceptable decision is reached.

I am most thankful to the many contributors for their willingness to participate and cooperate in this endeavor. The valuable information they present and their lucid, well-organized discussions are the foundation stones for this volume.

To Hassan Najafi, my departmental chairman, I express deep gratitude for his encouragement in this undertaking and for his constant support, vision, and wisdom in developing the Section of Thoracic Surgery at our institution.

And to Carroll Cann, medical editor of the W. B. Saunders Co., I extend heartfelt appreciation and admiration for his frequent advice concerning the many problems of producing a book. His competence and ready availability, coupled with an unflagging and deft guidance, provided a pleasant journey in the completion of this work.

C. FREDERICK KITTLE, M.D.

CONTENTS

I

The Management of Zenker's Diverticulum

There is no satisfactory explanation as to why the name Ludlow is not used for the eponym for pharyngoesophageal diverticulum. After all, Abraham Ludlow was the first to describe this lesion (1767): "A Case of obstructed Deglutition, from a preternatural Dilatation of, and Bag formed in, the Pharynx; in a Letter from Mr. Ludlow, Surgeon, at Bristol, to Dr. William Hunter. Read Aug, 27, 1764 (sic)." (Fig. 1.)

In succeeding years, others wrote about this abnormality, but it remained for Friedrich Albert Zenker to establish eponymic fame when he and von Ziemssen (1877) presented 34 patients with this diverticulum, discussing its etiology, pathology, and symptoms. They were pessimistic about treatment: "The radical cure of diverticulum of the esophagus by operative procedure from without is—at the present time—one of our vain wishes."

Early efforts at treatment consisted of washing out the sac, tube feeding, bougienage, attempted obliteration of the pouch with silver nitrate, or faradization. Nicoladoni (1877) was apparently the first to operate on a pharyngeal diverticulum. The patient was a four-year-old child. In his procedure, he established an external fistula, thus allowing the contents of the diverticulum to drain to the outside, as had been previously suggested by Sir Charles Bell. Unfortunately, the patient died six days after surgery.

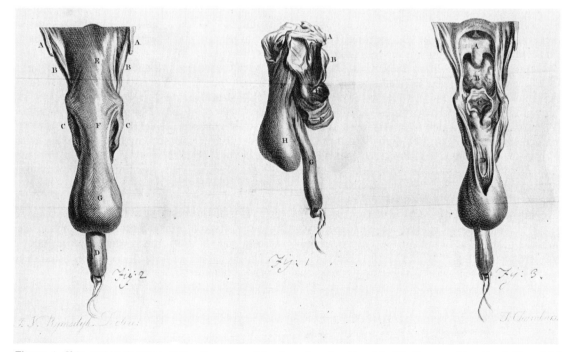

Figure 1. Side and back views of the pharynx and the "praeternatural bag" in "R. D. a considerable distiller of this city, near sixty years of age." Drawn by the famous Dutch medical artist Jan van Rymsdyk. Specimen 0.43 in the Hunterian Museum, Glasgow Royal Infirmary. (Plate 5, Ludlow, 1767.)

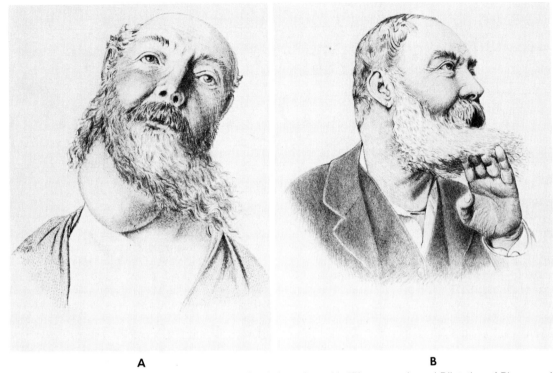

A   **B**

Figure 2. Pre and postoperative sketches of Mr. Wheeler's patient with "Pharyngocele and Dilatation of Pharynx with Existing Diverticulum at Lower Portion of Pharynx, Lying Posterior to the Oesophagus." Note that the first patient successfully operated on presented with Zenker's diverticulum on the right side! (1886).

Niehans of Berne attempted a one-stage excision of an esophageal diverticulum (1884) without success. The removal of a diverticulum was done with scissors in 1885 by a Dublin surgeon, Wheeler (1886). He operated on a 57-year-old male who presented with a right-sided pharyngeal diverticulum, which he termed an *aneurysma herniosa of the pharynx*. This was excised and closed by direct suture and the patient recovered uneventfully (Fig. 2).

Many other surgeons followed with reports of successful repairs for this diverticulum, each with some difference in operative technique. One of the more unusual operations was described by Girard (1896), who inverted the diverticulum into the lumen of the esophagus, a technique later revived by Bevan (1917).

To reduce the incidence of postoperative complications, the two-stage method of repair was introduced by Goldman (1909). Numerous modifications followed. Diverticulopexy or sacculopexy was proposed by Schmid (1912) and subsequently done by Hill (1918). In 1917 Mosher introduced an endoscopic method of treatment, popularized by Dohlman, "cutting the common wall" between the esophagus and the diverticulum.

Gradually the importance of the cricopharyngeus muscle was recognized. Jackson (1915) called attention to this structure, and in 1926 he clearly stated: "It is my opinion, based on oesophagoscopic studies, that it is the barrier presented to the advance of the bolus by the unrelaxed cricopharyngeus that is the functional factor that herniates the pharyngeal wall, thus creating the pharyngeal diverticulum.

With over a century of operative experience, no other structure or abnormality of the entire body has had so many different procedures devised for its treatment—and still the controversy continues.

1

The Management of Zenker's Diverticulum: Diverticulectomy

W. Spencer Payne, M.D.
Peter C. Pairolero, M.D.
Jeffrey M. Piehler, M.D.

Although pharyngoesophageal diverticulum has been appreciated clinically for more than 200 years,[8] its management still is controversial. Over the past century, a variety of techniques have been suggested, but only a few persist in current practice: (1) one-stage transcervical diverticulectomy with or without cricopharyngeal myotomy,[10, 14] (2) myotomy alone,[3, 12] (3) myotomy and diverticulopexy,[1] and (4) transoral endoscopic diathermic division of the common septum between the hypopharyngeal sac and upper esophagus.[2, 5, 13]

At the Mayo Clinic a one-stage transcervical diverticulectomy was first employed by W. J. Mayo and was subsequently modified and refined by S. W. Harrington and O. T. Clagett.[9] In recent decades we have added the use of a stapling device for diverticulectomy,[4] myotomy alone for small diverticula, and myotomy as an adjunct to diverticulectomy for more advanced diverticula.[10]

Since the Mayo Clinic experience is almost entirely confined to one-stage diverticulectomy, we will limit the present discussion to that and refer the reader to reports of others who champion diverticulopexy[1] or endoscopic diathermic treatment.[2, 5, 13]

ETIOLOGY

The cause of pharyngoesophageal diverticulum is not known. That it is an acquired problem, not congenital, seems almost certain, because the youngest patient in our series of more than 800 was 28 years of age. The diagnosis usually is made in the sixth through ninth decades of life (Fig. 1–1).

A variety of motility disturbances have been postulated as causes, ranging from a hypertensive cricopharyngeal (upper esophageal) sphincter[11] to an achalasia-type disorder in which the upper esophagus fails to relax on swallowing.[12] Specific manometric study of pharyngoesophageal motility does not confirm either of these mechanisms. Indeed, the only mechanism that we have been able to define is best described as "cricopharyngeal incoordination," in which there is premature contraction of the upper esophageal sphincter during pharyngeal contraction.[3] Even this abnormality is not observed with every swallow, but it is seen with over 60% of swallows among all patients studied. Furthermore, such motility disturbances have been seen in every patient studied, regardless of diverticulum size or duration of symptoms. Other workers have not been able to confirm this Mayo Clinic motility observation. Nonetheless, the use of cricopharyngeal myotomy rests on the hypothesis that malfunction of the upper esophageal sphincter has some etiologic relation to the genesis of diverticula in this region.

CLINICAL FEATURES

The chief symptoms and findings in patients with Zenker's diverticulum are those of high cervical obstruction to swallowing with consequent retention and regurgitation of ingested solids and liquids. Deglutition may be noisy, breath foul, and nutrition impaired; and with respiratory aspiration, suppurative lung disease may be evident. More subtle presentations include only asthma or chronic cough, fever of unknown origin, weight loss, or just cervical dysphagia without regurgitation. Regardless of initial symptoms, the condition is progressive in respect to diverticula size and to the number, frequency, and severity of symptoms and complications. Although the chief complications are nutritional and respiratory, the social implications are often dominant and not infrequently are the patient's chief reason for seeking medical attention.

Because of the progressive nature of this condition and its potentially serious and lethal

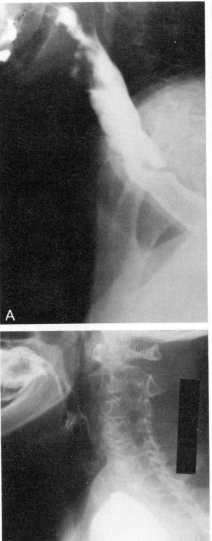

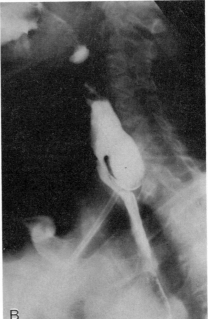

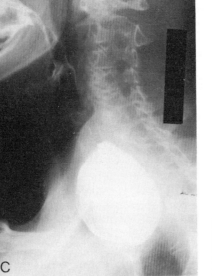

Figure 1–1. Pharyngoesophageal diverticula (lateral radiographic views): *A*, small; *B*, moderate; *C*, large. (From Payne WS: Esophageal diverticula. In Shields TW (ed): General Thoracic Surgery, 2nd ed. Philadelphia, Lea & Febiger, 1983, p. 859.)

consequences if untreated, we recommend surgical treatment whenever it is detected. Often, physicians are reluctant to permit operations on elderly patients. However, the recurrent hypoxic episodes associated with acute respiratory aspiration can prove serious or even fatal for those with compromised cerebral or coronary circulation. Furthermore, the risk associated with surgical intervention is so small that it should not be a significant factor in patient selection. Perforations of Zenker's diverticula, whether resulting from instrumen-

tation, foreign body ingestion, or external trauma, should be considered as emergencies requiring immediate surgical intervention.

Recurrent diverticula, though uncommon, constitute a special problem because of the severity of their symptoms and complications and also because of surgical risk. Indeed, in our experience[6] these are the most taxing and technically demanding diverticula.

Less well appreciated is the incidence of primary squamous cell carcinoma in chronic, neglected Zenker's diverticulum: It appears to

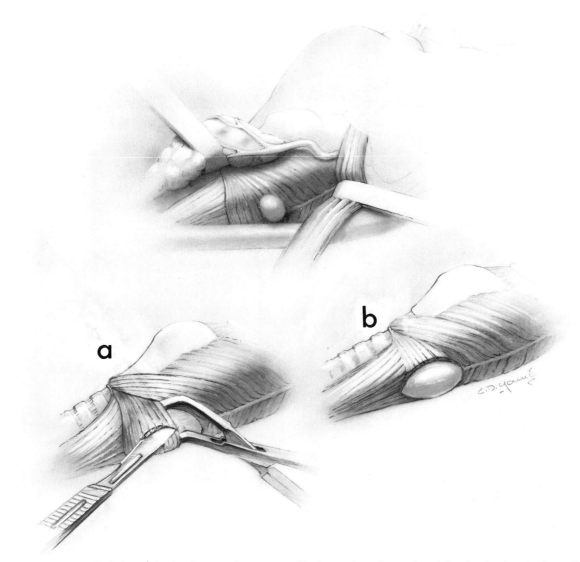

Figure 1–2. Technique of cricopharyngeal myotomy. Myotomy alone is employed for the treatment of small pharyngoesophageal diverticula. Surgical exposure of the retropharyngeal space is gained through an oblique left cervical incision oriented along the anterior border of the sternomastoid muscle (not shown). Retraction of the sternomastoid and carotid sheath laterally and of the thyroid, pharynx, and larynx medially provides necessary exposure of the diverticulum, which is located at the level at which the omohyoid crosses the surgical field. *Top,* Note that the omohyoid (at upper center of drawing) is retracted cephalad to show the diverticulum.

After connective tissue is dissected from mucosal sac to identify the defect in posterior pharyngeal wall *(a)*, a right-angle forceps is used to develop a dissection plane inferiorly between the muscularis and the mucosa. With a scalpel, a posterior midline extramucosal myotomy is effected from the neck of the small sac inferiorly for a distance of 3 cm. Retraction of the ends of the cut muscle *(b)* exposes an almond-shaped diffuse bulge of mucosa. A small Penrose drain is brought from the region of the myotomy and retropharyngeal space through the lower end of the cervical wound to the outside, and the platysma and skin are closed in layers around the drain. (From Payne WS: Esophageal diverticula. In Shields TW (ed): General Thoracic Surgery, 2nd ed. Philadelphia, Lea & Febiger, 1983, p. 859.)

be greater than in the general population.[7] Although carcinoma may develop in association with any esophageal diverticulum, it does not occur with such frequency as to constitute a major threat. On the other hand, diverticulectomy is preventive and has been curative in a few patients with in situ and early invasive diverticular malignancy.[7]

Finally, we offer a plea for early and prompt one-stage pharyngoesophageal diverticulectomy in the seriously ill patient with nutritional depletion or respiratory sepsis. Early operation restores the integrity of the swallowing mechanism and prevents continued respiratory soiling; antibiotics, chest physiotherapy, and parenteral alimentation then become more effective. There does not seem to be a place for gastrostomy or other nondefinitive delaying tactics in management of these seriously ill patients; it has been shown that the basic problem can be rectified by a definitive one-stage procedure effected with greater speed and safety than gastrostomy alone.

SURGICAL PROCEDURES

Cricopharyngeal Myotomy and Exposure of Diverticulum
(Fig. 1–2)

With the patient under general anesthesia and supine, and an endotracheal tube in place, the neck is prepared and draped from the chin to below the clavicles. A skin incision is made along the anterior border of the left sterno-mastoid muscle from the level of the hyoid bone to a point two fingerbreadths above the clavicle. The sternomastoid is retracted laterally to expose the strap muscles and the omohyoid. By blunt and sharp dissection, the retropharyngeal space is entered just cephalad to the omohyoid muscle. Goiter retractors draw the carotid sheath and its contents laterally and the larynx anteriorly and to the right. The cervical vertebral bodies form the floor of the space entered; the pharynx and esophagus are in front. The neck of the diverticulum is consistently just at the level of the upper border of the omohyoid as it crosses the anterior triangle of the neck to dip behind the sternomastoid muscle. A band retractor placed over the omohyoid to retract it caudally exposes the entire diverticulum.

One-stage Pharyngoesophageal Diverticulectomy with Myotomy
(Fig. 1–3)

The diverticular tip is grasped with an Allis forceps; and by sharp and blunt dissection, the diverticulum is separated from the back wall of the esophagus and retracted cephalad until its neck is identified. At this point, it is convenient and safe to have the anesthesiologist insert an esophageal stethoscope (28-F catheter) down the esophagus. Having direct vision, the surgeon can assist the progress of this tube past the diverticulum and into the upper portion of the esophagus.

The mucosal sac thus mobilized is seen to be ensheathed in a coat, 3 to 4 mm thick, of connective tissue and sparse attenuated muscle fibers. This coat is circumcised about the neck of the diverticulum, both to define the muscular defect in the pharynx through which the sac protrudes and to expose the neck of the mucosal sac for subsequent amputation. When this dissection is completed, there should be a collar of submucosa, 1 cm wide, clearly visible around the neck of the diverticulum. A posterior midline cricopharyngeal myotomy now can be effected, extramucosally, just below the neck of the diverticulum.

Blunt dissection with a right-angle forceps develops a dissection plane inferiorly between muscularis and mucosa. With the forceps in place, the muscle to be divided is put under tension and distracted away from mucosa for safe division by scissors or scalpel. This maneuver is repeated until a midline extramucosal myotomy, vertical and 3 to 4 cm long, is accomplished just below the neck of the diverticulum and until it is certain that all intervening muscle fibers are divided.

Up to this point, the esophageal stethoscope has served as a palpable landmark for the pharynx and esophagus. Now traction on the diverticulum, applied in preparation for its amputation, can compromise the lumen of the esophagus. The indwelling esophageal catheter is some protection against that. In an earlier period, we simply cross-clamped the neck of the diverticulum at the proposed point of division and, using a cut-and-sew technique,

---

Figure 1–3. One-stage pharyngoesophageal diverticulectomy with myotomy. This procedure is employed in the management of medium- and large-sized diverticula. *Top,* Medium-sized diverticulum exposed through left cervical incision, as for myotomy alone. Note that the omohyoid has been retracted cephalad and the diverticulum has been dissected out to its neck and its apex held cephalad. *a,* A right-angle forceps is used to develop a dissection plane between the muscularis and the mucosa just below the neck of the sac, in preparation for extramucosal myotomy with scalpel. *b,* After a 3-cm vertical myotomy is completed, the neck of the mucosal sac appears to have widened. *c,* With a 28-F catheter in the esophagus, a curved clamp is placed across the neck of the diverticulum at right angles to the long axis of the esophagus at the point of planned amputation. By a cut-and-sew technique, the sac is amputated stepwise and closed with fine vascular silk (5–0) placed so that tied knots are within the esophageal lumen. Alternatively, a stapling device can be used. *d,* Diverticulectomy and closure are completed. *e,* Vertical absorbable sutures are placed in the edges of the muscular defect after myotomy and diverticulectomy. *f,* This completed transverse closure provides a muscular layer closure over the mucosal suture line, which further minimizes leakage without restitution of the circopharyngeus. Drainage and closure are effected as with myotomy alone. (From Payne WS: Esophageal diverticula. In Shields TW (ed): General Thoracic Surgery, 2nd ed. Philadelphia, Lea & Febiger, 1983, p. 859.)

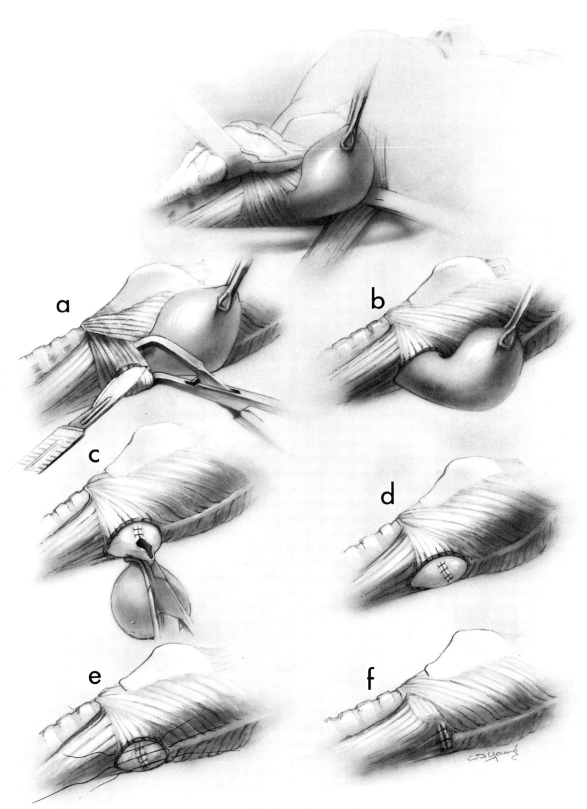

Figure 1–3. *See legend on opposite page*

divided the neck and closed it with 5–0 interrupted silk sutures. During the past 17 years, however, we have utilized the TA30 stapling device to effect closure; and we prefer it for both speed and accuracy of closure. Whichever technique is used, the axis of the amputation closure should be at right angles to the long axis of the esophagus. Thus, if a stricture is created (despite the indwelling catheter), it will be a short stricture and one more easily amenable to bougienage.

After amputation of the diverticulum, we have found it desirable to cover the mucosal closure with muscularis to prevent leakage. No leaks have occurred since we have adopted that precaution. This closure is effected by approximating the muscularis transversely and extramucosally with interrupted 3–0 absorbable suture material. No matter how dry the surgical field or how secure the suture line, we have never regretted the placement of two small cigarette-size Penrose drains in the retropharyngeal space, adjacent to the repair and leading to the outside through the lower end of the cervical incision, which is closed in layers with buried and absorbable suture material. The esophageal tube is removed and not replaced. Other than a wound dressing and a simple peripheral intravenous line for fluid administration, the patient is free of impediment on return to his room after the operative procedure has been completed.

On the day after the operation, a contrast roentgenogram of the esophagus is obtained. If there is no leakage, the oral diet is resumed and is rapidly upgraded to a solid, general diet during the next 72 hours. At that point, drainage tubes are shortened and removed if drainage is minimal. The patient is dismissed on the fourth postoperative day and may immediately resume full and normal activities as comfort permits.

Table 1–1. Complications and Recurrence following One-stage Pharyngoesophageal Diverticulectomy in 888 Mayo Clinic Cases, 1944–1978

Result	No. of Patients	% of Series
Morbidity		
Vocal cord paralysis	28	3.1
Wound infection	27	3.0
with fistula	16	1.8
Mortality	11	1.2
Recurrence	32	3.6

RESULTS

From 1944 through 1978, a series of 888 patients with Zenker's diverticulum underwent one-stage pharyngoesophageal diverticulectomy, with or without cricopharyngeal myotomy. The early and late results have been gratifying (Tables 1–1 and 1–2).

We reviewed the records of 70 randomized patients operated on since cricopharyngeal myotomy was added to diverticulectomy.[10] There were no deaths in this recent experience and no leaks when the procedure was performed as described. The results at follow-up 2 to 7 years postoperatively were essentially identical in respect to diverticular recurrence and vocal cord paralysis, whether or not myotomy was performed. There was one instance of leakage in the initial patient of the series, whose muscularis was not brought over the mucosal repair after diverticulectomy and myotomy. In all subsequent patients, muscle closure was done and no leakage was evident.

Although it is difficult to justify myotomy as an adjunct to diverticulectomy on the basis of this small series, we continue to employ it because we have noted less difficulty with

Table 1–2. Late Results (5–14 Years[a]) of One-stage Pharyngoesophageal Diverticulectomy[b]

Result		No. of Patients	% of Series
Highly satisfactory	Excellent	135	82 ⎫
	Good	18	11 ⎬ 93
Improved but symptomatic	Fair	5	3
Recurrence established	Poor	6	4
Total		164	100

[a]Identical with results in 888 patients at follow-up ranging from 1 to 20 years.
[b]Modified from Welsh GF, Payne WS: The present status of one-stage pharnygo-esophageal diverticulectomy. Surg Clin North Am 53:953, 1973.

swallowing in the face of anatomic recurrence and a decreased leakage rate when details of the operation were carried out thoroughly. Also, of nine additional patients with small diverticula treated by myotomy alone, seven had excellent results, but two had poor results, with diverticular progression sufficient to justify diverticulectomy.

Vocal paralysis, when it occurs after diverticular surgery, is unilateral and nearly always temporary. It results not from division of the recurrent laryngeal nerve but from traction. Recovery usually is complete by 6 to 12 months. Postoperative leakage with cervical cutaneous fistula did not prove to be a serious problem. With the drainage provided, all fistulas closed spontaneously in a week to 10 days.

Although not devoid of problems, diverticulectomy—with or without myotomy—is attended by minimal morbidity and mortality and has provided long-term satisfactory results in 93% of patients operated on.

References

1. Belsey R: Functional disease of the esophagus. J Thorac Cardiovasc Surg 52:164, 1966.
2. Dohlman G, Mattsson O: The endoscopic operation for hypopharyngeal diverticula: a roentgencinematographic study. Arch Otolaryngol 71:744, 1960.
3. Ellis FH Jr, Schlegel JF, Lynch VP, et al: Cricopharyngeal myotomy for pharyngo-esophageal diverticulum. Ann Surg 170:340, 1969.
4. Hoehn JG, Payne WS: Resection of pharyngoesophageal diverticulum using stapling device. Mayo Clin Proc 44:738, 1969.
5. Holinger PH, Schild JA: The Zenker's (hypopharyngeal) diverticulum. Ann Otol Rhinol Laryngol 78:679, 1969.
6. Huang B-S, Payne WS, Cameron AJ: Surgical management for recurrent pharyngoesophageal (Zenker's) diverticulum. Ann Thor Surg 37:189, 1984.
7. Huang B-S, Unni KK, Payne WS: Long-term survival following diverticulectomy for cancer in pharyngoesophageal (Zenker's) diverticulum. Ann Thor Surg 38:207, 1984.
8. Ludlow A: A case of obstructed deglutition, from a preternatural dilatation of, and bag formed in, the pharynx. Med Observ Inquir 3:85, 1767.
9. Payne WS, Clagett OT: Pharyngeal and esophageal diverticula. Curr Probl Surg p 3, 1965.
10. Payne WS, Reynolds RR: Surgical treatment of pharyngoesophageal diverticulum (Zenker's diverticulum). Surg Rounds 5:18, 1982.
11. Smiley TB, Caves PK, Porter DC: Relationship between posterior pharyngeal pouch and hiatus hernia. Thorax 25:725, 1970.
12. Sutherland HD: Cricopharyngeal achalasia. J Thorac Cardiovasc Surg 43:114, 1962.
13. Van Overbeek JJM: The Hypopharyngeal Diverticulum. Endoscopic Treatment and Manometry. Assen/Amsterdam, Van Gorcum, 1977.
14. Welsh GF, Payne WS: The present status of one-stage pharyngo-esophageal diverticulectomy. Surg Clin North Am 53:953, 1973.

2

The Management of Zenker's Diverticulum: Cricopharyngeal Myotomy

F. Henry Ellis, Jr., M.D., Ph.D.

Protrusion of the pharyngeal mucosa posteriorly between the oblique fibers of the inferior constrictor muscle of the pharynx and the transverse fibers of the cricopharyngeus muscle leads to a condition known as pharyngoesophageal (or Zenker's) diverticulum. First described in 1767 by Ludlow,[1] the condition gained association with Zenker's name in 1877 when he and von Ziemssen[2] collected 29 cases from the literature and added 5 of their own. They were the first workers to describe the nature of this diverticulum in detail, accurately identifying its anatomic location and theorizing about its cause. Primarily a condition of the elderly, pharyngoesophageal diverticulum is encountered more frequently now than in past years because of the increased longevity of the population.

ETIOLOGY

Although the cause of pharyngoesophageal diverticulum remains controversial, much has been learned about its nature since the introduction of esophageal manometry as a diagnostic tool. An understanding of the cause of upper esophageal pouches is pertinent to selection of proper therapy.

In 1919, Kelly[3] suggested that spasm occurred at the entrance of the esophagus in patients with the disease that became known later in Great Britain as Paterson-Kelly syndrome and in this country as Plummer-Vinson syndrome. Since Kelly's first observation, a variety of proposals have been offered to explain abnormalities of function of this portion of the esophagus. In addition to Kelly, a number of others have emphasized the role of cricopharyngeal spasm in certain disorders of swallowing. In 1946, Lahey[4] directed his attention to the cricopharyngeus muscle, implicating it in the cause of esophageal diverticulum and

advised forceful dilation of the muscle and surgical excision. Negus[5, 6] also advised dilation in patients with upper esophageal pouches although he considered cricopharyngeal incoordination, rather than spasm, to be the cause of the condition.

Delayed relaxation of the upper esophageal sphincter (UES) was considered an important mechanism by Cross and associates.[7] A related concept is that of cricopharyngeal achalasia in which, theoretically, the sphincter fails to relax. As early as 1926, Jackson and Shallow[8] postulated such a mechanism as being responsible for pharyngoesophageal diverticulum. Asherson[9] is usually given credit for introducing the term *cricopharyngeal achalasia* in 1950 as applied to various neuromuscular disorders affecting the cricopharyngeus muscle. Sutherland[10] revived the term in 1962 and implicated this mechanism in the development of pharyngoesophageal diverticulum.

Hunt and associates[11] and Smiley and coworkers[12] postulated that gastroesophageal reflux leads to cricopharyngeal spasm, which, in turn, results in the development of pharyngoesophageal diverticulum. This concept is based on the reported high incidence of hiatus hernia, 97% in one series,[13] occurring in association with Zenker's diverticulum. However, neither in my experience[14] nor in that of others are there data to support this view.[15, 16]

A more appealing explanation assigns primacy to incoordination of cricopharyngeal function as the cause of pharyngoesophageal diverticulum. Ardran and Kemp[17] in 1961, based on their radiographic studies of the upper food passages, proposed that premature contraction of the UES was the cause of upper esophageal dysphagia. Lund[18] has also described similar findings in instances of pharyngoesophageal diverticulum. The esophageal manometric studies carried out by myself and my colleagues[14, 19] in patients with pharyngoesophageal diverticula have supported the concept of premature contraction of the UES based on a high percentage of swallows in patients with upper esophageal pouches, a finding confirmed by others.[20–23] Recently, however, the concept has been called into question by Knuff and associates,[24] so the matter is far from settled.

The incoordination documented by esophageal manometry is characterized by premature relaxation and contraction of the UES so that the pharynx contracts against a closed sphincter, resulting in increased luminal pressures proximal to it. It is postulated that this increased pressure leads to outpouching of the mucosa and the development of a diverticulum. This concept is pertinent to my preference for cricopharyngeal myotomy as the treatment of choice for patients with pharyngoesophageal diverticula. In addition to incoordination of the UES, resting pressures of the sphincter in patients with upper esophageal pouches are slightly lower than normal. There is, therefore, no "spasm" in patients with upper esophageal pouches. Furthermore, the sphincter relaxes in response to swallowing in these patients, so that cricopharyngeal achalasia is not present.

TREATMENT

Early progressive enlargement characterizes the life history of pharyngoesophageal diverticulum. As the diverticulum enlarges, the upper esophageal pouch gives rise to dysphagia, noisy swallowing, regurgitation, and aspiration. Treatment is surgical and should be initiated when symptoms occur. Early surgical efforts employed before the turn of the century included extirpation, invagination of the diverticulum into the esophagus, and diverticulopexy, not all of which were successful. The first successful operation was a two-stage pharyngoesophageal diverticulectomy carried out by Goldmann[25] in 1909, although Mayo is generally credited with its development in the United States. This procedure was championed for many years, most recently by Lahey and Warren.[26] The one-stage operation favored earlier by Harrington[27] has gradually replaced the two-stage procedure and is now the most commonly employed technique. The largest reported series of one-stage pharyngoesophageal diverticulectomies is that by Welsh and Payne[28] from the Mayo Clinic, which included 809 patients with a 1.4% mortality rate. Residual or recurrent diverticula were detected in 3.3% of patients. Among those followed

from 5 to 14 years, 18% still experienced varying degrees of difficulty in swallowing. As a result, these workers now advise the performance of cricopharyngeal myotomy at the time of diverticulectomy.

The concept of purposely weakening the UES is not a new one. Reference has already been made to the use of forceful dilation in the management of patients with pharyngoesophageal diverticulum. Division of the septum or common wall between the esophagus and the diverticulum by endoscopic diathermy has been used by Dohlman and Mattsson[29] and is still preferred by some European otorhinolaryngologists.[30] The procedure of cricopharyngeal myotomy was a natural consequence of the introduction by Asherson of the term *achalasia* as applied to various neuromuscular disorders affecting the cricopharyngeal muscle. Whereas Harrison[31] employed cricopharyngeal myotomy combined with inversion of the diverticulum in three patients who had pharyngeal pouches, Sutherland[10] was, perhaps, the first to use the technique alone in patients with this condition. Subsequently, Davis and associates[32] and Blakeley and colleagues[33] each reported the cases of two patients with pharyngeal pouches successfully treated by cricopharyngeal myotomy. The most extensive experience with this technique is that of Belsey,[34] who in 1966 reported its use in 32 patients with pharyngoesophageal diverticulum, most of whom had diverticulopexy performed at the same time.

Others have advocated the use of cricopharyngeal myotomy whenever diverticulectomy is performed, as recurrences have been reported with diverticulectomy alone. I believe that cricopharyngeal myotomy is a successful procedure for patients with small-sized or medium-sized pouches. Those with pouches larger than 4 to 5 cm in diameter should have diverticulectomy performed, and recent experience with a diverticulum with excessive peridiverticular inflammation has influenced me to include this finding as an indication for excision.

TECHNIQUE OF CRICOPHARYNGEAL MYOTOMY

The technique of cricopharyngeal myotomy is illustrated in Figure 2–1. Access to the posterior pharyngoesophageal area is obtained through a left oblique or transverse cervical incision bordering the anterior edge of the sternocleidomastoid muscle. Retraction of the carotid sheath laterally and the trachea' and

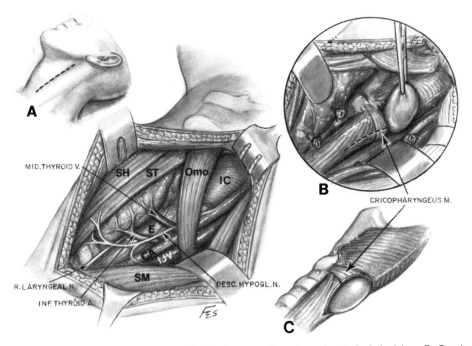

Figure 2–1. Operative field for performance of cricopharyngeal myotomy *(center)*. *A,* Incision. *B,* Omohyoid, middle thyroid vein, and inferior thyroid artery have been divided, the thyroid and trachea have been retracted, and the diverticulum has been freed. Dotted line indicates site of proposed myotomy. *C,* Appearance of completed myotomy. *SH* = sternohyoid; *ST* = sternothyroid; *Omo* = omohyoid; *IC* = inferior pharyngeal constrictor muscle; *E* = esophagus; *CA* = carotid artery; *SM* = sternocleidomastoid muscle; *IJV* = internal jugular vein. (From Ellis FH Jr, Crozier RE: Cervical esophageal dysphagia: indications for and results of cricopharyngeal myotomy. Ann Surg 194:284, 1981.)

larynx anteriorly and medially exposes the diverticulum. Access to this area may be facilitated by division of the inferior thyroid artery, the omohyoid muscle, and the facial vein. The diverticulum is freed to its neck, thereby exposing the transverse fibers of the cricopharyngeus muscle bordering the inferior margin of the neck of the diverticulum. After these muscles are identified, a right-angle clamp is insinuated beneath the transverse fibers of the cricopharyngeus muscle, and they are incised carefully. Because the length of the UES is somewhat longer than the width of the muscle, the incision extends onto the cervical esophagus for several centimeters so that the entire incision measures between 4 and 5 cm. After myotomy, esophageal and cricopharyngeus muscles are dissected from the underlying mucosa for about half the circumference of the mucosal tube to allow the mucosa to protrude freely through the incision. A longer incision, including the pharyngeal musculature and the cervical esophageal musculature caudad to the level of the clavicle, has been advocated by Orringer,[35] but I consider this unnecessary and in fact potentially harmful. After completion of the myotomy, the cervical wound is closed with interrupted sutures without drainage. The

patient is allowed free oral feedings immediately and is discharged from the hospital within a few days.

RESULTS

In 1969, my colleagues and I[19] reported on 18 patients with upper esophageal pouches who underwent cricopharyngeal myotomy. Four had diverticulopexy in addition, and four had diverticulectomy. All but one were improved by the operation. In a more recent report involving 28 patients undergoing cricopharyngeal myotomy at the Lahey Clinic,[36] 14 had a pharyngoesophageal diverticulum, which was recurrent in 4 in whom diverticulectomy had been performed previously elsewhere. One patient with a recurrent pharyngoesophageal diverticulum who exhibited considerable periesophageal fibrosis had persistent symptoms after operation and ultimately required diverticulectomy. All the rest have been relieved of their symptoms.

Radiographs of the esophagus obtained when the patient is about to be discharged from the hospital will reveal that the diverticulum either is no longer identifiable or is

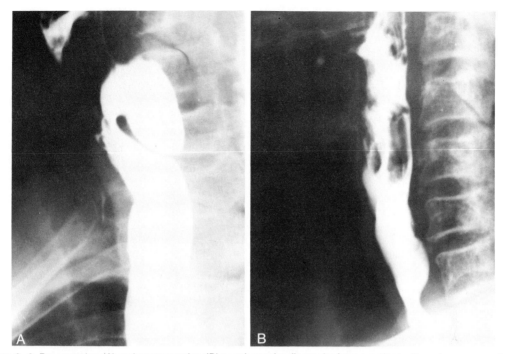

Figure 2–2. Preoperative *(A)* and postoperative *(B)* esophageal radiographs from a patient with a pharyngoesophageal diverticulum of the type pictured in Figure 1. (From Ellis FH Jr, Crozier RE: Cervical esophageal dysphagia: indications for and results of cricopharyngeal myotomy. Ann Surg 194:285, 1981.)

considerably smaller than before operation (Fig. 2–2). Postoperative manometric studies disclose an approximately 55% reduction in resting pressures at the UES in addition to a shortening of the high-pressure zone by more than one third, for an average reduction in length of 1.4 cm.[14]

CONCLUSIONS

The uniformly good results I have obtained using a limited cricopharyngeal myotomy (4 to 5 cm in length) in patients with pharyngoesophageal diverticulum of 4 to 5 cm or less in diameter supports use of this limited procedure in the symptomatic management of this problem. Diverticulectomy should be reserved for patients whose diverticula are in excess of 4 to 5 cm in diameter and for those who have considerable periesophageal fibrosis. Whether or not diverticulopexy has a role in the treatment of patients with upper esophageal pouches with or without myotomy has not been settled, in my opinion, but its use should probably be restricted to diverticula that are unusually large when excision is contraindicated.

References

1. Ludlow A: A case of obstructed deglutition, from a preternatural dilatation of, and bag formed in, the pharynx. Med Soc Phys 3:85–101, 1767.
2. Zenker FA, von Ziemssen H: Krankheiten des Oesophagus. In von Ziemssen H (ed): Handbuch der Speciellen Pathologie und Therapie, Vol 7 (suppl). Leipzig, FCW Vogel, 1877, p 1–87.
3. Kelly AB: Spasm at entrance of oesophagus. J Laryngol Otol 34:285–289, 1919.
4. Lahey FH: Pharyngo-esophageal diverticulum; its management and complications. Ann Surg 124:617–636, 1946.
5. Negus VE: Pharyngeal diverticula: observations on their evolution and treatment. Br J Surg 38:129–146, 1950.
6. Negus VE: The etiology of pharyngeal diverticula. Bull Johns Hopkins Hosp 101:209–223, 1957.
7. Cross FS, Johnson GF, Gerein AN: Esophageal diverticula: associated neuromuscular changes in the esophagus. Arch Surg 83:525–533, 1961.
8. Jackson C, Shallow TA: Diverticula of oesophagus: pulsion, traction, malignant and congenital. Ann Surg 83:1–19, 1926.
9. Asherson N: Achalasia of cricopharyngeal sphincter: record of cases, with profile pharyngograms. J Laryngol Otol 64:747–758, 1950.
10. Sutherland HD: Cricopharyngeal achalasia. J Thorac Cardiovasc Surg 43:114–126, 1962.
11. Hunt PS, Connell AM, Smiley TB: The cricopharyngeal sphincter in gastric reflux. Gut 11:303–306, 1970.

12. Smiley TB, Caves PK, Porter DC: Relationship between posterior pharyngeal pouch and hiatus hernia. Thorax 25:725–731, 1970.
13. Worman LW: Pharyngoesophageal diverticulum—excision or incision? (Editorial.) Surgery 87:236–237, 1980.
14. Ellis FH Jr, Crozier RE: Cervical esophageal dysphagia: indications for and results of cricopharyngeal myotomy. Ann Surg 194:279–289, 1981.
15. Stanciu C, Bennett JR: Upper oesophageal sphincter yield pressure in normal subjects and in patients with gastroesophageal reflux. Thorax 29:459–462, 1974.
16. Berte LE, Winans CS: Lower-esophageal sphincter function does not determine resting upper-esophageal sphincter pressure. Am J Dig Dis 27:877–880, 1977.
17. Ardran GM, Kemp FH: The radiography of the lower lateral food channels. J Laryngol Otol 75:358–370, 1961.
18. Lund WS: A study of the cricopharyngeal sphincter in man and in the dog. Ann R Coll Surg Engl 37:225–246, 1965.
19. Ellis FH Jr, Schlegel JF, Lynch VP, Payne WS: Cricopharyngeal myotomy for pharyngo-esophageal diverticulum. Ann Surg 170:340–349, 1969.
20. Hurwitz AL, Nelson JA, Haddad JK: Oropharyngeal dysphagia: manometric and cine-esophagraphic findings. Am J Dig Dis 20:313–324, 1975.
21. Frasson P, Ancona E, Tremolada C, et al: The importance of extramucosal sphincter myotomy in the treatment of upper and lower oesophageal diverticula. Surg It 6:139–147, 1976.
22. Lichter I: Motor disorder in pharyngoesophageal pouch. J Thorac Cardiovasc Surg 76:272–275, 1978.
23. Borrie J, Wilson RL: Oesophageal diverticula: principles of management and appraisal of classification. Thorax 35:759–767, 1980.
24. Knuff TE, Benjamin SB, Castell DO: Pharyngoesophageal (Zenker's) diverticulum: a reappraisal. Gastroenterology 82:734–736, 1982.
25. Goldmann EE: Die zweizeitige Operation von Pulsionsdivertikeln der Speiseröhre. Beitr Klin Chir 61:741–749, 1909.
26. Lahey FH, Warren KW: Esophageal diverticula. Surg Gynecol Obstet 98:1–28, 1954.
27. Harrington SW: Pulsion diverticula of hypopharynx: a review of forty-one cases in which operation was performed and a report of two cases. Surg Gynecol Obstet 69:364–373, 1939.
28. Welsh GF, Payne WS: Present status of one-stage pharyngo-esophageal diverticulectomy. Surg Clin North Am 53:953–958, 1973.
29. Dohlman G, Mattsson O: The endoscopic operation for hypopharyngeal diverticula: a roentgencinematographic study. Arch Otolaryngol 71:744–752, 1960.
30. Overbeek JJM van: The Hypopharyngeal Diverticulum: Endoscopic Treatment and Manometry. Assen, Amsterdam, Van Gorcum, 1977.
31. Harrison MS: The aetiology, diagnosis and surgical treatment of pharyngeal diverticula. J Laryngol Otol 72:523–534, 1958.
32. Davis MV, Mitchel BF Jr, Adam M: Cricopharyngeal achalasia: variant of hypopharyngeal diverticulum syndrome. Texas J Med 62:47–49, 1966.
33. Blakeley WR, Garety EJ, Smith DE: Section of the cricopharyngeus muscle for dysphagia. Arch Surg 96:745–762, 1968.
34. Belsey R: Functional disease of the esophagus. J Thorac Cardiovasc Surg 52:164–188, 1966.
35. Orringer MB: Extended cervical esophagomyotomy for cricopharyngeal dysfunction. J Thorac Cardiovasc Surg 80:669–678, 1980.
36. Ellis FH Jr: Cervical esophageal dysphagia: indications for and results of cricopharyngeal myotomy. In Najarian JS (ed): Advances in Gastrointestinal Surgery. Chicago, Year Book Medical Publishers, 1984, pp 47–55.

3

The Management of Zenker's Diverticulum: Cricopharyngeal Myotomy and Diverticulopexy

Alex G. Little, M.D.
David B. Skinner, M.D.

A Zenker's diverticulum—also known as a pharyngoesophageal diverticulum because of its anatomic location at the pharyngoesophageal junction—is an acquired diverticulum of the esophagus. The diverticular sac is composed solely of mucosa, with no muscle fibers in its wall; the condition is consequently described as a false diverticulum. The neck of this mucosal diverticular sac protrudes through a triangle-shaped bare area between the oblique fibers of the inferior constrictor muscle of the pharynx and the transverse fibers of the cricopharyngeus muscle, the upper esophageal sphincter (Fig. 3–1). The diverticulum itself lies in the prevertebral space, usually predominantly to the left of the midline, posterior to the pharynx and the proximal esophagus.

Although Ludlow was the first to describe this entity in 1767, Zenker's name became permanently associated with it following his more thorough description in 1877.[1, 2] This is the most commonly encountered esophageal diverticulum, perhaps because it is more likely to be associated with clinically important symptoms than are either mid-esophageal or epiphrenic diverticula. It is more common in males than in females but shows no racial predilection and, as a reflection of its acquired nature, is rarely found in patients under the age of 50 years.

PATHOGENESIS

The basic pathogenesis of this problem has not been conclusively demonstrated, although it clearly is related to a functional disorder of the cricopharyngeus muscle or upper esophageal sphincter. The effect of this muscular dysfunction is to produce an obstruction against, or resistance to, pharyngeal contractions at the level of the upper esophageal sphincter. This results in high pressures at the pharyngoesophageal junction, which produce a posterior "blowout" of the pharyngeal mucosa between the inferior pharyngeal constrictor and the cricopharyngeus, where there is no supporting or buttressing muscular protection. Because of this pathogenetic mechanism, a Zenker's diverticulum is classified as a pulsion diverticulum.

In theory, the muscle or sphincter dysfunction may be due to achalasia or failure of relaxation of the sphincter, muscular spasm with hypertensive sphincter pressures, or premature sphincter closure following pharyngeal contraction. Although some investigators have occasionally found hypertensive or high-pressure sphincters, this has not been a consistent

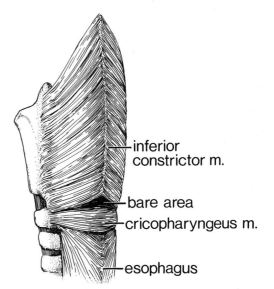

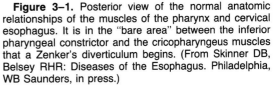

Figure 3–1. Posterior view of the normal anatomic relationships of the muscles of the pharynx and cervical esophagus. It is in the "bare area" between the inferior pharyngeal constrictor and the cricopharyngeus muscles that a Zenker's diverticulum begins. (From Skinner DB, Belsey RHR: Diseases of the Esophagus. Philadelphia, WB Saunders, in press.)

observation. Extensive work has been done by Ellis, who has recently reported an experience with 20 consecutive patients in all of whom careful manometric examination documented discoordination between pharyngeal contraction and cricopharyngeal relaxation.[3] An example of this type of discoordination is demonstrated in Figure 3–2. In the normal or physiologic situation, the pharyngeal contraction coincides exactly with the cricopharyngeal relaxation, so that there is no resistance to the pharyngeal propulsive wave. In the patient with a Zenker's diverticulum, cricopharyngeal relaxation, although complete, actually precedes the pharyngeal contraction, and the cricopharyngeus begins to contract as the pharyngeal pressure wave arrives (see Fig. 3–2). This produces a functional obstruction against the pharyngeal propulsive drive, and high pressures result. The discoordination is most convincingly demonstrated wih high-speed mano-

metric recordings, which allow precise judgment about the relative timing of pharyngeal and upper esophageal sphincter activities.

An intriguing speculation that is still debated is the possibility of an etiologic relationship between gastroesophageal reflux and Zenker's diverticulum. Ronald Belsey, a pioneer in investigations of esophageal disease, has emphasized the teleological hypothesis that the abnormality of cricopharyngeal function in these patients serves as the final protective barrier, when the cardia is incompetent, against regurgitation of refluxed gastric contents from the esophagus into the pharynx and subsequent aspiration.[4] Unfortunately, the arguments for this possible relationship are based on the incidence of hiatal hernias in various series of patients with Zenker's diverticulum or the presence of typical symptoms of gastroesophageal reflux, or both, rather than on objective evaluation of gastroesophageal reflux with pH

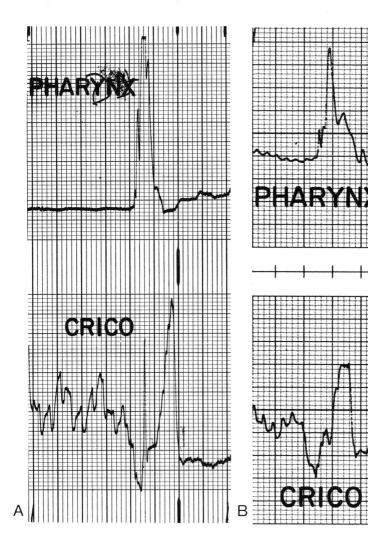

Figure 3–2. Manometric tracings obtained using a perfused catheter with the station pull-through technique. The upper channel shows events in the pharynx; the lower channel shows simultaneous events within the cricopharyngeus. *A,* Normal tracing. Cricopharyngeal relaxation coincides with the pharyngeal contraction. *B,* Tracing obtained in a patient with Zenker's diverticulum. Cricopharyngeal relaxation precedes the pharyngeal contraction, which now coincides with the post-relaxation cricopharyngeal contraction.

testing. In our experience, 6 of 13 patients had hiatal hernias evident on radiographs, and 4 of 5 patients undergoing pH testing were shown to have pathologic gastroesophageal reflux. Only 2 of our 13 patients (15%), however, required surgery for therapy of gastroesophageal reflux. It appears that although the incidence of gastroesophageal reflux is high in patients with Zenker's diverticulum, some patients clearly do not have pathologic reflux. Furthermore, only a few of those patients with reflux will require antireflux surgery.

CLINICAL ASPECTS

Dysphagia is the most prominent and frequent symptom of Zenker's diverticulum. Formerly it was thought that the dysphagia was caused by pressure on the cervical esophagus, with resulting obstruction, by an enlarged, food-filled diverticulum. Documentation of the cricopharyngeal dysfunction and of the occurrence of dysphagia in patients with very small diverticula makes it clear that the difficulty in swallowing results from the functional obstruction at the level of the upper esophageal sphincter. The other commonly noted symptom is regurgitation of food from the diverticulum into the patient's pharynx and mouth. The regurgitated material consists of undigested food, and the patient may actually be able to recognize bits of chewed material. Differentiation from regurgitation of stomach contents is possible because of the absence of bile or acid. Pulmonary aspiration of regurgitated material causes symptoms ranging from nocturnal cough to actual pneumonia.

Decay of stagnant food within the diverticular sac causes a constant foul odor and "bad breath." A gurgling sound associated with swallowing, presumably resulting from the sloshing about of material within the sac, may be noted by the patient. Symptoms of gastroesophageal reflux, particularly heartburn, are uncommon but should be sought for because surgical therapy for a Zenker's diverticulum diminishes the competency of the upper esophageal sphincter. Such diminished competency will increase the possibility of aspiration of refluxed gastric contents.

Physical examination of these patients is usually unremarkable and discloses no specific abnormality. Palpation may reveal a neck mass and, if the diverticulum is large enough, can produce a succussion splash as the diverticular contents are compressed.

The diagnosis is established with a barium contrast x-ray film (Fig. 3–3). Even if the diagnosis seems secure on clinical grounds, a barium study should be obtained for confirmation and to evaluate the distal esophagus, stomach, and duodenum for associated disease. When ordering the x-ray study, the clinician must specify that views of the cervical esophagus are required; otherwise the radiographic examination may be directed at the thoracic esophagus, and the diverticulum will escape detection. Endoscopy is not absolutely required unless there is a suspicion of distal disease. Flexible endoscopy is relatively safe, and examination of the interior of the diverticulum for ulceration or occult carcinoma is useful, but it is unusual to be able to pass the scope beyond the diverticulum itself. Rigid endoscopy is hazardous because the scope will have a tendency to enter and perforate the diverticulum.

Esophageal function tests, particularly manometric examination, are useful for defining the physiologic disorder producing the diverticulum and will aid in evaluating surgical results; however, these tests are not required for diagnosis. Objective documentation of gastroesophageal reflux with pH monitoring of the distal esophagus will help to define the true relationship between Zenker's diverticulum and reflux and will identify patients with incompetent cardias and increased risk of aspiration.

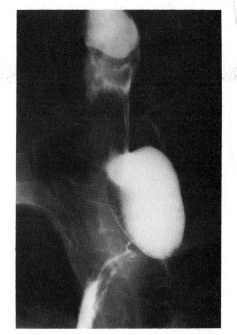

Figure 3–3. Typical barium contrast film in a patient with a Zenker's diverticulum.

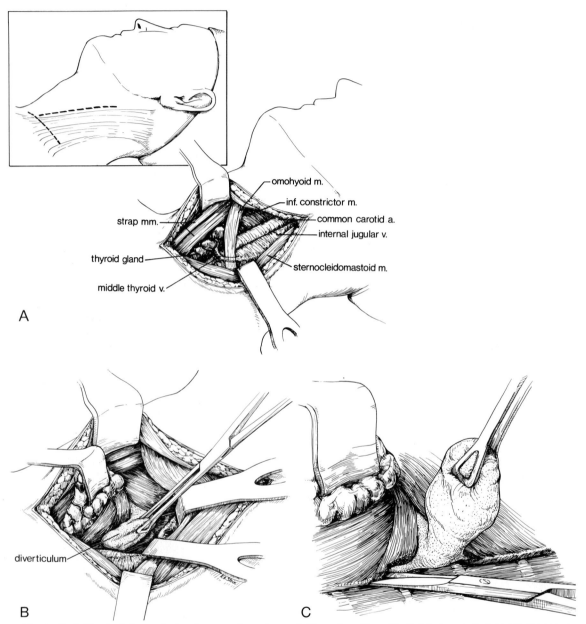

Figure 3–4. The technique of cricopharyngeal myotomy. *A,* Two alternative skin incisions are depicted in the insert. Adequate exposure is possible with either. The incision is usually made in the left neck, as the sac is most often on that side, but the operation can easily be done through a right-sided approach. *B,* With the carotid sheath retracted laterally and the thyroid gland medially, the prevertebral space is entered. The diverticulum can be identified lying posteriorly and, usually, to the left of the proximal esophagus. The sac should be grasped and dissected free from surrounding structures, and its neck clearly identified. *C,* The myotomy is best performed with blunt-tip scissors, as they will tend to push the mucosa away from the overlying muscle. The myotomy is extended a short distance above the diverticular neck and for 3 to 4 cm distally to ensure complete division of the cricopharyngeus. (From Skinner DB, Belsey RHR: Diseases of the Esophagus. Philadelphia, WB Saunders, in press.)

TREATMENT

The early attempts at surgical treatment of this problem followed the first successful resection in 1892 by von Bergmann* and were directed toward simple excision of the diverticulum, that is, diverticulectomy, with closure of the mucosal defect.[5] This procedure was abandoned because of a high rate of leak along the suture line and was replaced by a complicated two-stage procedure that called for initial suspension of the diverticulum from the cervical incision so that any leak following subsequent excision would produce an esophagocutaneous fistula. A return to the technique of single-stage excision came in the 1950s, perhaps because of the availability and use of antibiotics, but this approach proved unsatisfactory because of an extremely high incidence of recurrence of both the diverticulum and the symptoms.[6] Belsey was one of the first to recognize that correction of the functional obstruction caused by the upper esophageal sphincter is essential for success.[4] He recommended and performed cricopharyngeal myotomy in his patients; this procedure has become the cornerstone of surgical therapy.

The details of cricopharyngeal myotomy are shown in Figure 3–4. It should be emphasized that complete division of the cricopharyngeal muscle fibers is required. To ensure complete division of the cricopharyngeus, the myotomy is usually extended a short distance distally, along the upper esophagus, and proximally onto the inferior pharyngeal constrictor musculature. A more extensive myotomy not only is unnecessary but may actually be harmful by interfering with postoperative pharyngeal function. The overall length of the final myotomy

*"First" scissors was actually by Wheeler in 1885 (Ed.)

need be no longer than 5 cm because the length of the manometrically identified upper esophageal high-pressure zone is only 3 to 5 cm. After the muscle is divided, it is dissected circumferentially from the mucosa to a sufficient degree to prevent the possibility of healing together of the raw muscle edges. Healing of the muscle in this fashion could lead to recurrence of the initial anatomic-physiologic disorder.

After completion of the myotomy, a tube is passed by the anesthesiologist through the patient's nose and into the upper esophagus. A bolus of air is rapidly injected through the tube to distend the esophagus. This serves two purposes: First, any small mucosal defect can be identified, by escaping air bubbles, and repaired. Second, distention of the mucosa makes any remaining muscle fibers more obvious and thereby helps ensure completeness of the myotomy.

Some difference of opinion exists with regard to the handling of the diverticulum after completion of the myotomy. In some instances the diverticulum will essentially disappear after completion of the myotomy as the underlying esophageal mucosa bulges out, and nothing specific need be done. Larger diverticula must be attended to; it has been our practice to suspend them from the prevertebral fascia, behind the pharynx, as shown in Figure 3–5. Sutures of 5–0 wire are used because of their low tissue reactivity. Stitches are passed through the prevertebral fascia and then, in mattress fashion, peripherally and through the full thickness of the diverticulum in a horseshoe pattern. This diverticulopexy both suspends the sac in upside-down fashion, thus promoting gravity drainage, and partly obliterates the lumen as the stitches are put through the full thickness of the diverticulum. A typical

Figure 3–5. The sac of the diverticulum is suspended upside-down from the prevertebral fascia, as shown. Full-thickness wire sutures are placed through the sac in mattress fashion to partly obliterate the lumen. (From Skinner DB, Belsey RHR: Diseases of the Esophagus. Philadelphia, WB Saunders, in press.)

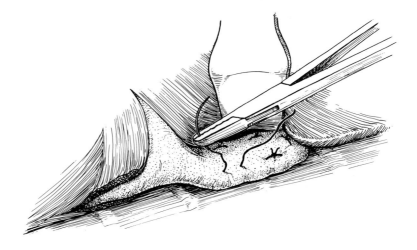

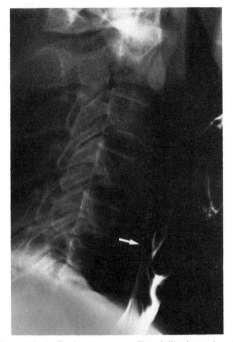

Figure 3–6. Barium contrast film, following cricopharyngeal myotomy and diverticulopexy, in the same patient as that in Figure 3–3. The arrow points to the barium in the suspended diverticulum, which is between the spine and the pharynx.

postoperative esophagogram, Figure 3–6, shows that no filling of the diverticulum takes place except for a small trickle of barium.

The alternative to diverticulopexy, when the sac is too large to ignore following cricopharyngeal myotomy, is to resect the diverticulum at its neck, either using a stapler or standard manual technique. This means an esophageal suture line will be present, and although ways of resuturing the muscle transversely to buttress the suture line have been devised, there will always be the risk of suture line leakage with the attendant morbidity. Diverticulopexy avoids all the potential problems associated with diverticulectomy, because there is no suture line. As a result, the patient can start oral intake the day after surgery, and only a short postoperative hospital convalescence is required.

RESULTS

Complete follow-up results are available for our 13 patients with Zenker's diverticulum treated with the technique of cricopharyngeal myotomy and diverticulopexy as described.

There has been no known anatomic recurrence; symptomatically, all patients have been satisfactorily relieved of dysphagia, with no late recrudescence. Patients commonly note a postoperative cough, which usually resolves in the first few days to weeks after surgery and may be correlated with documentation of aspiration of small amounts of barium at the postoperative radiographic examination. This is probably due to a transient pharyngeal discoordination and has not persisted or been the cause of any important problem in any of our patients.

We believe that if there is a clinical suspicion of concomitant gastroesophageal reflux, objective documentation should be obtained. If confirmed, the reflux should be treated according to standard criteria, which means that surgery will be required only if medical treatment fails to control symptoms, or if reflux complications such as stricture or ulcerative esophagitis occur. Five of our patients had associated gastroesophageal reflux, documented in four by objective pH testing and suggested in one by the combination of typical reflux symptoms and the presence of radiographic reflux. Three of these patients required only medical management for control of mild reflux symptoms after correction of the upper esophageal abnormality. One patient had a reflux-induced stricture of the distal esophagus at time of initial presentation; this required operative dilatation and performance of an antireflux procedure 1 week following cricopharyngeal myotomy and diverticulopexy. One additional patient is awaiting performance of an elective antireflux procedure required for persistent symptoms and ulcerative esophagitis, despite intensive medical therapy.

References

1. Ludlow A: A case of obstructed deglutition, from a preternatural dilatation of, and bag formed in, the pharynx. Med Soc Phys, 3:85–101, 1767.
2. Zenker FA, von Ziemssen H: Krankheiten des Oesophagus. In von Ziemssen H (ed.): Handbuch der Speciellen Pathologie und Therapie, Vol 7. Leipzig, FCW Vogel, 1877.
3. Ellis FH, Crozier RE: Cervical esophageal dysphagia. Indications for the results of cricopharyngeal myotomy. Ann Surg 194:279–289, 1981.
4. Belsey R: Functional disease of the esophagus. J Thorac Cardiovasc Surg 52:164–188, 1966.
5. von Bergmann E: Ueber den Oesophagusdivertikel und seine Behandlung. Arch Klin Chir 43:1, 1892.
6. Skinner DB: Discussion of Ref. 3, Ellis and Crozier, 1981 (ref. 3).

4

The Management of Zenker's Diverticulum: The Utilization of Intra-operative Manometry

C. Dale Mercer, M.D.
Lucius D. Hill, M.D.

Esophageal diverticula are blind pouches or pockets originating from the lining of the esophagus. These diverticula are classified according to anatomy, histology, and pathophysiology (see Table 4–1). Pharyngoesophageal diverticulum is an acquired, false, pulsion-type herniation of pharyngeal mucosa penetrating through the potential weak area between the lowermost fibers of the inferior pharyngeal constrictor muscle and the upper fibers of the cricopharyngeus muscle. Alternate names for the condition are hypopharyngeal diverticulum, Zenker's diverticulum, pharyngocele, pharyngeal pouch, and retrocricoid diverticulum.

This condition was first elegantly described by Ludlow[1] in 1767, more than a century prior to Zenker's description of 34 similar cases.[2] Ludlow's patient unfortunately succumbed two weeks following a variety of therapeutic efforts intended to clear the obstruction, which included attempted dilatation with a bullet on a string, dilatation with whalebone bougies, and ingestion by the patient of a half-pound of mercury, presumably in order to dilate the esophagus.[3] Ludlow correctly identified the pathophysiologic development and anatomic features of the disorder from his detailed autopsy studies of this single case. Fortunately, since then the surgical management of pharyngoesophageal diverticulum has evolved into a more effective treatment associated with minimal morbidity and mortality. However, controversy still exists over the pathophysiology and the surgical management of this condition.

INCIDENCE, ANATOMY, AND PATHOPHYSIOLOGY

A number of studies utilizing upper gastrointestinal x-ray examination in patients with other gastrointestinal problems have revealed the incidence of pharyngoesophageal diverticulum to be in the range of 0.07% to 0.11%.[4, 5] However, in patients with dysphagia the incidence increases to 1.8%.[6] This form of esophageal diverticulum is the most common type, accounting for 63% of the cases.[7] It is encountered usually in patients over 50 years of age and only rarely in those under 30. Males predominate in a 3:1 ratio.[8]

Table 4–1. Classification of Esophageal Diverticula

Differentiating Feature	Type	Description
Anatomy	Pharyngoesophageal (Zenker's)	Potentially weak area between lower fibers of inferior pharyngeal constrictor and upper fibers of cricopharyngeus
	Midesophageal	Midesophagus
	Epiphrenic	Distal esophagus
Histology	True	All layers of esophageal wall present in diverticulum
	False	Diverticular wall consisting of mucosa and submucosa only
Pathophysiology	Pulsion	Secondary to segmental area of elevated intraluminal pressure
	Traction	Secondary to tug from surrounding structure, e.g., chronically inflamed carinal lymph nodes

Much speculation exists regarding the possible mechanisms of development of pharyngoesophageal diverticulum. The constant site of origin is suggestive of a congenitally weakened anatomic area that allows slow development of the sac over many years. This weakened area is in the midline posteriorly between the oblique fiber of the inferior pharyngeal constrictor muscle and the transverse fibers of the cricopharyngeus muscle. This triangular area was initially described by Killian in 1908.[9] Keith[10] showed that the inferior pharyngeal constrictor and the cricopharyngeus had two different functions. The former is one of the main muscles used in the coordinated act of forcing the swallowed bolus of food from the pharynx into the esophagus. The latter serves as a sphincter for the esophageal orifice. Familial occurrences[11] and a number of case reports[12, 13] also provide suggestive evidence that this may be a congenital condition.

Most investigators believe that a physiologic abnormality of the cricopharyngeus results in focal elevations of intraluminal pressure that cause pharyngeal mucosa to "pout" outward through the potential weakness at Killian's triangle. The evidence for elevated cricopharyngeal pressures or dysmotility is contradictory, possibly because the manometric studies for measuring pressures and peristalsis in the upper esophageal sphincter are not standardized;[14] moreover, all such studies are subject to recording infidelities.[15] Negus[16] showed that in patients with pharyngoesophageal diverticulum, relaxation of the upper esophageal sphincter occurred normally but not at the correct time in the swallowing sequence. Other workers have implicated cricopharyngeal spasm, either resulting from elevated pressures intrinsic to the muscle itself[17, 18] or secondary to gastroesophageal reflux.[19] Winans[20] used a special arrangement of manometric catheters that measured the differences in pressure recordings secondary to axial and radial asymmetry of the sphincter; with this system he was unable to confirm the suspected increase in pressure in the upper sphincter. Ellis[21–23] has shown that the pressure in the upper esophageal sphincter is actually lower in patients with pharyngoesophageal diverticulum (37.2 ± 4.8 mm Hg) than in normals (55.9 ± 5 mm Hg), but that there is an abnormal temporal relationship between pharyngeal contraction and cricopharyngeal relaxation and contraction in these patients. This finding of a premature contraction has not been confirmed in other laboratories.[24, 25] We have also been unable to identify premature cricopharyngeal contrac-

tion as the cause for development of these diverticula.

SYMPTOMS

Symptoms related to pharyngoesophageal diverticulum result from the size of the sac, the size of its orifice, and the degree of extrinsic esophageal compression. Three stages of development are identified by Lahey,[26] and the symptoms relate to the stage of development. In the *first stage*, a small protrusion of mucosa and submucosa forms an asymptomatic bulge. In the *second stage,* the diverticulum is bigger, with the orifice of the pouch lying in the plane of the normal posterior wall of the pharynx. Since a direct pathway still exists for the bolus of food to pass into the esophagus, symptoms result only from accumulation of food and fluid in the diverticulum. These early symptoms include dryness of the throat and a foreign body sensation after meals. Regurgitation and aspiration may occur after eating or drinking and are especially severe at night. As the diverticulum enlarges, the esophagus becomes displaced, until, in the *third stage,* the diverticular orifice lies in the plane of the normally oriented esophagus, and the plane of the esophageal orifice lies parallel to its longitudinal axis. Food and saliva now preferentially enter the diverticulum and pass into the esophagus only as a result of overflow from the diverticulum. Obstructive esophageal symptoms develop, and dysphagia becomes progressively worse. As the nocturnal aspiration continues, pulmonary complications predominate and overshadow gastrointestinal symptoms, commonly resulting in delayed diagnosis. Chronic bronchitis, bronchiectasis, lung abscess, and aspiration pneumonia have all been observed with large diverticula.[27]

Other symptoms include noisy deglutition, halitosis, hoarseness due to compression of the recurrent laryngeal nerve,[28] and, in severe cases, malnutrition. Pills may lodge in the diverticulum, resulting in decreased drug bioavailability.[29] Rare complications include squamous cell carcinoma in the diverticulum[30] and esophagotracheal fistula formation.[31]

Table 4–2 lists, in order of frequency, the signs and symptoms found in our series of 10 patients.

Physical examination is usually unremarkable unless a large diverticulum is palpable as a soft mass. In one of our patients, the diverticulum was so large that it was readily visible as a left-sided neck swelling (Fig. 4–1).

Table 4–2. Signs and Symptoms in 10 Patients with Pharyngoesophageal Diverticulum*

Sign or Symptom	No. of Patients
Dysphagia	10
Aspiration	4
Regurgitation	3
Halitosis	1
Weight loss	1
Neck swelling	1

*Few, if any, patients complain of noisy deglutition (Cooper's sign), but this is generally present in every patient, often before dysphagia is noted (Ed.).

DIAGNOSIS

The pharyngoesophageal diverticulum is best demonstrated by barium x-ray examination (Fig. 4–2). Anteroposterior, lateral, and oblique views and cineradiography[32] are necessary to visualize fully the diverticulum, the diverticular orifice, and the esophagus, and to exclude esophageal web formation. Small diverticula may be obscured by barium in the esophagus or may otherwise escape detection because they empty barium so rapidly. In these situations and with a suggestive history, we have utilized standard radionuclide esophageal scintigraphy (Fig. 4–3B), which is a sensitive method of demonstrating retention of the radioisotope in the esophagus. We have found that this technique is also useful in diagnosis of a variety of other esophageal motor disorders.[33]

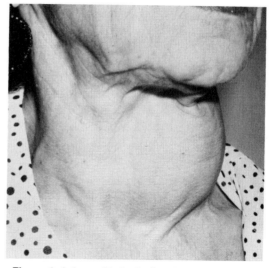

Figure 4–1. Large Zenker's diverticulum presenting as a soft, left-sided neck mass.

Endoscopic examination is hazardous if a large diverticulum is present, since the scope will pass easily into the diverticulum. An inexperienced endoscopist may confuse this thin-walled structure with the esophagus, and attempts to identify the lumen distally can result in perforation of the diverticular wall.

TREATMENT

Only symptomatic diverticula require treatment, which must be surgical. Some investigators have advocated dilatation of the upper

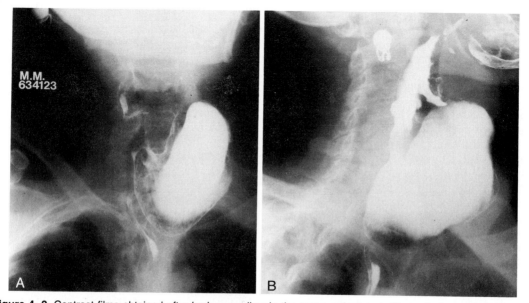

Figure 4–2. Contrast films obtained after barium swallow in the same patient as in Figure 4–1 revealed a large left-sided pharyngoesophageal diverticulum. *A*, Posteroanterior projection. *B*, Lateral projection.

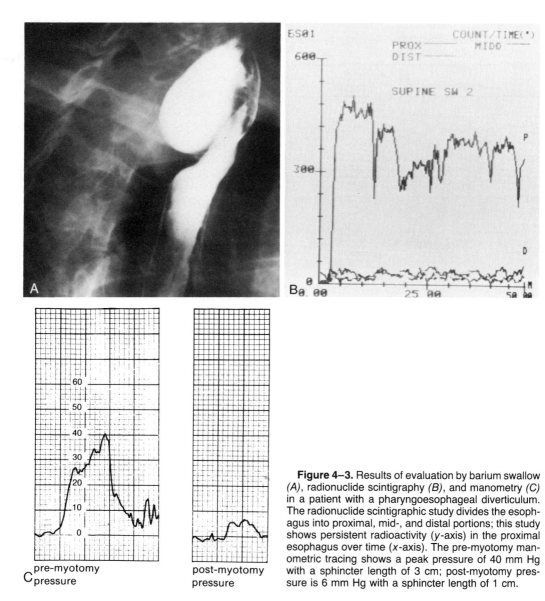

Figure 4–3. Results of evaluation by barium swallow (A), radionuclide scintigraphy (B), and manometry (C) in a patient with a pharyngoesophageal diverticulum. The radionuclide scintigraphic study divides the esophagus into proximal, mid-, and distal portions; this study shows persistent radioactivity (y-axis) in the proximal esophagus over time (x-axis). The pre-myotomy manometric tracing shows a peak pressure of 40 mm Hg with a sphincter length of 3 cm; post-myotomy pressure is 6 mm Hg with a sphincter length of 1 cm.

esophageal sphincter segment for small symptomatic diverticula, but we have not found this to be efficacious. Elective treatment carried out prior to development of chronic respiratory symptoms and malnutrition has the most favorable results. Once complications occur, urgent surgery is necessary; if a perforation is present, the surgical procedure should be performed on an emergency basis.

The surgical management of these diverticula has changed considerably over the years since Ludlow's first description and treatment. Initial attempts[35] at creating an esophagocutaneous fistula with the diverticulum resulted in the death of the patient. Since then, a variety of surgical procedures have been carried out, but not all have been successful. The earliest

procedures included one-stage extirpation, invagination, and diverticulopexy. However, the early morbidity and mortality were high, prompting development of a two-stage diverticulectomy[36, 37] in which the diverticulum was isolated and sewn inverted under the skin incision. This allowed the fascial planes in the neck to become sealed; subsequently, at a second operation, the sac was removed. Other operations included invagination of the sac,[38] partial excision plus invagination,[39] diverticulopexy,[40] and resection of the proximal esophagus with primary anastomosis.[41] Today's method of one-stage diverticulectomy, pioneered by Harrington,[42] has been found to be safe and highly successful. Stapling devices have also been used for the excision of the diverticulum.[43, 44] The use of cricopharyngeal myotomy[22]—in addition to diverticulectomy for large diverticula,[45] as a primary procedure[46] for small diverticula, or as an adjunct to diverticulopexy[47]—has been found to reduce the incidence of recurrence.[48] Endoscopic technique for division of the wall between the esophagus and the diverticulum has also been described,[49] but this has not gained widespread acceptance.

We have utilized exclusively the one-stage diverticulectomy with cricopharyngeal myotomy. We have demonstrated that intraoperative manometry is useful in surgery for motor disorders of the esophagus,[50] and we have incorporated this technique in our approach to the management of pharyngoesophageal diverticulum.

OPERATIVE TECHNIQUE

We prefer to use prophylactic antibiotics (Ampicillin) prior to surgery since we routinely open the diverticulum and palpate the sphincter from within the esophageal lumen. Nutritional repletion is necessary only when malnutrition is identified. Pulmonary toilet and antibiotics are required prior to surgery if aspiration has been a significant problem.

A modified nasogastric sump tube in which the second lumen has a recording orifice 12 cm from the tip is utilized as a manometric catheter and is inserted preoperatively for intraoperative sphincter pressure measurement. General anesthesia is induced, and a left oblique cervical skin incision is made along the anterior border of the sternocleidomastoid muscle, beginning at the clavicle and ending at the level of the hyoid bone. The sternocleidomastoid muscle is retracted laterally to expose the anterior belly of the omohyoid muscle, which is then cut. The middle thyroid vein is exposed, ligated, and divided if necessary to facilitate upward retraction of the thyroid gland. The carotid sheath is retracted laterally, and the inferior thyroid artery arising from the thyrocervical trunk is divided between ligatures if it interferes with exposure. The recurrent laryngeal nerve must be identified and carefully preserved throughout the procedure. The esophagus is now easily identified anterior to the prevertebral fascia, and the diverticulum is freed from surrounding tissue.

Prior to excision of the diverticulum, the manometric catheter is withdrawn slowly through the upper esophageal sphincter to measure the pressure and the length of the high-pressure zone (see Fig. 4–3C). The sac is now dissected down to its neck. The apex of the sac is opened, and the surgeon's finger is inserted to identify the sphincter. A myotomy is performed by dividing the longitudinal and circular muscle layers caudad up to the diverticulum over a distance of 2 to 3 cm. The divided muscle is dissected away from approximately one half of the circumference of the mucosal tube. Care must be taken not to enter the mucosa of the esophagus. Digital palpation of the sphincter is again performed. The redundant diverticulum is excised, making sure to leave enough mucosa to prevent stricture. The mucosa is closed with a running suture of 3–0 chromic, and the muscle layer is carefully reapproximated with 3–0 silk.

Following closure, the manometric catheter is again drawn through the sphincter. If a high-pressure zone still exists distally, the myotomy is continued caudally until the manometric recording confirms the transection of the entire sphincter musculature (see Fig. 4–3C). A small drain is brought out from the retropharyngeal space, and the wound is closed. The nasogastric tube is removed 24 hours following surgery, and the patient is started on oral liquids. The drain is removed after 36 to 48 hours, or when drainage is minimal. A soft diet may be started at home 1 week later.

RESULTS

With the operative technique described, incorporating intraoperative manometry, our results have been excellent. Since 1979, we have utilized this procedure in 10 patients with pharyngoesophageal diverticulum. The average age at operation in this series was 70.6 years (range 56–94 years); there were eight male and two female patients.

There was no mortality in our series, and none of our patients experienced complications of fistula formation, stenosis, or recurrence of diverticulum. The only complication was transient hoarseness in a patient following resection of a giant diverticulum (see Fig. 4–1). The hoarseness persisted for 1 month postoperatively but then gradually resolved.

The average follow-up period was 24 months (range 1–60 months). Results of pre- and postoperative manometric studies are given in Table 4–3; both sphincter pressure and length of the high-pressure zone were considerably reduced following myotomy.

Table 4–3. Results of Manometric Studies Before and After
Surgical Correction of Pharyngoesophageal Diverticulum[a]

	Pre-Myotomy		Post-Myotomy	
	Mean	*Range*	*Mean*	*Range*
Sphincter pressure (mm Hg)	40	35–50	9	6–15
Sphincter length (cm)	3	2–4	0.5	0.2–1.0

[a]In 10 patients.

CONCLUSIONS

Our series utilizing intraoperative manometry is small, but our excellent results indicate the value of this method in determining the required extent of myotomy. Cricopharyngeal myotomy alone without excision of the sac may be adequate therapy for a small diverticulum, especially if intraoperative manometry objectively identifies complete transection of the sphincter. We have used diverticulectomy in all of our patients, however, because the diverticulum was 4 to 5 cm in diameter in each case. The addition of intraoperative manometry assures that the entire sphincter has been divided, thus preventing recurrence of the diverticulum.

References

1. Ludlow A: A case of obstructed deglutition, from a preternatural dilatation of, and bag formed in, the pharynx. Med Observ Inquir 3:85–101, 1767.
2. Zenker FA, von Ziemssen H: Krankheiten des Oesophagus. *In* von Ziemssen H (ed): Handbuch der Speciellen Pathologie und Therapie, Vol 7 (suppl). Leipzig, FCW Vogel, 1877.
3. Chitwood WR Jr: Ludlow's esophageal diverticulum: a preternatural bag. Surgery 85:549–553, 1979.
4. Shallow TA, Clerf LH: One stage pharyngeal diverticulectomy: improved technique and analysis of 186 cases. Surg Gynecol Obstet 86:317–322, 1948.
5. Wheeler D: Diverticula of the foregut. Radiology 49:476–481, 1947.
6. MacMillan AS: Statistical study of diseases of the esophagus. Surg Gynecol Obstet 60:394, 1935.
7. Postlethwait RW: Diverticula of the esophagus. In Surgery of the Esophagus. New York, Appleton-Century-Crofts, 1979.
8. Harrington SW: The surgical treatment of pulsion diverticula of the thoracic esophagus. Ann Surg 129:606–618, 1949.
9. Killian G: La boudre de l'oesophage. Ann Mal Oreille Larynx. 34:1, 1908. Cited by Moersch HJ, Judd ES: Surg Gynecol Obstet 58:781, 1934.
10. Keith A: On the origin and nature of hernia. Br J Surg 11:455, 1924.
11. Groves LK: Pharyngoesophageal diverticulum in each of three sisters, report of cases. Cleve Clin Q 35:207, 1968.
12. Brintnall ES, Kridelbaugh WW: Congenital diverticulum of the posterior hypopharynx simulating atresia of the esophagus. Ann Surg 131:564, 1950.
13. Nelson AR: Congenital true esophageal diverticulum. Report of a case unassociated with other esophagotracheal abnormality. Ann Surg 145:258, 1957.
14. Welch RW, Luckmann K, Ricks PM, et al.: Manometry of the normal upper esophageal sphincter and its alterations in laryngectomy. J Clin Invest 63:1036–1041, 1979.
15. Dodds WJ, Stef JJ, Hogan WJ: Factors determining pressure measurement accuracy by intraluminal esophageal manometry. Gastroenterology 70:117–123, 1976.
16. Negus VE: The etiology of pharyngeal diverticula. Bull Johns Hopkins Hosp 101:209, 1957.
17. Cross FS, Johnson GF, Gerein AN: Esophageal diverticula, associated neuromuscular changes in the esophagus. Arch Surg 83:525, 1961.
18. Cross FS: Esophageal diverticula related neuromuscular problems. Ann Otol Rhinol Laryngol 77:914, 1968.
19. Smiley TB, Caves PK, Porter DC: Relationship between posterior pharyngeal pouch and hiatus hernia. Thorax 25:725, 1970.
20. Winans CS: The pharyngeal closure mechanism: a manometric study. Gastroenterology 63:768, 1972.
21. Ellis FH, Crozier RE: Cervical esophageal dysphagia. Indications for and results of cricopharyngeal myotomy. Ann Surg 194:279, 1981.
22. Ellis FH, Schlegel JF, Lynch VP, Payne WS: Cricopharyngeal myotomy for pharyngoesophageal diverticulum. Ann Surg 170:340, 1969.
23. Ellis FH Jr: Pharyngoesophageal diverticula and cricopharyngeal incoordination. Mod Treat 7:1098, 1970.
24. Pederson SA, Hansen JB, Alstrup P: Pharyngoesophageal diverticula—a manometric follow-up study of ten cases treated by diverticulectomy. Scand J Thorac Cardiovasc Surg 7:87, 1973.
25. Knuff TE, Benjamin SB, Castell DO: Pharyngoesophageal (Zenker's) diverticulum: a reappraisal. Gastroenterology 82:734, 1982.
26. Lahey FH, Warren KW: Esophageal diverticula. Surg Gynecol Obstet 98:1–28, 1954.
27. Hawes LE, Walker JH: Severe pulmonary disease subsequent to Zenker's diverticulum. N. Engl J Med 253:209, 1955.
28. Becker H, Ungeheuer E: Zur Klinik and Therapie des Oesophagusdivertikels. Med Klin 65:589–594, 1970.
29. Baron SH: Zenker's diverticulum as a cause for loss of drug availability: a "new" complication. Am J Gastroenterol 77:152–153, 1982.
30. Som ML, Deitel M: Carcinoma in a large pharyngoesophageal diverticulum. Arch Surg 94:35, 1967.

31. Stanford W, Barloon TJ, Lu CC: Esophagotracheal fistula from a pharyngoesophageal diverticulum. Chest 84:229–231, 1983.
32. Ekberg O, Nylander G: Lateral diverticula from the pharyngoesophageal area. Radiology 146:117–122, 1983.
33. Russell C, Hill LD, Pope C, et al: Radionuclide transit: a sensitive test of esophageal dysfunction. Gastroenterology 75:1248, 1980.
34. Negus VE: Pharyngeal diverticula. Observations on their evolution and treatment. Br J Surg 38:129–146, 1950.
35. Nicoladoni K: Study of the operative treatment of diverticula of the esophagus (Ein Beitrag zur operativen Behandlung der Oesophagusdivertikel). Wien Med Wochenschr 27:605–631, 1877. Cited by Saint JH: Arch Surg 19:53, 1929.
36. Lahey FH: Esophageal diverticulum. JAMA 101:994, 1933.
37. Goldmann EE: Die zweizeitige Operation von Pulsionsdivertikeln der Speiseröhre. Beitr Klin Chir 61:741–749, 1909.
38. Girard C: Du traitement des diverticules de l'oesophage. Cong Fr Chir 10:392, 1896. Cited by Saint JH: Arch Surg 19:23, 1929.
39. Bevan AD: Diverticula of the esophagus. JAMA 76:285, 1921.
40. Schmid HH: Vorschlag eines einfachen Operationsverfahrens zur Behandlung des Oesophagusdivertikels. Wein Klin Wochenschr 25:487–488, 1912.
41. Weisel W, Pink JJ, Fitzsimmons JJ: Upper esophageal resection and reanastomosis to pharynx. Surgery 38:723, 1955.
42. Harrington SW: Pulsion diverticula of hypopharynx: a review of forty-one cases in which operation was performed and a report of two cases. Surg Gynecol Obstet 69:364–373, 1939.
43. Hoelm JG, Payne WS: Resection of pharyngoesophageal diverticulum using stapling device. Mayo Clin Proc 44:738–741, 1969.
44. Vered IY, Rosen G, Resnick S: Excision of Zenker's diverticulum using autosuture technique. Laryngoscope 92:1081–1082, 1982.
45. Cross FS, Johnson GF, Gerein AN: Esophageal diverticula: associated neuromuscular changes in the esophagus. Arch Surg 83:525–533, 1961.
46. Sutherland HD: Cricopharyngeal achalasia. J Thorac Cardiovasc Surg 43:114–126, 1962.
47. Belsey R: Functional disease of the esophagus. J Thorac Cardiovasc Surg 52:164–188, 1966.
48. Worman LW: Pharyngoesophageal diverticulum—excision or incision? Surgery 87:236–237, 1980.
49. Dohlman G, Mattsson O: The endoscopic operation for hypopharyngeal diverticula, a roentgencinematographic study. Arch Otolaryngol 71:744, 1960.
50. Hill LD, Asplund CM, Roberts PN: Intraoperative manometry: Adjunct to surgery for esophageal motility disorders. Am J Surg 147:171–174, 1984.

5

The Management of Zenker's Diverticulum: Endoscopic Diverticulotomy (the Dohlman Procedure)

Jos. J. M. van Overbeek, M.D.
Paul E. Hoeksema, M.D.

In 1964 we started to treat Zenker's diverticulum endoscopically, using the procedure described by Dohlman.[1, 2] We believe that our experience bears out the advantages of endoscopic management and the good results that can be obtained with this approach.[3] Although the first endoscopic surgical treatments were carried out in the United States by Mosher,[4] the literature indicates that this method has not become popular there.

The principle of endoscopic surgical treatment is that the septum between the diverticulum and the esophagus is divided to allow a more ample overflow from diverticulum to esophagus. The cricopharyngeal muscle located in the upper part of the septum is severed at the same time. Division of the septum is accomplished through the scope, and the risks associated with the transcutaneous approach are avoided.

ETIOLOGY AND DIAGNOSIS

Much discussion in the literature concerning Zenker's diverticulum is related to the etiology of this condition. Various theories have been propounded, but no single conclusion is generally accepted. Important in the pathogenesis is the presence of the triangle of Killian as a weak spot in the posterior wall of the pharyngoesophageal segment between the propulsive oblique fibers of the inferior constrictor muscle and the horizontal fibers of the cricopharyngeal muscle with a sphincter function in the esophageal inlet. At precisely this level the food bolus must be passed from the wide, funnel-shaped hypopharynx through the relatively narrow esophageal inlet.

Anatomic studies in nonaffected persons have shown us the presence of local variations in the pharyngoesophageal segment. For example, the triangle of Killian is often particularly large. We believe that an anatomic predisposition plays a prominent role in the mucosal herniation. Such a predisposition is supported by the familial occurrence of these relatively rare diverticula; our series of 303 patients included two brothers and one male patient whose mother also had a Zenker's diverticulum confirmed on radiographs.

Zenker's diverticulum is rarely seen in persons under 40 years. Age, therefore, is undoubtedly also of importance in the etiology.

There is no apparent reason for the fact that Zenker's diverticulum is more than twice as frequent in males as in females. However, the size of the laryngeal skeleton can perhaps explain this sex predilection. Age and sex distributions in our series are shown in Figure 5–1.

By simultaneous intraluminal pressure registrations we have obtained sufficient indications to reject the theory of a disorder in temporal coordination between hypopharynx and sphincter as a cause of diverticulum formation. We have also been unable to corroborate this hypothesis by measurements indicating increased resting sphincter pressure or insufficient sphincter relaxation.[5]

The diagnosis of Zenker's diverticulum is established by barium swallow radiography. A Zenker's diverticulum is readily visible in a lateral or an oblique projection. Barium x-ray films can show widely varying features in the same patients depending on the moment of exposure during deglutition (Fig. 5–2).

It is generally assumed that chronic irritation and inflammation of the diverticular wall, as a result of food retention, are factors predisposing to carcinoma in a Zenker's diverticulum. Data on the incidence vary, but we believe it

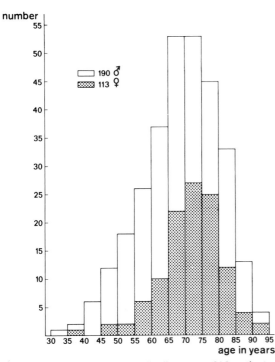

Figure 5–1. Age and sex distribution in 303 patients with Zenker's diverticulum.

goscopy in the presence of a verified Zenker's diverticulum. We have seen only one patient with a carcinoma in the pouch, which was treated with diverticulectomy and radiotherapy.

PATIENT SELECTION AND CLASSIFICATION OF LESIONS

At our institution, Zenker's diverticulum has been managed endoscopically since 1964. From 1964 to 1983, 304 patients with diverticula were admitted to our clinic; except for the patient with a carcinoma in the pouch, all were considered suitable candidates for endoscopic management, despite significant variation in lesion size, age, severity of symptoms, and so forth. Nine of our patients were suffering from a recurrent diverticulum after previous surgical diverticulectomy elsewhere.

We have classified the diverticula in our series into three groups according to size, as shown in Table 5–1. The "yardstick" used in this classification is the vertebral column posterior to the diverticulum on the radiograph.

to be a rare complication with an incidence of 0.05% or less. On radiographs, such a carcinoma can be seen as a filling defect in the contrast medium. A filling defect in the diverticulum is usually caused by food retention, but if the defect is consistently seen on radiographs taken at certain intervals, then the possibility of carcinoma should be considered. In our opinion the suspicion of carcinoma is in fact the only indication for diagnostic esopha-

OPERATIVE TECHNIQUE

The procedure is carried out either with general anesthesia or with local anesthesia and diazepam given intravenously. The relatively mild stress imposed by local anesthesia is an important advantage in older patients, whose general condition may be poor. However, we prefer general anesthesia, particularly for first-time treatment, because muscle relaxants can

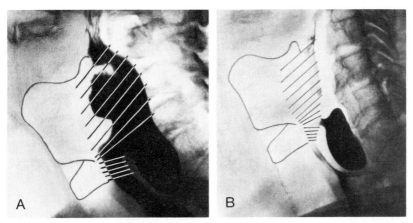

Figure 5–2. Radiographs of a Zenker's diverticulum, in which the inferior constrictor muscle and the cricopharyngeal muscle have been outlined. *A*, During the passage of contrast medium, hypopharynx and diverticulum form a single mass, and the esophagus is in line with the hypopharynx. *B*, After passage, the muscles contract and the diverticulum is "tied off" from the hypopharyngeal lumen. Contraction of the cricopharyngeal muscle alters the position of the esophageal inlet.

Table 5–1. Classification of Zenker's Diverticulum in 303 Patients

Size	No. of Patients
Small (<1 vertebral body)	35
Medium	228
Large (>3 vertebral bodies)	40
Total	303

then be given to relax the pharyngoesophageal sphincter. With relaxation, the esophageal inlet is open and can be more readily identified.

Locating the esophageal inlet and severing the tissue bridge to the proper extent requires experience and is in fact the most difficult part of the procedure. To facilitate location of the esophageal inlet during endoscopy, the patient is asked to swallow a metallic pellet attached to a black thread the night before the endoscopic procedure. On the day of the operation, radiofluoroscopy is carried out in order to locate the pellet. Even when the pellet lies in the diverticulum, the thread can still be a useful aid in locating the esophageal inlet, because in such cases esophagoscopy often discloses that a loop of the thread lies in the inlet.

Initially we used an esophagoscope with an electrocautery smoke exhaust canal within its wall. This scope is now used only when treatment must be done under local anesthesia. If there is food retention, the diverticulum is first emptied by suction to allow careful examination of the diverticular wall. When the tip of the scope is placed in the esophageal inlet, the spur between diverticulum and esophagus is exposed properly. With an insulated forceps the spur is grasped in the midline, and electrocoagulation is carried out. The diathermic knife is then used to cut through the center of the coagulated tissue.

With the increase in the number of patients with this disorder, the technique and instruments used have improved. In 1981 we started to apply a microendoscopic procedure with a specially designed scope (Fig. 5–3) and an operating microscope. The special scope is 25 cm long, with a divided end. Channels in both lateral walls permit introduction of light conductors. Once the scope is adjusted and fixed to the chest support, the light conductors are replaced by cannulas for continuous suction drainage. This is necessary to remove the smoke of electrocoagulation or the steam and disagreeable odor associated with the use of the carbon dioxide (CO_2) laser.

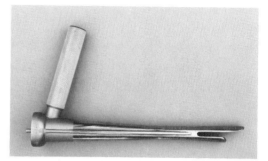

Figure 5–3. Lateral view of the scope applied for severance of the tissue bridge between esophagus and diverticulum under microscopic control.

Although endoscopic skill is required, exposure of the tissue bridge with the aid of the double-lipped scope generally poses no special problems. Once the longer (upper) lip of the scope is in position behind the arytenoids, the larynx is lifted and at the same time the scope is advanced. In many cases the upper lip enters the esophageal inlet almost automatically. The shorter lip finds its way into the ample lumen of the diverticulum without difficulty, and the tissue bridge is in effect caught between the two lips. Once the spur is in focus, the chest support is attached to the scope. In order to avoid restriction of respiration excursions of the chest we prefer to fix the support on a platform mounted over the patient's chest (Fig. 5–4). The operating microscope with a conventional 40-cm objective affords a splendid overview of the bridge to be severed (Fig. 5–5A). General anesthesia is necessary for microendoscopic surgery. When there is objection to general anesthesia owing to the patient's condition, the endoscopic procedure is performed with local anesthesia using esopha-

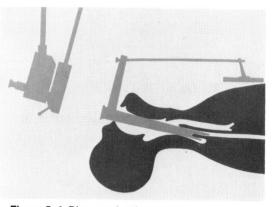

Figure 5–4. Diagram showing the scope in position and the CO_2 laser micromanipulator coupled with the operating microscope.

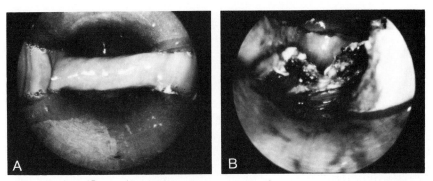

Figure 5–5. Microendoscopic views. *A,* The tissue bridge between esophagus and diverticulum. *B,* After severance with the CO_2 laser.

goscopy and the electrocoagulation technique, without preadjustment of the operating microscope. In microendoscopic surgery very precise severance of the tissue bridge between esophagus and diverticulum is feasible, using either electrocoagulation, with insulated-shaft microsurgical instruments, or CO_2 laser.[6]

In the past few years we have increasingly utilized the CO_2 laser, because it appears to cause less tissue necrosis and to produce less cicatricial tissue. Initially we feared that the complications of emphysema and mediastinitis might occur more frequently than with the more familiar technique of electrocoagulation, but this has not proved to be the case. Both with electrocoagulation and with the CO_2 laser, the wound edges as a rule separate immediately, resulting in a wedge-shaped excision (Fig. 5–5*B*). This separation is caused by retraction of the severed cricopharyngeal muscle fibers, which are readily identifiable through the microscope. In microendoscopic surgery for Zenker's diverticulum we use an output of 35 watts for severance of the tissue bridge. Wet "patties" are placed in the esophagus and the diverticulum. With the CO_2 laser the procedure has sometimes caused slightly greater blood loss than with electrocoagulation. When the bleeding is copious and cannot be arrested with the laser, brief electrocoagulation via an insulated suction drain is effective. Our impression is that patients treated with the CO_2 laser suffered less pain during the first postoperative day and consequently were able to take food more readily. After the operation all patients are given antibiotics and liquid food for 1 week.

In patients with very large diverticula, we prefer to sever the spur in two or three separate applications of the laser. After six weeks we evaluate the need for continued cutting by barium swallow radiographs and by the patient's reported subjective sensation of symp-

tomatic relief. In an occasional case there is radiologic evidence of a residual diverticulum, but the patient is usually asymptomatic postoperatively. Repetition of the procedure is always possible, but with a small residual spur, no further treatment is required if the patient has no discomfort (Fig. 5–6). Although diagnostic radiologic studies are indispensable in the postoperative phase and during the follow-up period, the importance of information obtained by such studies should not be overestimated. The patient's subjective sense of well-being is at least as important a criterion of successful treatment.

RESULTS

In 79% of our patients the minimum follow-up period has been of 2 years' duration, and, as far as we know, none of our patients has since sought treatment elsewhere. Of the 303 patients, 276 (91%) are highly satisfied and 26 (8.6%) are fairly satisfied with the result obtained. Although one patient died two days postoperatively of cardiac failure, the complications we observed were mostly not serious, and our complication rate was very low (Table 5–2). Our experience indicates that the risk of mediastinitis is smaller than often suggested in the presence of adhesions between diverticulum and the posterior esophageal wall. Radiologic follow-up studies revealed no essential difference between results with the electrocoagulation technique and those with the CO_2 laser.

CONCLUSIONS

Our results obtained over many years with endoscopic management of Zenker's diverticulum have prompted us to continue to use this

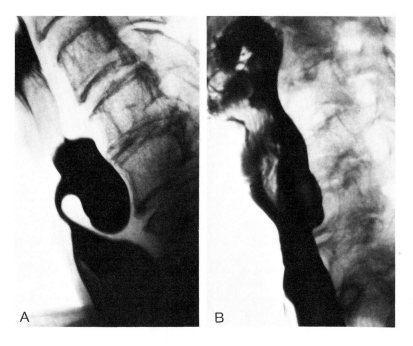

Figure 5–6. Radiographs before *(A)* and after *(B)* microendoscopic treatment of a medium-sized diverticulum.

approach and to further perfect the techniques involved. Exposure of the tissue bridge between esophagus and diverticulum, with the aid of the specially designed double-lipped scope and facilities for fixation as described, poses no significant problems. The use of the operating microscope has allowed great improvement in endoscopic surgical treatment. Very precise severance of the spur is feasible using a CO_2 laser or insulated-shaft microsurgical instruments for electrocautery. The magnification makes it possible to identify the nature of the tissue in the plane of severance and to follow the separation of the muscle fibers. Hemorrhage, if it occurs, can be arrested without causing more than minimal tissue damage.

It is somewhat surprising that endoscopic management of Zenker's diverticulum has failed to become more popular. An important advantage of endoscopic treatment is that it can be carried out in patients whose general condition is poor. The procedure requires experience, but we believe experience is likewise important in the transcutaneous approach.

In view of our results in 303 patients, we feel justified in maintaining that endoscopic surgical management of Zenker's diverticulum can be regarded as a safe and effective method of treatment. The risk of complications with this method is minimal with our techniques as described.

ACKNOWLEDGMENTS

The authors wish to thank the technicians A. de Jong and H. Leever as well as photographer M. Goslinga.

Table 5–2. Complications and Their Outcome Following Endoscopic Treatment of Zenker's Diverticulum in 303 Patients

Complication	No. of Patients[a]	Outcome
Mediastinitis	5	Cured by conservative therapy
Hemorrhage	4	Endoscopically controlled
Esophagotracheal fistula	1	Closed spontaneously within 3 weeks
Emphysema	9	Only temporary, in the neck
Tendency to stenosis	8	Satisfactory results following endoscopic dilations
Death	1	At 2 days postoperatively from cardiac failure

[a]More than one complication occurred in 3 patients.

References

1. Dohlman G: Endoscopic operations for hypopharyngeal diverticula. *In* Proceedings of the Fourth International Congress on Otolaryngology, London, 1949, pp 715–717.
2. Dohlman G, Mattson O: The endoscopic operation for hypopharyngeal diverticula. Arch Otolaryngol 71: 744–752, 1960.
3. Overbeek JJM van, Hoeksema PE: Endoscopic treatment of the hypopharyngeal diverticulum: 211 cases. Laryngoscope 92:88–91, 1982.
4. Mosher HP: Webs and pouches of the esophagus, their diagnosis and treatment. Surg Gynecol Obstet 25:175–187, 1917.
5. Overbeek JJM van: The Hypopharyngeal Diverticulum. Endoscopic Treatment and Manometry. Assen, Amsterdam, Van Gorcum, 1977.
6. Overbeek JJM van, Hoeksema PE, Edens E: Microendoscopic surgery of the hypopharyngeal diverticulum using electrocoagulation or carbon dioxide laser. Ann Otol Rhinol Laryngol 93:34–36, 1984.

6

The Management of Zenker's Diverticulum: Endoscopic (Dohlman) Diverticulotomy

James E. Rejowski, M.D.
Lauren D. Holinger, M.D.

In the United States, traditional treatment of the hypopharyngeal (Zenker's) diverticulum has been single-stage transcutaneous diverticulectomy. Complications following this procedure include mediastinitis, vocal cord paralysis, esophageal stenosis, fistula, and recurrent or persistent diverticulum. Endoscopic (Dohlman) diverticulotomy, widely used throughout Europe, is relatively straightforward and efficacious. In our experience, transoral management of these diverticula has allowed symptomatic relief with a low incidence of complications. The following discussion presents indications, techniques, and results of endoscopic management, as well as the history, related anatomy, etiology, symptoms, and methods of diagnosis of this interesting disorder.

INDICATIONS

The hypopharyngeal (Zenker's) diverticulum is an uncommon and interesting entity with a classic symptom complex. Because it is primarily a disease of the elderly, its incidence in the United States has increased with the aging of our population. The respiratory and deglutitory symptoms and complications often require surgical intervention. Cricopharyngeal myotomy alone or as a supplemental procedure to diverticulectomy has been recommended to prevent recurrence. Endoscopic diverticulotomy (including cricopharyngeal myotomy), although not a new procedure, represents an effective method of treatment, with relief of dysphagia and aspiration. It is particularly suitable for the elderly debilitated patient with multiple medical problems who is at increased risk with a more prolonged procedure requiring general anesthesia.

HISTORICAL ASPECTS

In 1764 Abraham Ludlow, an English surgeon, presented "a case of obstructive deglutition from a preternatural dilatation of, and bag formed in, the pharynx."[1] His 60-year-old patient suffered progressive and ultimately fatal dysphagia and regurgitation. At autopsy a large hypopharyngeal diverticulum was visualized extending into the thoracic cavity between the esophageal and prevertebral fascia. It was not until 1877 that esophageal diverticula were classified by Zenker.[2] The hypopharyngeal diverticulum has since borne his name.

Evolution of the surgical treatment of hypopharyngeal diverticula began in 1877 when Nicoladoni successfully established a fistula from an esophageal pouch to the skin.[1] In 1884 Niehaus performed the first excision of a sac in a patient operated on for a goiter. A two-stage transcervical approach with initial sac ligation and, 2 weeks later, sac division, was employed in 1909 by Goldman;[3] this technique was later widely used by Lahey and Warren.[4] In 1932, as an alternative to diverticulectomy, a cricopharyngeal myotomy without diverticulectomy was performed by Siefert, with successful results.[3]

Endoscopic diverticulotomy, a transoral division of the septum between the esophageal lumen and the diverticulum, was described in 1917 by Mosher.[3, 5] He used a punch forceps to excise this septum successfully in six patients. However, he abandoned the technique when fatal mediastinitis occurred in the seventh patient. In 1960, Dohlman[6] reported results that demonstrated the safety and efficacy of endoscopic diverticulotomy. He used a specially designed double-lipped esophagoscope (Fig. 6–1) and electrocautery to divide the septum. No severe complications or deaths

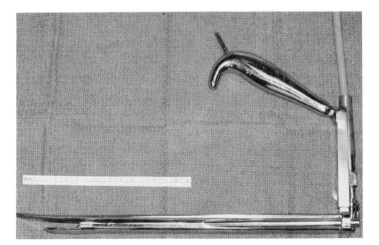

Figure 6–1. Dohlman endoscope.

were reported in 100 operations. Holinger[7, 8] was able to duplicate Dohlman's results, confirming the efficacy and safety of the technique. Currently, diverticulotomy is considered the treatment of choice in Europe.[9]

RELATED ANATOMY AND PATHOGENESIS

The hypopharyngeal diverticulum has been considered a pseudodiverticulum of mucosa and submucosa herniating through Killian's dehiscence in the posterior hypopharyngeal wall. The borders of Killian's triangle are the oblique fibers of the inferior pharyngeal constrictor muscle superiorly and the transverse fibers of the cricopharyngeus muscle inferiorly. The consistent anatomic location and increasing prevalence of Zenker's diverticulum in the elderly suggests that prolonged neuromuscular dysfunction is a primary etiologic factor.

The cricopharyngeus muscle functions as the upper esophageal sphincter. It is normally closed to prevent inspiration of air into the esophagus. Deglutition involves a voluntary oral phase followed by an involuntary pharyngoesophageal phase. A highly coordinated reflex mechanism (mediated through the vagus nerve and pharyngeal plexus) allows cricopharyngeal muscle relaxation synchronous with contraction of the pharyngeal constrictors. Recontraction of the cricopharyngeus initiates the esophageal peristaltic wave. Disturbance of this complicated sequence or timing (such as in cricopharyngeal muscle spasm, premature contraction, delayed relaxation with a second swallow against a closed sphincter, or achalasia) has been considered to be responsible for hypopharyngeal diverticulum formation.[10] In such circumstances, pharyngeal forces exerted against a closed sphincter would eventually cause a herniation through the congenitally weakened area above.

Progressive weakening of the prevertebral fascia with loss of support and anterior migration of the larynx has also been considered to be responsible for cricopharyngeal dysfunction and diverticulum formation.[11] Although manometric studies have resulted in conflicting evidence,[10, 12] premature contraction and hypertrophy of the cricopharyngeus has been demonstrated by Ellis.[10]

Extramucosal myotomy without resection of the sac has been reported to be effective in the management of Zenker's diverticulum;[13] this too suggests an important role of the cricopharyngeus in the pathogenesis of sac formation. Concomitant esophageal disorders, such as gastroesophageal reflux, may also contribute to the formation of hypopharyngeal diverticula.[14]

SYMPTOMS

Hypopharyngeal diverticula usually occur in males over age 60 years. Pulmonary and obstructive symptoms are related to the underlying motility disorder as well as to the size and mass effect of the sac. Slowly progressive dysphagia is a frequent symptom; often it has been present for more than 10 years. Food impaction, gurgling (especially at night), foreign body sensation in the postcricoid area, choking, and a constant desire to clear the throat are common. Successive swallows are necessary for deglutition. Regurgitation of undigested food when supine and nocturnal coughing spells due to aspiration of sac contents are frequent. Borborygmi may occur with swallowing. Decomposition of food within the sac causes fetid breath. Hoarseness from recurrent laryngeal nerve compression is sometimes seen with large diverticula. Acute esophageal obstruction from impaction of a meat bolus occurs infrequently; in such cases the patient usually relates an antecedent history of dysphagia and weight loss. The rare occurrence of carcinoma within the sac is suggested by expectoration of blood-tinged saliva or persistent pain.[15]

Indirect laryngoscopy may reveal pooling of secretions in the hypopharynx. Rarely, an enlargement is palpable in the supraclavicular area; compression may cause coughing owing to expression of fluid into the airway. Patients with a diverticulum of long standing may develop malnutrition, bronchiectasis, and lung abscess.

DIAGNOSIS

The diagnosis is confirmed radiographically. An air–fluid level within the pouch may be evident on routine posteroanterior and lateral chest x-ray films. A barium contrast study demonstrates the sac projecting posterior and slightly lateral to the esopharyngeal lumen, usually to the left. The thickness of the septum demonstrated on the lateral view is due to the bulk of the cricopharyngeus muscle (Fig. 6–2).

MANAGEMENT

Diverticulectomy

Diverticulopexy with inversion and suspension of the sac and *two-stage diverticulectomy* have had their proponents in the past.[4] In the United States the most common procedure currently is a *single-stage diverticulectomy with cricopharyngeal myotomy*. The principles of this procedure are as follows. Following a collar incision, the left carotid sheath is identified and retracted posteriorly. The omohyoid muscle is divided and the larynx rotated to the right. The recurrent laryngeal nerve is identified and preserved. Placement of an esophagoscope within the sac facilitates identification. The sac is dissected free and amputated, and the mucosa is carefully closed with absorbable

sutures or using a surgical stapling device. An esophageal (Maloney) dilator prevents excessive resection of mucosa with subsequent stenosis. It also facilitates cricopharyngeal myotomy, which is done in all cases. The wound is drained and closed. Oral intake is resumed 1 week postoperatively.

Reported results are satisfactory, but complications such as injury to the recurrent laryngeal nerve, fistula, wound infection, hematoma, or persistent or recurrent diverticulum may occur.[16-18] Repeat operation to resect a recurrent diverticulum (Table 6–1) is difficult and significantly increases the risk of injury to the recurrent laryngeal nerve.

Endoscopic Diverticulotomy

Patients with Zenker's diverticulum are usually elderly, often having concomitant medical problems contraindicating a longer procedure under general anesthesia. Management of such patients includes immediate correction of dehydration and electrolyte imbalance and of the sequelae of aspiration and the eventual treatment of the diverticulum itself. Such intervention is initially directed to relief of the esophageal obstruction and to prevention of recurrent aspiration.

Endoscopic diverticulotomy effectively removes the septum (common wall) from between the diverticulum and the esophagus to create one common lumen. The cricopharyngeus muscle is severed with division of the septum. Although complete anatomic removal of the sac is not accomplished (nor should it be attempted), the anterior wall of the diverticulum is effectively lowered. This eliminates overflow of sac contents into the larynx. Instead, contents of the diverticulum spill asymptomatically into the cervical esophagus below the level of the cricopharyngeus (Fig. 6–3). The procedure immediately eliminates overflow from the diverticulum into the larynx, providing early restoration of integrity of the swallowing mechanism with minimal physical manipulation. Division of the cricopharyngeus muscle alleviates the underlying cause of the dysphagia; pulmonary sequelae resolve rapidly. A postoperative barium study demonstrates the remnant of the diverticulum emptying readily into the esophagus on a second swallow.

Either general or topical anesthesia may be employed. Insertion of an esophagoscope permits evacuation of retained secretions from the

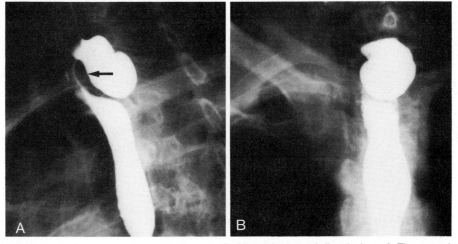

Figure 6–2. Barium esophagograms demonstrating a typical hypopharyngeal diverticulum. *A,* The arrow indicates the septum, containing the cricopharyngeus muscle, which separates the diverticulum from the cervical esophagus. *B,* AP view.

hypopharynx and contents of the diverticulum and allows careful examination to rule out the presence of carcinoma. The esophagoscope is withdrawn, and the double-beaked endoscope is inserted: the anterior lip into the esophagus, the posterior lip into the diverticulum. This brings the septum (containing the cricopharyngeus muscle) clearly into view suspended across the central portion of the field. An alligator forceps (Fig. 6–4) with insulated shaft is used to grasp the septum in the midline for a distance of 2.5 to 3 cm. A coagulating current is applied until the tissue is visibly cauterized. The forceps is removed and the insulating spatula is passed into the diverticulum posterior to the coagulated portion of the septum. The cauterized portion of the septum is incised using a blade with mixed cutting and coagulating current. This incision divides the cricopharyngeus muscle as well as the septum. Bleeding at the cut ends of the tissue is minimal and is easily controlled with electrocautery or

the application of surgical gel (Gelfoam). Complete division of a septum longer than 3 cm is contraindicated because of the associated risk of a leak into the mediastinum. If necessary, further division can be done at a later date.[19] The lateral pull of the cricopharyngeus opens the sac into the esophagus. Use of the operating microscope facilitates accurate division of the septum; this instrument is routinely used when the septum is divided with the laser.[20]

The procedure usually takes only a few minutes, in contrast to the considerably longer external cervical approach. Oral intake is begun 48 hours postoperatively. The patient is monitored carefully for fever, chest pain, tachycardia, and subcutaneous emphysema. Broad-spectrum parenteral antibiotics are administered. Clear liquids are begun on the third postoperative day, a soft diet on the fifth. Patients are usually discharged on the fifth postoperative day.

Table 6–1. Incidence of Complications Following Transcervical Diverticulectomy in Reported Series

| | | Incidence of Complications (%) | | |
Series	No. of Patients	*RLN*[a] *Palsy*	*Fistula*	*Recurrent Diverticulum*
Kuhn et al[18] (1977)	26	4	4	4
Todd[16] (1974)	48	19	19	13
Welsh and Payne[17] (1973)	809	2.8	1.4	3.3

[a] Recurrent laryngeal nerve.

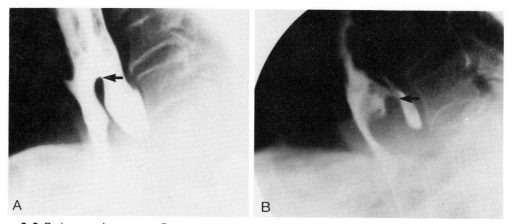

Figure 6–3. Barium esophagograms. Preoperatively *(A)*, the septum is high *(arrow)*. Contents of the diverticulum may overflow into the larynx. Postoperatively *(B)*, the septum is effectively lowered *(arrow)*, allowing fluids to spill asymptomatically from the diverticulum into the esophagus.

Dramatic symptomatic relief occurs at once following endoscopic diverticulotomy. Morbidity is minimal (Table 6–2). Dohlman[6] reported no severe complications in 39 patients (100 operations). Mediastinitis occurred twice in Holinger and Jensik's series of 43 patients.[8] One case was due to severe postoperative vomiting, and the other from too-aggressive division of the septum. Both patients recovered following external drainage. Todd[16] performed 75 diverticulotomies in 58 patients and obtained satisfactory results in 38 patients (65%) following the first procedure; 17 patients had repeat diverticulotomy (overall success rate, 84%). No deaths occurred; one case each of mediastinitis and hemorrhage developed. Asymptomatic surgical emphysema and stenosis requiring dilatations developed in three and two cases, respectively. Trible[5] re-

ported improvement in 24 of 25 patients with no mortality, mediastinitis, or hemorrhage.

Van Overbeek and Hoeksema have used the endoscopic technique in several hundred patients with excellent results and minimal complications.[19] Their three cases of mediastinitis responded to conservative management. Two patients had postoperative hemorrhage, which required a repeat endoscopic procedure for control. There was one instance of tracheoesophageal fistula (due to defective insulation of the cautery apparatus), which closed spontaneously.

CONCLUSIONS

The hypopharyngeal (Zenker's) diverticulum can cause significant morbidity in elderly patients. Although complications of the tradi-

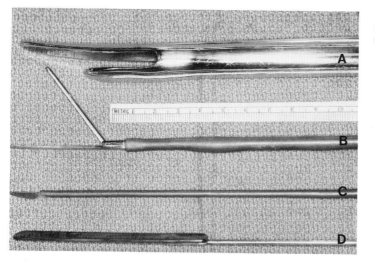

Figure 6–4. Dohlman diverticulotomy instruments. *A*, Endoscope; *B*, alligator forceps; *C*, blade; *D*, insulating spatula.

Table 6–2. Results of Endoscopic Diverticulotomy in Reported Series

Series	No. of Patients	% of Patients with Resolution of Symptoms	Incidence of Mediastinitis (%)	No. of Deaths
van Overbeek[19] (1982)	211	91.5	1.4	1
Trible[5] (1975)	25	96	0	0
Todd[16] (1974)	58	84	3.4	0
Holinger and Schild[17] (1969)	43		4.6	0
Dohlman[6] (1960)	39		0	0

tional external approach for diverticulectomy (vocal cord paralysis, fistula, and recurrent diverticulum) are infrequent, they represent difficult management problems when they occur. A prolonged operation is undesirable in elderly, debilitated patients with concurrent medical diseases.

Endoscopic diverticulotomy is a rapid, effective, and safe technique for management of hypopharyngeal diverticula. The incidence of mediastinal infection is low. Resection of the sac neither is necessary nor should be attempted, since division of the septum and cricopharyngeus muscle allows emptying from the pouch into the esophagus. This alleviates the dysphagia and prevents overflow of the secretions into the larynx, which is the cause of pulmonary complications. Endoscopic diverticulotomy is an effective alternative to diverticulectomy accomplished through an external approach and is particularly suitable for elderly patients with multi-system diseases who are at greater risk with prolonged procedures and general anesthesia.

References

1. Chitwood WR Jr: Esophageal diverticulum: a preternatural bag. Surgery 85:549–553, 1979.
2. Zenker FA, von Ziemssen H: Krankheit des Oesophagus. In von Ziemssen H (ed): Handbuch der Speciellen Pathologie und Therapie. Vol 7 (suppl). Leipzig, FCW Vogel, 1877.
3. White, Irving L: Severe complication of a Zenker's diverticulum with endoscopic diverticulotomy rescue. Laryngoscope 91:708–719, 1981.
4. Lahey FH, Warren KW: Esophageal diverticula. Surg Gynecol Obstet 98:1–28, 1954.
5. Trible, WM: The surgical treatment of Zenker's diverticulum: endoscopic vs. external operation. South Med J 68:1260–1262, 1975.
6. Dohlman G: The endoscopic operation for hypopharyngeal diverticula. Arch Otolaryngol 71:744–752, 1960.
7. Holinger PH, Schild JA: The Zenker's (hypopharyngeal) diverticulum. Ann Otol Rhinol Laryngol 78:679–688, 1969.
8. Holinger PH, Jensik RJ: Halting the progress of Zenker's diverticula. Geriatrics 28:133–137, 1973.
9. Overbeek JJM van: The Hypopharyngeal Diverticulum. Endoscopic Treatment and Manometry. Assen, Amsterdam, Van Gorcum, 1977.
10. Ellis FH Jr, Schlegel JF, Lynch VP, Payne WS: Cricopharyngeal myotomy for pharyngo-esophageal diverticulum. Ann Surg 170:342–350, 1969.
11. Dorsey JM, Randolph DA: Long-term evaluation of pharyngo-esophageal diverticulectomy. Ann Surg 173:680–685, 1971.
12. Knuff TE, Benjamin SB, Castell DO: Pharyngoesophageal (Zenker's) diverticulum: a reappraisal. Gastroenterology 82:734–736, 1982.
13. Zuckerbraun L, Bahna MS: Cricopharyngeus myotomy as the only treatment for Zenker diverticulum. Ann Otol 88:798–803, 1979.
14. Delahunty JE, Margulies SI, Alonso WA, Knudson DH: The relationship of reflux esophagitis to pharyngeal pouch (Zenker's diverticulum) formation. Laryngoscope 81:570–577, 1971.
15. Donald PJ, Huffman DI: Carcinoma in a Zenker's diverticulum. Head Neck Surg 2:71–75, 1979.
16. Todd GB: The treatment of pharyngeal pouch. J Laryngol Otol 88:307–315, 1974.
17. Welsh GF, Payne WS: The present status of one-stage pharyngo-esophageal diverticulectomy. Surg Clin North Am 53:953–958, 1973.
18. Kuhn FA, Sessions DG, Ogura JH: Hypopharyngeal diverticulum. Laryngoscope 87:147–153, 1977.
19. Overbeek JJM van, Hoeksema PE: Endoscopic treatment of the hypopharyngeal diverticulum: 211 cases. Laryngoscope 92:88–91, 1982.
20. Overbeek JJM van, Hoeksema PE, Edens ET: Microendoscopic surgery of the hypopharyngeal diverticulum using electrocoagulation or the carbon dioxide laser. Ann Otol Rhinol Laryngol 93:34–36, 1984.

II

The Surgical Management of Recurrent or Persistent Pneumothorax

Air in the chest, or *empyema of air in the pleura,* as pneumothorax was termed originally, was not considered very significant by ancient physicians. As examples, both Hippocrates and Galen were well aware of the pleural space and some of its diseases because of the high incidence of purulent empyema in their times. Hippocrates accurately described the *how, when,* and *why* of opening the pleural space for treatment of empyema. He also recommended the introduction of air into the chest to relieve pleuritic pain. The splashing sound now termed hippocratic succussion was noted by him, but he did not appreciate the fact that air, in addition to pleural fluid, must be present to produce this noise.

Penetrating wounds of the chest obviously caused air in the chest, but such wounds generally attracted attention only when subcutaneous emphysema was present; this situation was termed emphysema of the chest. The surgical dogma for many centuries was that stab wounds and even sucking wounds of the chest could be managed solely by wound care and were rarely fatal. If emphysema of the chest was present, then one or several incisions might be needed to "let the air escape."

By the 18th century the technique of thoracentesis in treating certain cases of empyema was fairly well recognized. Hewson (1767) noted that in some patients occasionally air, not fluid, was aspirated by *"paracentesis thoracis"* and that removal of the air alone resulted in clinical relief of the patient's dyspnea. Further experiments by Hewson with rabbits conclusively showed the harmful effects of air in the pleural cavity. Previously Alexander Munro the younger (1697–1767) had stated in his lectures that air should be removed in certain instances of "empyema of air in the pleura" if the patient had extreme dyspnea.

Itard (1803) was the first to suggest the term pneumothorax; others recommended pneumato-thorax or pneuma-thorax. If mediastinal shift was present, it was called *tense* or *valvular* pneumothorax. Gradually, pneumothorax with various modifying adjectives has become the accepted terminology.

Air in the pleural cavity and collapse of the lung were noted at autopsy during the 17th and 18th centuries. In the majority of instances these were accompanied by inflammatory lung disease, particularly tuberculosis. The clinical findings of pneumothorax were described by Laennec (1819), who also suggested that it was caused by rupture of an emphysematous bleb. However, the accurate and definitive diagnosis of pneumothorax, particularly when small, became possible only after development of the x-ray. In 1901 Martin presented the first "skiagram" showing a pneumothorax, although the picture was taken after the patient's death!

In the second half of the 19th century the high incidence of tuberculosis in the population and its frequent complication of pneumothorax quite naturally led to the teaching that when pneumothorax occurred, tuberculosis was the most likely etiology. The beneficial effect of pneumothorax in treating tuberculosis was suggested by Forlanini in 1882. The existing attitude toward traumatic pneumothorax and the therapeutic effect of pneumothorax in tuberculosis led to a casual attitude toward the clinical importance of pneumothorax, regardless of its etiology.

It was not until 1926 that Miller gave a clearcut anatomic description of emphysematous blebs and bullae and their distinction from congenital cysts. Early in this century it became increasingly evident that pneumothorax could and did occur in nontuberculous patients. When this type of pneumothorax became chronic, treatment to produce a symphysis of the pleural surfaces was attempted by poudrage (Spengler, 1906). In these early efforts silver nitrate, hypertonic glucose, the patient's blood, and many other substances were injected into the pleural space.

Lockwood (1928), in discussing a paper about recurrent spontaneous pneumothorax, asked, and quite properly: "Why could not the lung be inflated and sutured and perhaps the opening located? That just occurred to me as a possibility." Such an operation was subsequently done by Bigger some time "prior to 1937." That *recurrent* spontaneous pneumothorax should be treated surgically was first emphasized in an article by Tyson and Crandall (1941). They described a patient with five episodes of pneumothorax who was operated on (1936) and a 5-cm. emphysematous bleb excised, but no pleural poudrage, abrasion, or pleurectomy was performed.

The onset of World War II focused attention on high altitude flying and its relation to pneumothorax. The rapid expansion of blebs and bullae (estimated at 30 times in the change from 15,000 to 60,000 feet!) demanded consideration of this situation in pilots (Dominy and Campbell, 1963). As a result, the indications for and value of an operative procedure to manage current and prevent future episodes of pneumothorax became established.

Despite the frequency of chronic recurrent pneumothorax and the great amount of attention it has received, controversy still exists regarding the "procedure of choice" for its surgical treatment.

Pleural abrasion, poudrage, or pleurectomy—which *is* preferable?

7

The Surgical Management of Recurrent or Persistent Pneumothorax: Abrasive Pleurodesis

Peter C. Pairolero, M.D.
W. Spencer Payne, M.D.

Air in the pleural cavity compressing the lung was first recognized as a clinical entity in 1803 by Itard;[1] he named this process *pneumothorax*. Sudden nontraumatic unexpected pulmonary collapse in an otherwise apparently healthy person was subsequently termed *spontaneous* pneumothorax.

ETIOLOGY

For many years, tuberculosis was considered the primary cause of spontaneous pneumothorax. Although DeVilliers in 1826 reported the first case of spontaneous pneumothorax secondary to rupture of a pulmonary bleb,[2] it was not until 1932 that Kjaergaard demonstrated that tuberculosis was an uncommon cause.[3] Since then, other studies have substantiated his findings,[4, 5] and many disease entities are now recognized that can result in pulmonary collapse, including pulmonary blebs, tuberculosis, cancer (both primary and metastatic), scleroderma, histiocytosis X, pneumoconiosis, diffuse interstitial pulmonary fibrosis, enterogenous cyst, pulmonary endometriosis (catamenial pneumothorax), tuberous sclerosis, and Marfan's syndrome.[5-8] Today, the majority of cases of spontaneous pneumothorax have been demonstrated by Dines and coworkers to result from rupture of small subpleural pulmonary blebs located most commonly in the apex of the lung.[7]

CLINICOPATHOLOGIC FEATURES

Spontaneous pneumothorax occurs most often in young adults, is five times more frequent in men than in women, and is slightly more common on the right side than on the left. Although strenuous exercise may precipitate pneumothorax, many episodes do occur during sleep or at rest. The most common symptoms are pain and dyspnea. Other signs and symptoms seen with more extensive pulmonary collapse include cyanosis, hypotension, and tachypnea. Unless advanced chronic obstructive pulmonary disease is present, death rarely occurs.[7]

SELECTION OF TREATMENT

From a practical point of view, the management of recurrent spontaneous pneumothorax should pose few problems irrespective of cause. The primary goal should be re-expansion of the lung. The mode of treatment indicated, however, depends upon the extent of pulmonary collapse, the cause of the collapse, and the number of episodes of collapse.

Conservative Management

BED REST

Spontaneous pneumothorax was for many years treated by bed rest alone. The period of hospitalization required was usually several weeks in duration. In some cases, many months would elapse before the lung re-expanded fully.

INTERCOSTAL TUBE THORACOSTOMY SUCTION

In the mid-1940s, intercostal tube thoracostomy suction was introduced; the use of this modality reduced the length of required hospitalization considerably.[9] Today, patients with a small apical pneumothorax can still be well managed with bed rest and restricted activity alone. Delayed pulmonary expansion, progressive pneumothorax, or the development of symptoms, however, indicates the need for the use of an intercostal suction catheter.

Selection of Tube Insertion Site. The site of insertion of the thoracostomy suction tube depends on the location of the pneumothorax. When pleural adhesions are absent, the second or third intercostal space anteriorly is usually appropriate. This point is chosen since it is situated close to the apex of the pleural cavity; with the patient in the recumbent position, this anterior location is more suitable for the evacuation of air. In women, an insertion site in the inframammary fold often avoids injury to the breast. In certain cases, other placement sites may be indicated—for example, supradiaphragmatic placement in a patient with subpulmonic pneumothorax.

Selection of Intercostal Tube. The choice of intercostal tube utilized varies among surgeons. Generally, small polyethylene catheters should be avoided since they limit air flow. We prefer a soft plastic catheter, size 20 to 24 F.

Pleurodesis for Prevention of Recurrence

The rate of recurrence of spontaneous pneumothorax varies in reported series but overall is approximately 50% after one episode and 80% after three.[10] Collapse of the contralateral lung occurs in approximately 15% of patients. Seremetis found the recurrence rate to be 49% with treatment by bed rest alone, 40% with treatment initially by bed rest and later by tube thoracostomy suction, and 38% with treatment primarily by tube suction.[11] Because of the high rate of recurrent pneumothorax, efforts at prevention are directed toward obliteration of the pleural space (pleurodesis).

DISADVANTAGES OF CHEMICAL PLEURODESIS

The first attempt to obliterate the pleural space to prevent recurrent pneumothorax was described by Spengler in 1906.[12] He demonstrated that when injected into the pleural cavity, silver nitrate produced a chemical pleuritis that resulted in delicate avascular adhesions between the pleural surfaces, which prevented pulmonary collapse. Since then, various other irritating chemicals have also been advocated, including tetracycline hydrochloride, talcum powder, iodoform, iodized oil, guaiacol, nitrogen mustard, and hypertonic glucose

solution; these chemicals are generally injected into the pleural cavity through a thoracentesis or tube thoracostomy. Such injections, however, have the disadvantage of being blind and imprecise, and with each of the chemicals used, results are often less than satisfactory, with effective pleurodesis being accomplished only in gravity-dependent areas of the thorax. In addition, multiple injections, which frequently are painful for the patient, are often necessary.

INDICATIONS FOR THORACOTOMY

For the aforementioned reasons, thoracotomy is usually necessary in patients with recurrent pneumothorax, not only to effect pleurodesis but also to enable control of the course of the air leak. Thoracotomy is indicated in patients who have (1) persistent air leak after 4 or 5 days; (2) failure of re-expansion of the lung; (3) borderline cardiopulmonary reserve; or (4) history of recurrent pneumothorax. At thoracotomy, either pleural abrasion or parietal pleurectomy can be done to achieve pleurodesis.

MANAGEMENT WITH ABRASIVE PLEURODESIS

In patients in whom thoracotomy is indicated, we prefer pleural abrasion over parietal pleurectomy for the following reasons: Abrasion can be performed through a limited thoracotomy; intraoperative and postoperative bleeding is minimal; empyema is rare; and nerve injury is eliminated.[13] Moreover, pleural abrasion results in filmy, elastic, avascular adhesions that can be readily divided if another thoracotomy becomes necessary. Also, abrasive pleurodesis is not associated with restrictive lung disease that is occasionally seen after parietal pleurectomy.

Technique

In the simplest cases involving only apical pulmonary collapse without entrapment, pleural abrasion can be carried out through a limited lateral axillary thoracotomy, which causes little postoperative discomfort or disfigurement. Any blebs or persistent air leaks can be managed either by suturing or by stapling through this incision without the need for more extensive thoracotomy. The operation is completed by simply abrading both the parietal and visceral pleurae with dry gauze until these surfaces become erythematous and telangiectatic. The thorax is then closed in the standard fashion after insertion of an intercostal drainage tube. Early ambulation is allowed following operation. Tube thoracostomy suction is continued until the air leak has stopped, usually by 48 to 72 hours postoperatively. The patient is generally dismissed from the hospital by the seventh postoperative day.

More extensive and persistent pneumothorax is better managed through a standard lateral thoracotomy, which provides access to all of the lung surface, since in many of these patients, bullous disease may not be confined to the lung apex. If pulmonary entrapment is encountered, decortication can be readily performed. Unexpected pulmonary pathologic findings, such as endometriosis or cancer, can also be managed more expediently.[8] Following re-expansion of the lung, dry gauze abrasion of both pleurae is performed and the thoracotomy is closed as described. Patients requiring pleurodesis for bilateral recurrent pneumothorax are best managed by the abrasive pleurodesis technique utilizing a median sternotomy approach rather than a bilateral sequential lateral thoracotomy.

Results

During the past few years, we have performed thoracotomy and pleural abrasion in approximately 100 patients with spontaneous pneumothorax, caused by a ruptured pulmonary bleb in most cases. There were no operative deaths nor any serious postoperative complications. Prolonged tube thoracostomy drainage was necessary in approximately 10% of patients. Recurrent ipsilateral pneumothorax following pleural abrasion was unusual and occurred in less than 2% of our patients.

We believe that pleural abrasion remains the operative procedure of choice in patients who require thoracotomy for control of spontaneous pneumothorax.

References

1. Itard JE: Sur le pneumo-thorax ou les congestions gazeuses qui se forment dans la poitrine, Thesis, Paris, 1803.
2. Devilliers A: Du Pneumothorax Déterminé par la Rupture de la Plèver et d'une Vésicule Aérienne Emphysémateuse. Thesis, Paris, 1826.
3. Kjaergaard H: Spontaneous pneumothorax in the apparently healthy. Acta Med Scand [Suppl] 43:1–159, 1932.
4. Ellis FH Jr, Carr DT: The problem of spontaneous pneumothorax. Med Clin North Am (Mayo Clinic Number):1065–1074, 1954.
5. Carr DT, Silver AW, Ellis FH Jr: Management of spontaneous pneumothorax with special reference to prognosis after various kinds of therapy. Proc Staff Meet Mayo Clin 38:103–109, 1963.
6. Dines DE, Clagett OT, Good CA: Nontuberculous pulmonary parenchymal conditions predisposing to spontaneous pneumothorax: Report of four cases. J Thorac Cardiovasc Surg 53:726–732, 1967.
7. Dines DE, Clagett OT,, Payne WS: Spontaneous pneumothorax in emphysema. Mayo Clin Proc 45:481–487, 1970.
8. Shearin RPN, Hepper NGG, Payne WS: Recurrent spontaneous pneumothorax concurrent with menses. Mayo Clin Proc 49:98–101, 1974.
9. Klassen KP, Meckstroth CV: Treatment of spontaneous pneumothorax: Prompt expansion with controlled thoracotomy tube suction. JAMA 182:1–5, 1962.
10. Gobbel WG Jr, Rhea WG Jr, Nelson IA, Daniel RA Jr: Spontaneous pneumothorax. J Thorac Cardiovasc Surg 46:331–345, 1963.
11. Seremetis MG: The management of spontaneous pneumothorax. Chest 57:65–68, 1970.
12. Spengler L: Zur chirurgie des pneumothorax. Beitr Klin Chir 49:68–89, 1906.
13. Clagett OT: The management of spontaneous pneumothorax (editorial). J Thorac Cardiovasc Surg 55:761–762, 1968.

8

The Surgical Management of Recurrent or Persistent Pneumothorax: Pleuroscopy and Talc Poudrage

Dov Weissberg, M.D.

The management of spontaneous pneumothorax is a matter of controversy. In most instances pneumothorax can be treated effectively by tube thoracostomy. When evacuation of air does not suffice and pneumothorax persists, or with recurrence following lung expansion, some surgeons favor an operative approach, choosing among pleural abrasion, pleurectomy, or excision of blebs;[1-4] others prefer instillation of one of the irritating substances causing pleural adhesions. Many pleural irritants have been used, including iodized oil, dextrose, human blood, caustics such as silver nitrate,[1] quinacrine (Atabrine),[5-7] tetracycline,[8-10] iodized talc,[11-19] and others.

REVIEW OF CLINICAL EXPERIENCE

Although the management of recurrent pneumothorax by *pleuroscopy* and *pleurodesis* was first suggested by Sattler in 1937,[20] this technique has not yet gained much popularity. In the majority of medical centers pleuroscopy is not used in the management of spontaneous pneumothorax, nor is it mentioned in this context in many textbooks,[21, 22] with some exceptions.[23] Yet a good direct look at the lung and pleura may enable disclosure of factors causing either persistence or recurrence of pneumothorax, and there is accumulating evidence that the information provided by pleuroscopy is of great value in the successful management of this affliction.

Babichev and colleagues[24] compared a group of 110 patients in whom spontaneous pneumothorax was managed without pleuroscopy with another group of 120 patients in whom pleuroscopy was performed and treatment was modified according to the findings. There were 34 recurrences in the first group and only 6 in the second group. Sukhanovsky and Konstantinova[25] have reviewed 67 cases of pneumothorax reported in the literature and found

significant pathologic changes in the pleura in 37 cases. They also reported on their own experience with 74 patients: Pleuroscopy was performed in 48 of the 74 patients, with finding of blebs in 31 and adhesions preventing reexpansion in 22. Treatment was modified according to these findings.

The use of pleuroscopy in the management of spontaneous pneumothorax was also evaluated and recommended by Swierenga and associates,[26] Keller and colleagues,[27] and Bloomberg.[28] The changing attitude toward the use of pleuroscopy in pneumothorax is reflected particularly well in the approach of Bloomberg.[28] As a rule, he treats spontaneous pneumothorax at its inception with tube thoracostomy. In the past, in patients in whom air leak persisted, he resorted to thoracotomy for finding and elimination of the causative factors. In later years he acknowledged the need for early pleuroscopy in order to define the abnormality. He now recommends pleuroscopy before thoracotomy in patients who have air leak lasting between 10 and 14 days. Our own experience confirms the correctness of Bloomberg's approach and indicates that persistent or recurrent pneumothorax requires pleuroscopy.[17, 19]

INDICATIONS

Persistent Pneumothorax. Persistent pneumothorax is defined as that lasting over 10 days despite uninterrupted treatment by tube thoracostomy with underwater seal, either with or without suction. In over 85% of our patients treated with tube drainage, the lung expanded completely within a few days and remained expanded. In such patients, pleuroscopy is not indicated. However, pleuroscopy should be carried out if the air leak continues for more than 10 days and the lung does not expand completely. This arbitrary routine of 10 days' waiting time is not crucial. Far more important are disclosure and elimination of the factors responsible for nonexpansion. For the purpose of investigation, then, pleuroscopy is invaluable.

Recurrent Pneumothorax. Pleuroscopy for a recurrent pneumothorax is recommended for the third episode (second recurrence on the same side) of pneumothorax involving 20% or more of the pleural space. Among patients with spontaneous pneumothorax treated on our service, 55% had only one episode of pneumothorax, 35% had two episodes on the same side, and only 10% had three episodes or more. Because 90% of patients experience pneumothorax only once or twice, it is not necessary to subject this majority to pleuroscopy. However, when pneumothorax appears for the third time on the same side, the reasons for recurrence must be sought.

PROCEDURE

On our service, pleuroscopy is performed under general endotracheal anesthesia, with the patient in the lateral decubitus position. A 3-cm incision is made in the midaxillary line at the fifth or sixth intercostal space. The incision is deepened, the parietal pleura is pierced with a hemostat, and the mediastinoscope is inserted. Fluid, if present, is aspirated. In an organized manner the entire lung surface and chest wall are inspected. Using this technique for either recurrent or persistent spontaneous pneumothorax, we found subpleural blebs or bullae in 65% of patients, adhesions preventing expansion in 15%, and inexpansible lung in 10% (see Precautions and Contraindications). The causes of inexpansibility included pulmonary fibrosis, inflammatory conditions affecting lung, atelectasis due to obstructing lesions, and thick pleura, which developed in some patients with long-standing pneumothorax. In another 10% of patients, no abnormalities were found, and the cause of persistence or recurrence could not be determined.

Following pleuroscopy, the pneumothorax is treated according to the findings.

Subpleural Blebs. If subpleural blebs are present, and no tear is seen, it is assumed that there had been a small rupture of a bleb, which healed spontaneously. If the lung is fully expansible and fills the pleural space during inflation by the anesthetist, 2 g of sterile iodized talc is sprinkled lightly over the entire pleural surface using an Asepto syringe (Fig. 8–1). This almost invariably causes obliteration of the pleural space by adhesions and

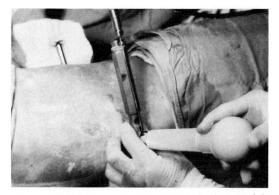

Figure 8–1. Talc insufflation through the lumen of the mediastinoscope.

prevents further recurrences of pneumothorax. The presence of a rent, with a small amount of air leaking, does not necessarily negate the possibility of a full lung expansion. While the pleuroscopist looks on, the lung is inflated by the anesthetist. If the lung expands completely despite the air leak, talc is insufflated, and two chest tubes are inserted and connected to the underwater seal with suction for 3 to 4 days. This keeps the lung expanded while the adhesions are forming and the rent closes. If the rent is large, and the lung does not expand well during inflation by the anesthetist, an operation with resection of all blebs should be considered. The finding of a large emphysematous bulla that has ruptured and caused the pneumothorax makes resection mandatory.

A 52-year-old man had chronic obstructive lung disease, pulmonary sarcoidosis, and multiple emphysematous blebs in both lungs. Over the 12 months prior to admission he suffered multiple episodes of pneumothorax on the left side, which were treated in various hospitals by tube thoracostomy. He was admitted to our service with another episode of pneumothorax. Under treatment with tube thoracostomy without suction the lung did not expand, and air leak through the tube continued. When the tube was connected to a suction of 20 cm H_2O, the air flow increased markedly, but the lung expanded. During the following week no change occurred: Air leak was massive, but the lung remained fully expanded. When suction was discontinued, the lung collapsed again, with diminished air leak (Fig. 8–2). Pleuroscopy was performed, disclosing several apical blebs, with a tear in one. The patient's pulmonary function was poor, and thoracotomy was inadvisable. Therefore, talc was insufflated and the pleural drain was connected to suction for 4 days. On the first post-pleuroscopy day the air leak decreased markedly, and on the second day it ceased. The pleural drain was removed on the fourth day. There were no recurrences during the following 7 years (Fig. 8–3).

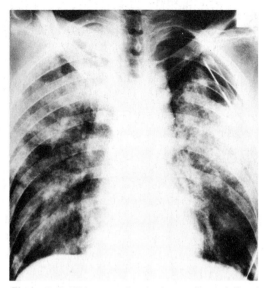

Figure 8–2. Without suction the lung collapsed, despite pleural drainage.

Adhesions. Although it is usually assumed that pneumothorax cannot occur in presence of adhesions, this is not always true. Irregularly scattered adhesions do not always prevent pneumothorax, and they may prevent complete expansion of the lung once pneumothorax has occurred. If such adhesions are present, they should be divided by means of diathermy. A sharp-pointed coagulation tip is applied intermittently to the adhesion bands, with careful coagulation of blood vessels be-

fore their division. Using this technique with care, we have not had any instances of serious bleeding. Nevertheless, blood for transfusion should always be available. After division of the disturbing adhesions, talc should be sprinkled lightly over the entire pleural surface.

A 68-year-old man with bullous emphysema was admitted because of spontaneous pneumothorax on the left side. Roentgenograms demonstrated a large pneumothorax and partial adhesions preventing total lung collapse (Fig. 8–4). A pleural drain was inserted and attached to an underwater seal, but the lung did not expand. Addition of suction resulted in greater air leak, and the lung remained collapsed. On pleuroscopy a small tear was seen in a bulla. The pleural adhesions were clearly demonstrated and were divided with a coagulating current. Talc was insufflated and suction was applied to the pleural drain for 4 days. The lung expanded immediately, and all air leak ceased on the second post-pleuroscopy day. During the following 5 years no relapses occurred (Fig. 8–5).

Absence of Abnormalities. If no underlying abnormalities are seen at pleuroscopy, as in 10% of our patients, talc insufflation is carried out, and a pleural drain is inserted and attached to an underwater seal with suction for 3 to 4 days. In such cases pneumothorax virtually never recurs.

PRECAUTIONS AND CONTRAINDICATIONS

Talc is a physical irritant capable of causing fibrosis and granuloma, which in serosa-lined surfaces amounts to adhesions. It is finely

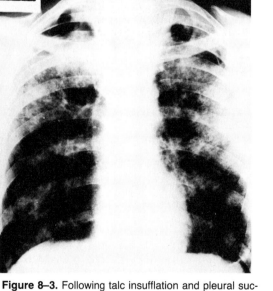

Figure 8–3. Following talc insufflation and pleural suction, the lung expanded and became adherent to the chest wall. The sarcoid infiltrates are clearly seen.

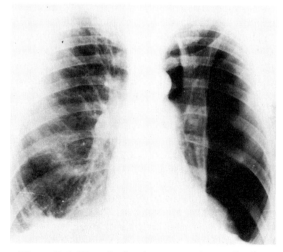

Figure 8–4. Pleural adhesions preventing total collapse of the left lung.

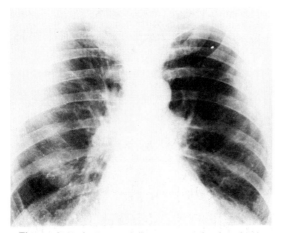

Figure 8–5. At 5-year follow-up examination the lung remains fully expanded.

powdered hydrous magnesium silicate with the general formula $Mg_6(Si_2O_5)_4(OH)_4$.[17, 29, 30] The formula may vary depending on the source from which the talc is obtained. Talc from various sources may contain contaminants such as asbestos, clay, chalk, quartz, and other minerals. Of these, asbestos is most dangerous, because of its ability to cause mesothelioma and bronchogenic cancer. Because of this association with malignant neoplasms, objections have been raised against the use of talc in humans. However, Kleinfeld and colleagues[31, 32] have shown in very convincing clinical studies that purified talc free of contaminants caused fibrosis and granuloma, not cancer. The results of their studies have been confirmed conclusively in animal experiments by Wagner and associates.[33] Judging from these and other studies,[34, 35] we consider *purified* talc safe for therapeutic use in humans. The talc that we use corresponds with the requirements of the British Pharmacopoeia.[29, 30] It is tested periodically, and does not contain asbestos.[17–19]

Whatever the indication, talc should be used very sparingly, because excessive amounts may cause granuloma and fibrothorax that will interfere with the physiologic expansion of the lung. In addition, rare instances of adult respiratory distress syndrome have been reported after instillation of 10 g of talc into the pleural cavity.[36] In actual practice no more than 2 g of talc should be insufflated for complete pleurodesis. In our hands this amount has been sufficient in the great majority of patients.

In presence of inexpansible lung, the use of talc is contraindicated. Whether inexpansibility is due to pachypleuritis or to primary lung disease causing atelectasis, no pleurodesis can be achieved when the lung cannot fill the pleural space. In such cases the cause of inexpansibility must be determined and appropriate treatment given if pneumothorax is to be managed effectively.

RESULTS

In our series of more than 200 patients, a single insufflation of talc gave excellent results with no recurrences of pneumothorax in 75%. Insignificant apical pneumothorax remained in 13% of patients, indicating *nearly* complete pleurodesis. In the 12% who suffered a recurrence, a second trial of talc insufflation was given, with excellent results in 80% of this group of initial failures. Only 20% of this small group, or 3% of all patients, developed further early or late recurrences. Very few of these patients needed a thoracotomy.

Complications

Complications of pleuroscopy and talc insufflation are remarkably few. Bleeding during the division of adhesions did not occur in our series, but this possibility must be kept in mind, and blood for transfusion should always be available. Another complication that may occur during division of these adhesions is related to their location. They are very commonly seen at the base of the blebs, and by their division, a rent in the bleb may be created. This occurred in five of our patients; all were treated by talc insufflation with tube drainage and suction, and all recovered. Should a large rent with uncontrollable air leak be created, a thoracotomy with resection of all blebs would be necessary.

Conclusions

In summary, pleuroscopy with talc pleurodesis is a very effective method of controlling recurrent and persistent pneumothorax. In our hands this method has been effective in 75% of patients at the first trial, and the success rate increased to 97% when treatment was repeated in the initially unsuccessful cases. Purified talc free of asbestos is safe for use in humans, when used sparingly. Open thoracotomy is unnecessary in the great majority of patients but should be used when a ruptured emphysematous bulla causes uncontrollable air leak.

References

1. Gaensler EA: Parietal pleurectomy for recurrent spontaneous pneumothorax. Surg Gynecol Obstet 102:293, 1956.
2. Baronofsky ID, Warden HG, Kaufman JL, et al: Bilateral therapy for unilateral spontaneous pneumothorax. J Thorac Surg 34:310, 1957.
3. Askew AR: Partial pleurectomy for recurrent pneumothorax. Br J Surg 63:203, 1976.
4. Deslauriers J, Beaulieu M, Després JP, et al: Transaxillary pleurectomy for treatment of spontaneous pneumothorax. Ann Thorac Surg 30:569, 1980.
5. Borda I, Krant M: Convulsions following intrapleural administration of quinacrine hydrochloride. JAMA 201:173, 1967.
6. Leff A, Hopewell PC, Costello J: Pleural effusion for malignancy. Ann Intern Med 88:532, 1978.
7. Austin EH, Flye MW: The treatment of recurrent malignant pleural effusion. Ann Thorac Surg 28:190, 1979.
8. Thorsrud GK: Pleural reaction to irritants. Acta Chir Scand (Suppl) 355:1, 1965.
9. Rubinson RM, Bolooki H: Intrapleural tetracycline for control of malignant pleural effusion: A preliminary report. South Med J 65:847, 1972.
10. Wallach HW: Intrapleural tetracycline for malignant pleural effusions. Chest 68:510, 1975.
11. Bethune N: Pleural poudrage. A new technique for the deliberate production of pleural adhesions as a preliminary to lobectomy. J Thorac Surg 4:251, 1935.
12. Haupt GJ, Camishion RC, Templeton JY III, et al: Treatment of malignant pleural effusion by talc poudrage. JAMA 172:918, 1960.
13. Camishion RC, Gibbon JH Jr, Nealon TF Jr: Talc poudrage in the treatment of pleural effusion due to cancer. Surg Clin North Am 42:1521, 1962.
14. Pearson FG, MacGregor DC: Talc poudrage for malignant pleural effusion. J Thorac Cardiovasc Surg 51:732, 1966.
15. Bloomberg AE: Thoracoscopy in diagnosis of pleural effusion. NY State J Med 70:1974, 1970.
16. Adler RH, Sayek I: Treatment of malignant pleural effusion: A method using tube thoracostomy and talc. Ann Thorac Surg 22:8, 1976.
17. Weissberg D, Kaufman M: Diagnostic and therapeutic pleuroscopy: Experience with 127 patients. Chest 78:732, 1980.
18. Weissberg D, Kaufman M, Zurkowski Z: Pleuroscopy in patients with pleural effusion and pleural masses. Ann Thorac Surg 29:205, 1980.
19. Weissberg D: Talc pleurodesis: A controversial issue. Poumon–Coeur 37:291, 1981.
20. Sattler A: Zur Behandlung des Spontanpneumothorax mit besonderer Berücksichtigung der Thorakoskopie. Bietr Klin Tuberk 89:395, 1937.
21. Sabiston DC, Spencer FC: Gibbon's Surgery of the Chest, 3rd ed. Philadelphia, WB Saunders, 1976.
22. Shields T: General Thoracic Surgery, 2nd ed. Philadelphia, Lea & Febiger, 1983.
23. Collis JL, Clarke DB, Smith RA: D'Abreu's Practice of Cardiothoracic Surgery, 4th ed. London, Edward Arnold, 1976.
24. Babichev SI, Chudnovsky PD, Katkovsky GB: The use of thoracoscopy in spontaneous nonspecific pneumothorax. Vestn Khir 101:50, 1968.
25. Sukhanovsky IVP, Konstantinova GD: Thoracoscopy in spontaneous pneumothorax. Vestn Khir 103:21, 1969.
26. Swierenga J, Wagenaar JPM, Bergstein PGM: The value of thoracoscopy in the diagnosis and treatment of diseases affecting the pleura and lung. Pneumonologie 151:11, 1974.
27. Keller R, Gutersohn J, Herzog H: The management of persistent pneumothorax by thoracoscopic procedures. Thoraxchirurgie 22:457, 1974.
28. Bloomberg AE: Thoracoscopy in perspective. Surg Gynecol Obstet 147:433, 1978.
29. British Pharmaceutical Codex. London, Pharmaceutical Press, 1973, p 492.
30. Martindale W: The Extra Pharmacopoeia, 27th ed. London, Pharmaceutical Press, 1977, p 455.
31. Kleinfeld M, Messite J, Kooyman O, et al: Mortality among talc miners and millers in New York State. Arch Environ Health 14:663, 1967.
32. Kleinfeld M, Messite J, Zaki MH: Mortality experiences among talc workers: A follow-up study. J Occup Med 16:345, 1974.
33. Wagner JC, Berry G, Cooke TJ, et al: Animal experiments with talc. Proceedings of the Fourth International Symposium on Inhaled Particles and Vapour, Edinburgh, Scotland, Sept 22–26, 1975. Oxford, Pergamon Press, 1977, pp 647–654.
34. Selikoff IJ, Bader RA, Bader ME: Asbestosis and neoplasia. Am J Med 42:487, 1967.
35. Editorial: Cosmetic talc powder. Lancet 1:1348, 1977.
36. Rinaldo JE, Owens GR, Rogers RM: Adult respiratory distress syndrome following intrapleural instillation of talc. J Thorac Cardiovasc Surg 85:523, 1983.

9

The Surgical Management of Recurrent or Persistent Pneumothorax: Pleurectomy

Robert M. Bojar, M.D.
C. Frederick Kittle, M.D.

Spontaneous pneumothorax remains a common problem confronting thoracic surgeons. The leading cause is rupture of either apical blebs in young adults or emphysematous blebs and bullae in older patients. Iatrogenic pneumothorax from complications of subclavian vein catheterization, thoracentesis, and from barotrauma during mechanical ventilation has recently become more prevalent. Other well-described but less common etiologies are listed in Table 9–1.

The size of the pneumothorax and its degree of symptomatology dictate the management of the patient. The small asymptomatic pneumothorax may be merely observed in anticipation of its resolution; a mildly symptomatic pneumothorax involving less than 20% of the pleural space may be aspirated. A larger pneumothorax, however, should be treated by tube thoracostomy and suction to effect the rapid evacuation of air and complete expansion of the lung. Although this method is generally successful, it is estimated that 10% to 20% of patients[29] will eventually come to thoracotomy because of recurrence or other concomitant problems indicating a "complicated pneumothorax." Such problems include tension pneumothorax, persistence of air leak for more than a week, failure of the lung to expand, associated hemothorax yielding more than 1000 cc of blood, bilateral synchronous or metachronous pneumothorax, associated lung pathology noted on the chest roentgenogram, chronic pneumothorax with trapped lung, and pneumothorax in patients with a potential job-related disability.

Numerous techniques exist for the surgical treatment of recurrent or complicated pneumothorax. Since the early 1900s, chemical pleurodesis has been utilized to effect pleural symphysis. There has been a resurgence of interest in this method, using talc, quinacrine, or tetracycline, owing to the success of these substances in the management of malignant pleural effusions. Bleb resection alone or combined with operative pleurodesis is often used. Gaensler in 1956[17] recommended pleurectomy to control recurrent pneumothorax; several groups have subsequently reported excellent results with it.

Table 9–1. Causes of Pneumothorax

Spontaneous: apical blebs
Iatrogenic
  Subclavian vein catheterization
  Surgical procedures
  Barotrauma
Trauma
Dissection of mediastinal air
Intrinsic lung disease
  Emphysematous blebs/bullae
  Tumors: primary and metastatic
  Infection
    Tuberculosis
    Fungal disease
    Pneumonia
    Abscess
  Other
    Cystic fibrosis
    Sarcoidosis
    Tuberous sclerosis
    Eosinophilic granuloma
    Alpha$_1$-antitrypsin deficiency
    Honeycomb lung
    Congenital and parasitic cysts
Other causes
  Connective tissue disorders
  Endometriosis

PATIENT POPULATION

From 1970 through 1982, 112 pleurectomies were performed in 106 patients for pneumothorax-related problems at Rush–Presbyterian–St. Luke's Medical Center. All patients underwent unilateral thoracotomy with stapling or oversewing of blebs and pleurectomy, except for one patient, who underwent bilateral pleurectomies through a median sternotomy. Five patients had a second pleurectomy for contralateral disease. Apical pleurectomy or pleurectomy of the upper portion of the

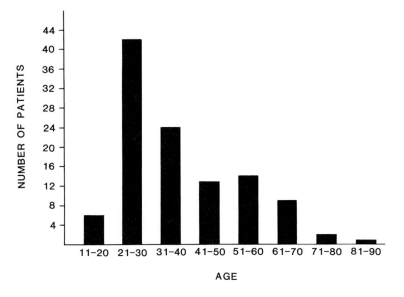

Figure 9–1. Age distribution of patients undergoing pleurectomy.

hemithorax was performed in 73 patients, total pleurectomy in 31, inferior pleurectomy in 2, and an unstated extent of pleurectomy in the remainder. There were 75 men and 36 women, giving a slightly greater than 2:1 sex ratio. The ages ranged from 17 to 82 years, with a mean age of 36 (Fig. 9–1) and a peak incidence in the 20- to 24-year age group; 50% of the patients were between the ages of 20 and 35.

INDICATIONS FOR SURGERY
(Table 9–2)

Among the indications for surgery were recurrence of pneumothorax in 73 patients and persistent air leak in 38. In this latter group, persistent leak developed in 28 patients during the first occurrence of pneumothorax, 5 during a recurrent episode, 2 subsequent to thoracentesis, and 2 following pulmonary resection. One patient had a hemopneumothorax necessitating operative intervention while an active air leak was still present. In 13 patients who had bilateral metachronous pneumothorax, thoracotomy was performed for recurrence on one side in 11 and for first contralateral occurrence in the other 2. Three patients of the 106 (2.8%) had bilateral synchronous pneumothorax, two patients had chronic pneumothorax with trapped lung, and three had abnormal pulmonary or mediastinal pathology (two with bullous disease and one with metastatic testicular germ cell tumor).

Table 9–2. Associated Disease and Indications for Pleurectomy

Associated Disease	No. Of Pleurectomies	Mean Patient Age (yr)	Recurrence	Indication Persistence[a]	Other
Spontaneous pneumothorax: apical bleb only	79	31	61	15	3
Chronic obstructive pulmonary disease with bullae	17[b]	57	7	7	3
Cancer	6	48	1	1	4
Metastatic disease	3	41			
Lung	2	58			
Mediastinal mass	1	35			
Tuberculosis	3	59	1	1	1
Eosinophilic granuloma	3	27	2	1	
Rheumatoid lung	1	22		1	
Sarcoid	1	30		1	
Staphylococcal pneumonia	1	27		1	
Marfan's syndrome	1	67	1		
Total	112	36	73	28	11

[a]Persistent air leak over 7 days during first occurrence of pneumothorax.
[b]16 patients; 2 pleurectomies in one patient via median sternotomy.

OPERATIVE TECHNIQUE

After the induction of general anesthesia and endotracheal intubation, the patient is placed in the lateral decubitus position with the involved side of the chest elevated 90 degrees. The upper arm is abducted 90 degrees and suspended on an arm rest with the elbow flexed 90 degrees, thus exposing the axilla. Unless an active air leak is present, the chest tube is removed prior to skin preparation to optimize sterility of the field. A lateral incision is made extending from below the breast to the anterior margin of the latissimus dorsi muscle, which is retracted posteriorly. The serratus anterior is incised through its fibers, with care being taken to identify and preserve the long thoracic nerve. The chest is entered in the fourth intercostal space. Dissection of the parietal pleura is usually done extrapleurally before entering the pleural space; this greatly facilitates dissection of the pleura itself. The lung is thoroughly inspected for blebs, which are either removed after stapling with the TA-30 stapler using 3.5-mm staples or excised and oversewn with 3–0 Dexon. The pleura is excised from the top half of the wound, at the apex, or in its entirety, depending on the extent of the disease and the ease of resection through the incision. If only an upper or apical pleurectomy is done, a pleural abrasion of the remaining parietal pleura is done. Apical and basal chest tubes are placed, and the wound is closed in layers. The chest tubes are removed when there is no air leak and the amount of drainage is less than 200 cc per day.

RESULTS

There appear to be three distinct groups of patients that come to thoracotomy for recurrent or complicated pneumothorax: Group I consists of young adults with apical blebs but no other pulmonary parenchymal disease; Group II consists of older patients with marked emphysematous changes, diffuse blebs, or bullae; and Group III, patients with miscellaneous underlying lung disease.

In our series, there were 79 patients in Group I with a mean age of 31 years. Apical blebs or scarring were encountered in every case. Two patients developed a spontaneous pneumothorax during pregnancy; one underwent thoracotomy during the third trimester for a second recurrence, and the other developed a pneumothorax just prior to delivery and underwent pleurectomy one week post partum for persistent air leak. Of these 79 patients, recurrent pneumothorax was the indication in 61. Fifteen patients had air leaks that persisted beyond 1 week during the first occurrence despite 20 cm of suction or the placement of additional chest tubes. The indications in the other three patients were hemopneumothorax yielding more than 1000 cc of blood, a first contralateral occurrence after a previous pleurectomy, and bilateral synchronous pneumothorax with nonexpansibility of one lung.

It is noteworthy that two patients in this group presented with recurrence following apical pleurectomy performed at other institutions. The first patient had undergone resection of apical blebs and apical pleurectomy 3 years previously and presented with a basilar space for which chest tube placement could not be accomplished. A lower lobe decortication and lower pleurectomy were successfully done. The other patient also had a basilar airspace and disruption of the apical staple line; because of failure of the lung to expand the patient was re-explored, the apex oversewn, and decortication done. Despite the inferior pleurectomy, a persistent air leak ensued, necessitating subsequent open drainage and decortication for empyema.

There was no mortality in Group I. Major morbidity occurred in four patients (5.1%). Two patients required re-exploration for hemothorax. One developed a wound infection that closed secondarily over 4 months. The patient with persistent air leak and empyema was noted above. Minor morbidity occurred in four patients (5.1%). These included a persistent air space that resolved spontaneously in several weeks, a persistent space and air leak that required use of a Heimlich valve for 2 weeks, and atelectasis from retained secretions that was successfully managed by bronchoscopy. One patient developed temporary anhidrosis of the ipsilateral arm and thorax without Horner's syndrome after an apical pleurectomy.

Group II in our series consisted of 16 patients with chronic obstructive pulmonary disease (COPD) and large bullae or diffuse blebs. The mean age was 57 years. Seven patients were operated upon for recurrence, seven for persistent air leak during the first occurrence, one for chronic pneumothorax with trapped lung, and one for large bullae noted on the chest x-ray film. One patient with recurrent unilateral pneumothorax and bilateral bullae underwent resection of bullae with bilateral pleurectomy through a median sternotomy. One patient in this group required repeated bronchoscopy and tracheostomy for pulmonary care.

The only mortality occurred in a 61-year-old man with advanced COPD in whom a chest tube was placed for right-sided pneumothorax. Owing to a persistent leak, he was transferred to our institution and arrived with massive subcutaneous emphysema, necessitating the immediate placement of chest tubes. He required mechanical ventilation and a contralateral tension pneumothorax developed, which responded to chest tube placement. At thoracotomy a large apical leak was found, and a total pleurectomy was performed on the right side. Although this terminated the air leak, respiratory failure persisted and the patient died 7 weeks later.

Group III in our series consisted of 16 patients with miscellaneous types of lung disease. There were three patients with eosinophilic granuloma (average age of 27 years). One had apical blebs; the other two had diffuse disease. One of these patients developed a right upper lobe abscess and recurrent sterile effusions. Three patients with tuberculosis were in an older age group (average age 59 years). Two had apical tuberculous nodules that were discovered incidentally. The third patient had a persistent air leak and airspace following thoracentesis for pleural effusion. A contralateral pneumothorax spontaneously developed. He underwent a pleurectomy and decortication for what proved to be a tuberculous empyema. A persistent air leak and basilar space necessitated re-exploration, lower lobe decortication, and subsequent open drainage.

Six patients with malignancy and pneumothorax were encountered. One patient with small cell carcinoma underwent a thoracentesis for malignant effusion with a resultant pleural laceration and persistent air leak requiring total pleurectomy; another had a persistent air leak from the minor fissure following right upper lobectomy for carcinoma. Two patients had spontaneous pneumothorax from metastatic sarcoma, and another had a persistent postoperative leak following extensive resection for metastatic hypernephroma. This patient underwent pleurectomy but required a Heimlich valve for 4 weeks for persistent air leak. The other patient was noted to have a superior mediastinal mass to which the lung ws adherent when the pneumothorax occurred. An anaplastic carcinoma consistent with germ cell tumor was found at thoracotomy.

Group III also included patients with Marfan's syndrome, sarcoidosis, and rheumatoid lung disease. One patient with Weber-Christian disease on high-dose steroids experienced recurrent staphylococcal pneumonia; a pneumatocele ruptured, producing a pneumothorax and persistent air leak. At thoracotomy, total pleurectomy and decortication were done. Disseminated intravascular coagulation (DIC) developed in the operating room, and the patient exsanguinated. Thus, in this group of 16 patients, there two major morbidities, one minor morbidity, and one hospital death.

For the entire series, there were two deaths (1.8%), seven major morbidities (6.2%), and five minor morbidities (4.4%) (Table 9–3). There have been no known recurrences among the 112 pleurectomies performed for pneumothorax.

PRINCIPLES OF MANAGEMENT

The asymptomatic patient with a pneumothorax involving less than 20% of the pleural space may be managed with restriction of activity, with the anticipated expansion of

Table 9–3. Complications Encountered in 112 Pleurectomies and Their Management

Complications	No. of Cases	Management
Major (6.2%)		
Hemothorax	2	Re-exploration
Persistent air leak and empyema	2	Re-exploration, decortication
Wound infection	1	Antibiotics, drainage
Lung abscess and recurrent effusions	1	Antibiotics and bronchoscopy; tube thoracostomy
Retained secretions	1	Bronchoscopy and tracheostomy
Minor (4.4%)		
Residual airspace	1	Observation
Persistent leak	2	Heimlich valve
Retained secretions	1	Bronchoscopy
Anhidrosis	1	Observation

1.25% of the lung volume daily.[20] Use of oxygen may speed resolution by increasing the gradient for nitrogen absorption. Although spontaneous resolution usually ensues, the potential exists for tension pneumothorax or failure of expansion with residual airspace, trapped lung, and empyema. Recurrence may result in intrathoracic hemorrhage from torn adhesions.

Patients with underlying lung disease, especially emphysema, tend to have pulmonary symptoms disproportionate to the extent of pneumothorax. These patients and those with pneumothorax involving more than 20% of pleural space should be managed by the insertion of an intercostal catheter placed to suction. Use of a flutter or Heimlich valve[8, 24] is satisfactory in allowing evacuation of air and has been utilized on an outpatient basis, although inadequate expansion and empyema have been described with this technique.[36]

Tube thoracostomy is generally successful in promoting expansion and terminating air leak, but an estimated 9% to 20% of patients managed in this way will require thoracotomy.[7, 27, 29] An air leak persisting over 1 week usually indicates more severe subpleural disease and necessitates further therapy. Even if the air leak seals and the chest tube is removed, the chances for a recurrence are 15% to 20%[27, 29, 31] and up to 80% for the second or third recurrence.[18] Therefore, most surgeons now recommend operation after the first recurrence. Improved results have also been obtained if early thoracotomy is performed for a large hemopneumothorax (more than 1000 cc of aspirate) by eliminating the potential for respiratory compromise, fibrothorax, and empyema.[13]

Bilateral synchronous pneumothorax occurs in approximately 5% to 7% of instances[15] and places the patient at great risk for respiratory embarrassment. With the documentation that patients undergoing median sternotomy recover pulmonary function more rapidly than those with lateral thoracotomies,[12] median sternotomy seems preferable to bilateral simultaneous[1] or staged thoracotomies to explore both pleural spaces for bilateral synchronous pneumothorax and to restore pulmonary function in the presence of bilateral bullous disease.[23] Although justifiable for bilateral metachronous pneumothorax, extending this approach to unilateral pneumothorax is questionable. Baronofsky[4] suggested in 1957 that patients with unilateral pneumothorax should undergo a bilateral procedure since contralateral blebs are present in 96% of patients. Other groups utilizing the sternotomy approach[19, 26] have confirmed these findings. However, since the incidence of contralateral pneumothorax is approximately 10% to 15%, an approach to both pleural cavities is unnecessary in 85% of patients.

The earliest approach to complicated pneumothorax-related problems was that of chemical pleurodesis. In the early 1900s, Spengler[32] introduced sodium nitrate and 30% dextrose; in 1935 Bethune[6] advocated talc. Among the myriad of agents that have been tried, talc,[38] quinacrine,[22] and tetracycline[33] have recently been recommended to induce pleural symphysis nonoperatively. Talc has not been extensively utilized owing to the possibility of its contamination with asbestos fibers and its production of uneven dense adhesions, granulomas, and chest wall tumors.[21] Success has been variable with these agents. In a recent series of 125 pleurectomies, 10 patients came to surgery following failed pleurodesis.[31]

Because of unsatisfactory results with previously used procedures, Gaensler[17] called attention to the efficacy of parietal pleurectomy for recurrent pneumothorax in 1956, utilizing it in patients with diffuse cystic disease. He emphasized its preference over other methods of pleurodesis. Thomas[34, 35] subsequently expanded its use to patients with localized blebs, emphasizing the necessity of subtotal pleurectomy to prevent most efficiently recurrent pneumothorax. Others[9, 25] have condemned this procedure because of concern over excessive blood loss and the difficulty of reoperation following pleurectomy. Clagett[9] has stated that pleural stripping "is certainly too radical a treatment and it must be condemned completely." Excellent results have been reported with bleb resection alone[16] or combined with operative pleurodesis,[25, 39] although a recent review found a recurrence rate of 2.3% in four different series of pleurodeses.[37] Others remain selective in their use of pleurectomy, utilizing it only when diffuse involvement makes wedge excision alone impossible.

The efficacy of pleurectomy in preventing recurrence of pneumothorax is unequivocal. Studies have shown uniform adherence of the pleural surfaces and inability to induce artificial pneumothorax after the procedure.[17] Review of 1313 pleurectomies[3, 5, 6, 11, 14, 18, 27, 28, 30, 31, 34, 35, 37] in 13 series since 1956 reveals only four known recurrences (0.3%). In our series of 112 pleurectomies, there have been no known recurrences, although two patients presented with basal recurrences following apical pleurectomy performed at other institutions. Studies have also dispelled the fear that pleurectomy might induce a fibrothorax with restrictive pulmonary function. There has been found to be no significant impairment of the mechanical efficacy of respiration[2] and little effect on pulmonary function tests after pleurectomy.[14, 17, 31, 37]

Mortality is rare following pleurectomy. In seven series since 1965 (Table 9–4)[3, 5, 7, 14, 27, 30, 31, 37] there have been only four mortalities in 1046 procedures. In our series, one operative death resulted from exsanguination from DIC in a very ill patient; another respirator-dependent patient with advanced COPD and persistent air leak died of respiratory failure 2 months following the procedure.

Major morbidity occurs in less than 5% in most series; this includes reoperation for hemothorax, persistent air leak, nonexpanding lung or empyema, and wound infection. Minor complications such as persistent air leak for more than 1 week that responds to valve drainage, small intrapleural airspace, delayed expansion, pleural effusion, need for aspiration bronchoscopies, and rib osteitis occur in about 5% of cases and are probably unrelated to the pleurectomy per se.

Thomas and Gebauer[34] stated in 1958 that subtotal pleurectomy was essential to prevent recurrence, emphasizing the stripping of the pleura from the chest wall except in the region of the mediastinum and diaphragm. Deslauriers and colleagues[14] felt that apical pleurectomy should suffice for patients with disease limited to the apex, since it can be easily performed through the limited exposure of the axillary incision. Weeden and Smith[37] noted a significant increase in the incidence of complications when a full pleurectomy was performed, but found that this correlated most directly with the high incidence of chronic obstructive lung disease in these patients. We found no difference in our results with use of either apical or subtotal pleurectomy. We

agree with the selective approach of Brooks[7] and Weeden and Smith[37] that an apical pleurectomy is sufficient in the presence of apical disease, but subtotal pleurectomy should be performed in the presence of diffuse subpleural disease not amenable to resection.

CONCLUSIONS

Review of our data suggests that the majority (70%) of patients coming to thoracotomy for pneumothorax-related problems are young adults with apical blebs unassociated with parenchymal lung disease. Recurrence and persistent air leak account for 95% of operative indications. A small axillary incision allowing bleb resection and apical pleurectomy should suffice to prevent recurrence with a minimum of complications.

In the older age group, pneumothorax most commonly results from emphysematous changes with diffuse subpleural disease (15% of cases). Resection of large blebs and bullae with performance of subtotal pleurectomy should be performed. Although we employed unilateral thoracotomy in nearly all of our patients, median sternotomy is an attractive and preferable approach to patients with bilateral bullous disease and compromised pulmonary function. This approach should also be considered in the management of bilateral simultaneous pneumothorax, but its application to all cases of unilateral pneumothorax is not recommended.

The third group represents a heterogenous population. In patients with diffuse subpleural disease, as with eosinophilic granuloma or metastatic sarcoma, where concomitant pulmonary resection is not feasible, subtotal pleurectomy should be performed.

It is interesting that no patient suffering

Table 9–4. Results of Nine Series of Pleurectomies

Series		No. of Pleurectomies	Hospital Mortality	Results (No. of Patients)		Recurrence
				Morbidity		
				Major	Minor	
Ruckley and McCormack[27]	(1966)	35	0	1	0	0
Brooks[7]	(1973)	33	0	3	1	0
Askew[3]	(1976)	103	0	7	4	1
Singh[30]	(1979)	50	0	0	2	0
Deslauriers et al[14]	(1980)	409	1	4	13[a]	2
Singh[31]	(1982)	125[b]	0	2	6	0
Behl and Holden[5]	(1983)	150	0	1	0	0
Weeden and Smith[37]	(1983)	241	3	9	39	1
Bojar and Kittle	(1985)	112	2	7	5	0
Total		1208[b]	6 (0.5%)	34 (2.8%)	70 (5.5%)	4 (0.3%)

[a]Excludes 32 patients with air–fluid levels that resolved spontaneously and atelectasis responding to chest physiotherapy.
[b]Includes the 50 patients from Singh's earlier series.

pneumothorax from attempted subclavian vein catheterization required thoracotomy for persistent leak. This suggests that in the absence of underlying subpleural or parenchymal disease, the pleura is able to seal, thereby allowing resolution of the pneumothorax.

With minimal morbidity and mortality associated with pleurectomy, and with negligible recurrence rates, our data and a review of the recent literature suggest that bleb resection with pleurectomy is an excellent choice in the management of recurrent and complicated pneumothorax.

References

1. Adkins PC, Smyth NPD: Bilateral simultaneous spontaneous pneumothorax. Dis Chest 37:702–704, 1960.
2. Andersen I, Poulsen T: Surgical treatment of spontaneous pneumothorax. Acta Chir Scand 118:105–112, 1959.
3. Askew AR: Parietal pleurectomy for recurrent pneumothorax. Brit J Surg 63:203–205, 1976.
4. Baronofsky ID, Warden HG, Kaufman JL, et al: Bilateral therapy for unilateral pneumothorax. J Thorac Surg 34:310–322, 1957.
5. Behl PR, Holden MP: Pleurectomy for recurrent pneumothorax. Chest 84:785, 1983.
6. Bethune N: Pleural poudrage—a new technic for the deliberate production of pleural adhesions as a preliminary to lobectomy. J Thorac Surg 4:251–261, 1935.
7. Brooks JW: Open thoracotomy in the management of spontaneous pneumothorax. Ann Surg 177:798–805, 1973.
8. Cannon WB, Mark JBD, Jamplis RW: Pneumothorax: A therapeutic update. Am J Surg 142:26–29, 1981.
9. Clagett OT: The management of spontaneous pneumothorax. J Thorac Cardiovasc Surg 55:761–762, 1968.
10. Clark TA, Hutchinson DE, Deaner RM, Fitchett VH: Spontaneous pneumothorax. Am J Surg 124:728–731, 1972.
11. Collins HA, Daniel RA Jr, Diveley WL: Parietal pleurectomy for spontaneous pneumothorax. Am Surg 29:844–849, 1963.
12. Cooper JD, Nelems JM, Pearson FG: Extended indications for median sternotomy in patients requiring pulmonary resection. Ann Thorac Surg 26:413–420, 1978.
13. Deaton WR, Johnston FR: Spontaneous hemopneumothorax. J Thorac Cardiovasc Surg 43:413–415, 1962.
14. Deslauriers J, Beaulieu M, Despres JP, et al.: Transaxillary pleurectomy for treatment of spontaneous pneumothorax. Ann Thorac Surg 30:569–574, 1980.
15. DeVries WC, Wolfe WG: The management of spontaneous pneumothorax and bullous emphysema. Surg Clin North Am 60:851–866, 1980.
16. Ferguson LJ, Imrie CW, Hutchinson J: Excision of bullae without pleurectomy in patients with spontaneous pneumothorax. Brit J Surg 68:214–216, 1981.
17. Gaensler EA: Parietal pleurectomy for recurrent spontaneous pneumothorax. Surg Gynecol Obst 102:293–308, 1956.
18. Gobbel WG Jr, Rhea WG Jr, Nelson IA, Daniel RA Jr: Spontaneous pneumothorax. J Thorac Cardiovasc Surg 46:331–345, 1963.
19. Kalnins I, Torda TA, Wright JS: Bilateral simultaneous pleurodesis by median sternotomy for spontaneous pneumothorax. Ann Thorac Surg 15:202–206, 1973.
20. Kircher LT Jr, Swartzel RL: Spontaneous pneumothorax and its treatment. JAMA 155:24–29, 1954.
21. Jackson JW, Bennett MH: Chest wall tumour following iodized talc pleurodesis. Thorax 28:788–793, 1977.
22. Larrieu AJ, Tyers GFO, Williams EN, et al: Intrapleural instillation of quinacrine for treatment of recurrent spontaneous pneumothorax. Ann Thorac Surg 28:146–150, 1979.
23. Lima O, Ramos L, DiBiasi P, et al: Median sternotomy for bilateral resection of emphysematous bullae. J Thorac Cardiovasc Surg 82:892–897, 1981.
24. Mercier C, Pagi A, Verdant A, et al: Outpatient management of intercostal tube drainage in spontaneous pneumothorax. Ann Thorac Surg 22:163–165, 1976.
25. Mills M, Baish BF: Spontaneous pneumothorax: A series of 400 cases. Ann Thorac Surg 1:286–293, 1965.
26. Neal JF, Vargas G, Smith DE, et al: Bilateral bleb excision through median sternotomy. Am J Surg 138:794–797, 1979.
27. Ruckley CV, McCormack RJM: The management of spontaneous pneumothorax. Thorax 21:139–144, 1966.
28. Saha O: Parietal pleurectomy for prevention of recurrent spontaneous pneumothorax. Brit J Dis Chest 58:78–84, 1964.
29. Seremetis MG: The management of spontaneous pneumothorax. Chest 57:65–68, 1970.
30. Singh SV: Current status of parietal pleurectomy in recurrent pneumothorax. Scand J Thorac Cardiovasc Surg 13:93–96, 1979.
31. Singh SV: The surgical treatment of spontaneous pneumothorax by parietal pleurectomy. Scand J Thorac Cardiovasc Surg 16:75–80, 1982.
32. Spengler L: Zur Chirurgie des Pneumothorax. Beitr Klin Chir 49:80, 1906.
33. Tassi GF, Fabio D, Chiodera PL, et al: Intrapleural tetracycline for recurrent pneumothorax. Chest 83:836, 1983.
34. Thomas PA, Gebauer PW: Pleurectomy for recurrent spontaneous pneumothorax. J Thorac Surg 35:111–117, 1958.
35. Thomas PA, Gebauer PW: Results and complications of pleurectomy for bullous emphysema and recurrent pneumothorax. J Thorac Cardiovasc Surg 39:194–201, 1960.
36. Vosi-Moykopf I, Haiderer O: Current views on the management of spontaneous pneumothorax. Surg Gynecol Obst 122:313–316, 1966.
37. Weeden D, Smith GH: Surgical experience in the management of spontaneous pneumothorax. Thorax 38:737–743, 1983.
38. Weissberg D: Disscussion of 14. Ann Thorac Surg 30:569–574, 1980.
39. Youmans CR Jr, Williams RD, McMinn MR, Derrick JR: Surgical management of spontaneous pneumothorax by bleb ligation and pleural dry sponge abrasion. Am J Surg 120:644–648, 1970.

III

Malignant Pleural Mesothelioma

Asbestos, the magic and mysterious mineral . . . so-called because it is unaffected by fire (from the Greek *asbestos* or inextinguishable), is a general term applied to any one of several silicates *if* it breaks into fibers when crushed. Impressed by the "unstainability and the resistance to pollution or defilement" of this mineral, others have suggested the word *amiantos*. In England "amianthus" was used until this century. It has been gradually replaced by asbestos, but today in France either *amiante* or *asbeste* is equally acceptable.

The unique properties of asbestos—flexibility, fire resistance, and virtual indestructibility—have fascinated and were utilized by humans for centuries. Pottery containing asbestos fibers mixed with clay has been found in Finland dating from 2500 B.C. and in Africa from the Stone Age. Plutarch (46–120 A.D.) mentioned fireproof lamp wicks used by the vestal virgins made of a woven mineral fiber from Cyprus. He also wrote of a rock producing "soft, petrous filaments like yarn" that can be made into "towels, nets and women's head coverings which cannot be burned by fire; but if they become soiled by use, their owners throw them into a blazing fire and take them out bright and clean." Incidentally, it was noted that the weavers wore masks to avoid inhaling the fibrous dust.

Both Herodotus (ca. 500 B.C.) and Pliny (ca. 50 A.D.) described shrouds of woven asbestos used in the cremation of nobility, the *linum vivum* or funeral dress of the kings.

Use of asbestos was episodic and occasional until the Industrial Revolution, when its singular features were found to be increasingly desirable for a myriad of industrial products. Its current use, chiefly in combination with other materials, is measured in the millions of tons annually, with the United States being the largest consumer.

The harmful effects of asbestos were noted as early as the first century by the Greeks and the Romans. The Greek geographer Strabo and the Roman naturalist Pliny both mentioned a sickness of the lungs in slaves who wove asbestos into cloth. But health hazards were of little concern then, and the advantages of the asbestos outweighed any sickness in slaves. The use of asbestos diminished greatly during the next 17 centuries until the Industrial Revolution. Then the desire to capitalize on and utilize the unique physical and chemical properties of asbestos completely overshadowed any memories, knowledge, or interest about its toxicity.

World War II, with its strenuous demands on manufacturing and industry, greatly increased the use of asbestos in the United States. The war's race with time postponed consideration of any health hazards that asbestos might present, and this continued during the postwar building boom.

A discussion of malignant mesothelioma must recognize three major problems, two that have been solved and one that remains unsolved.

Problem 1. Does such an entity as mesothelioma exist?

The term *mesothelioma* was coined by Woolley (1902): "It seems wise, therefore, to call this tumor a 'mesothelioma,' . . . (since) we call serous membranes and their derivatives mesothelium." At this time pleural tumors had been noted but were designated by such names as endothelioma, carcinosarcoma, and papillomatosis. Klemperer and Rabin (1931) classified pleural tumors into fibrous and epithelial types and also stated that the term mesothelioma ". . . be accepted to designate all the diffuse neoplasms of the pleura that arise from the mesothelium, whether they appear to be composed of epithelium, connective tissue, or both." No association with asbestos was recognized.

Others, however, steadfastly denied the diagnosis of mesothelioma, insisting that

". . . tumours in the serous membranes have often been mistakenly called primary 'endotheliomas' or 'mesotheliomas,' when they were really only secondary growths from undetected primary tumors elsewhere" (Willis, 1972). With further study by many pathologists, mesothelioma has become a recognized entity.

Problem 2. Is there a causal relationship between asbestos and mesothelioma?

Attention in modern times was first directed to the harmful effects of asbestos by Murray (1907), who associated this mineral with pulmonary fibrosis causing the death of a man he had autopsied in 1899. Auribault also recorded numerous deaths among workers in a French asbestos spinning mill and asbestos factory (1906). Cooke (1924) described the autopsy findings in a 33-year-old female asbestos worker and attributed her death directly to asbestos exposure. His papers were the turning point in the acceptance of the pathogenicity of asbestos and introduced a new term, "asbestosis" (1927).

Mallory and colleagues (1947) discussed an asbestos worker with a pleural and pericardial mesothelioma, although no relationship with asbestos was suggested. Weiss (1953) reported on 32 patients with asbestosis, three with malignant tumors of the pleura and six with cancer of the lung. Other accounts of mesothelioma quickly followed, but it remained for Wagner and coworkers (1960) to link the high incidence of mesothelioma in the Cape Province of South Africa with asbestos exposure. Wagner subsequently demonstrated that mesothelioma could be produced by implanting asbestos dust into the pleural cavities of rats (1962).

It is now established that the inhalation or ingestion of asbestos can cause mesothelioma, although it is also recognized that this substance is probably not the sole cause of this malignancy.

Problem 3. What can be done to improve the clinical treatment of malignant pleural mesothelioma?

Much attention has been devoted to the management of this malignancy. One of the most recent publications (Law and colleagues, 1984) evaluates three forms of therapy (surgery, chemotherapy, and radiotherapy in 52 patients) against no treatment (64 patients). They conclude that "There was no significant difference in survival between treatment groups or between treated and untreated patients. . . ."

Frustration, confusion, and controversy—all of these exist about therapy for malignant pleural mesothelioma. There is a wide spectrum of opinions and much remains to be done.

10

Malignant Pleural Mesothelioma: A Nonsurgical Problem

Ralph J. Lewis, M.D.

In the past, mesothelioma was a rare lesion. Recently, its incidence has been increasing significantly.[1] Because of the close proximity of an asbestos factory, this lesion occurs with even greater frequency in our area than elsewhere. Between 1930 and 1950, almost no precautions were taken nor was protection offered to the factory workers against asbestos exposure; in fact, so numerous were the free-floating white asbestos flakes that patients have described the interior of the plant as resembling a snowstorm. Asbestos particles were carried home on the workers' clothing and skin, exposing their families. Moreover, children were permitted to play on the asbestos dump outside the factory.

The lesion acquired from asbestos exposure was diffuse mixed pleural mesothelioma, which causes a slow and painful death by suffocation. Another form of the disease, solitary pedunculated mesothelioma, appears to be a different variant and has a relatively good prognosis with resection.[2] We have seen several patients with this isolated lesion who did not have a definite history of asbestos exposure. However, all of our patients with diffuse mixed mesothelioma either worked in the asbestos factory or were relatives of employees. It is our contention that diffuse mixed mesothelioma is not affected favorably by surgical resection.

Initially, we hoped and believed that early diagnosis followed by surgical resection would lead to improved survival, but our results have been very disappointing. This tumor has proved to be a relentless, progressive, lethal lesion that appears 20 to 40 years after exposure—the duration of which may be as brief as 6 to 8 weeks.[3]

PATIENT POPULATION

The total number of patients seen in our area with diffuse mixed mesothelioma is 186. Of these, 112 patients had pleural mesothelioma; however, there were also 74 patients who had peritoneal mesothelioma, most of whom were treated by general surgeons.

Since 1970, we have evaluated 62 consecutive patients with diffuse mixed pleural mesothelioma. All had been exposed to crocidolite, amosite, or chrysotile asbestos fibers for varying periods of time. Each patient had annual roentgenograms to determine the change, if any, in pulmonary fibrosis from the previous year. When suspicious roentgenographic changes were noted, patients were referred for further evaluation.

In our study, there were 49 men and 13 women, who ranged in age from 38 to 80 years. The lesion occurred in the right hemithorax in 35 patients and in the left hemithorax in 27. Sixty patients worked in the asbestos factory; the other two patients lived in the surrounding city. Three patients were admitted in a terminal state and died within 7 to 20 days. In the remaining 59 patients, survival ranged from 2 to 24 months.

Survival rates according to treatment regimen were as follows: For 14 patients who received neither radiation therapy nor chemotherapy following tissue diagnosis, average survival was 9.6 months. For 43 patients who received only chemotherapy, average survival was 10.8 months. In five patients, resection was attempted because the lesion was visualized early at thoracoscopy; these patients survived an average of 6.8 months.

DIAGNOSIS

Because asbestosis occurs much more commonly than mesothelioma, biopsy for definitive differentiation of these two diseases is mandatory. The prognosis and also the amount of financial compensation awarded to the patient and family by the employer (more than 16,000 lawsuits are currently pending against the asbestos factory) depend upon this differentiation. Therefore, every patient in our series had a tissue diagnosis.

Early in our experience, tissue was obtained

by thoracotomy because of our enthusiastic anticipation of a curative resection. We soon learned that a curative resection or even a significant debulking procedure was not possible in these patients. Mini-thoracotomy next became the procedure of choice and then thoracoscopy.[4] Recently, we have been successful with percutaneous needle biopsy.

Each of our patients was considered a possible candidate for resection, and we have always been prepared to proceed with a resection when the findings were favorable; unfortunately, this was seldom the case. In our group of 62 consecutive patients, 5 underwent a formal thoracotomy with resection, 9 a mini-thoracotomy, 33 a thoracoscopy, and 14 a thoracentesis. In no instance was bronchoscopy positive, and in only one patient did mediastinoscopy return malignant tissue. In two patients, thoracoscopy was initially negative, but both eventually went on to develop mesothelioma. Nevertheless, we still consider thoracoscopy to be a very rewarding procedure with a very high diagnostic yield. Whenever a needle biopsy is negative, we proceed to thoracoscopy.

For percutaneous needle biopsy, pleural fluid was aspirated with a small-size needle (No. 21), in order to decrease the likelihood of neoplastic invasion of the chest wall. The pleural fluid was submitted for cytologic examination and for determination of hyaluronic acid content. Thoracoscopy was carried out by a technique described earlier in the literature.[4] If no free space was present, a mini-thoracotomy was performed. Multiple tissue samples were submitted for frozen section examination. In some patients, a trapped lung and loculated areas containing fluid were encountered. Biopsy specimens from these sites usually revealed diffuse mixed mesothelioma.

CLINICAL EXPERIENCE: CASE REPORTS

Patient 1. A 46-year-old woman had never worked in the asbestos factory but, as a child, had washed the clothes of her mother, who worked there. She developed a dull, nagging pain in the left lower chest area over many months. Serial x-ray films over the course of several months revealed progressive blunting of the left costophrenic angle (Fig. 10–1, *A* and *B*). Because of the history of asbestos exposure, thoracoscopy was performed; a diagnosis of mesothelioma was confirmed.

Because of the patient's young age, her otherwise excellent health, and apparently limited disease,

resection was advised. At thoracotomy, however, voluminous deposits of mesothelioma were found invading the diaphragm, parietal pleura, and apex of the chest and lung. Diaphragmatic resection, pleurectomy, and a partial lung resection were performed (Fig. 10–1*C*). Chemotherapy and radiotherapy were given postoperatively.

The patient survived 15 months. The last 10 months were characterized by severe weakness, progressive deterioration, debilitation, and intractable pain; the quality of life was very poor.

Patient 2. A 42-year-old male was the attorney for the employees of the asbestos factory. He had been a college athlete and always enjoyed excellent health. When he was 18 years old, he worked in the asbestos factory for only 8 weeks during his summer vacation.

The patient presented with shortness of breath and a massive bloody pleural effusion (Fig. 10–2*A*). Thoracoscopy was negative for malignancy, but mesothelioma was strongly suspected, and under subsequent observation, the lung never cleared completely. Within 3 months the patient developed a gelatinous mass in the thoracic cavity. Thoracentesis returned malignant mesothelioma (Fig. 10–2*B*).

The patient was advised against surgical intervention but elected to undergo a debulking procedure at another institution. This procedure was aborted because of massive hemorrhage, and assisted ventilation was required for a prolonged period of time. He died 4 months following surgery.

Patient 3. A 48-year-old asbestos factory employee had had pain in the right costophrenic area for 1 month. A chest roentgenogram revealed a lesion in the right costophrenic angle. The patient underwent a right pneumonectomy, complete pleural stripping, partial resection of the diaphragm, instillation of a chemotherapeutic agent, and postoperative cobalt therapy. He died 5 months following operation. Postmortem examination revealed diffuse mixed mesothelioma involving both pleural cavities and the peritoneal cavity.

Patient 4. A 47-year-old man was employed as a stock boy in the asbestos factory for only 4 months 25 years before the onset of right chest pain He underwent a right pleurectomy and decortication and died 12 months later. Postmortem examination revealed involvement of both pleural cavities and of the peritoneal cavity by advanced invasive, diffuse mixed mesothelioma.

Patient 5. A 42-year-old woman presented with nagging right chest pain. She had never worked in the asbestos factory but had played on the asbestos dump as a child. Roentgenograms suggested mesothelioma. After further evaluation, the patient underwent a right decortication and pleurectomy. She died 6 months later of diffuse mixed mesothelioma involving the peritoneal and both thoracic cavities.

Patient 6. A 62-year-old woman was employed as a secretary in the asbestos factory research department for 40 years. Because of persistent, nag-

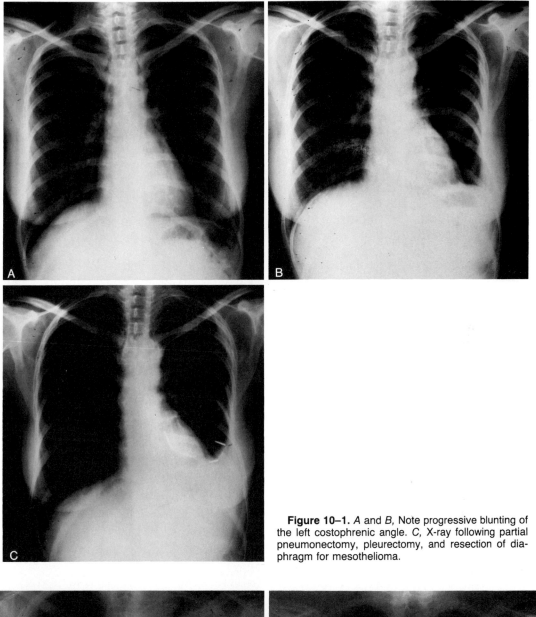

Figure 10–1. *A* and *B,* Note progressive blunting of the left costophrenic angle. *C,* X-ray following partial pneumonectomy, pleurectomy, and resection of diaphragm for mesothelioma.

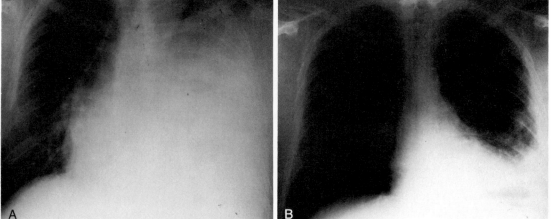

Figure 10–2. *A,* Massive left-sided pleural effusion. *B,* Persistent pleural effusion with blunting of costophrenic angle.

ging right chest pain, a chest roentgenogram was made and revealed right pleural thickening (Fig. 10–3*A*). On closer evaluation, irregularity along the diaphragm and fullness of the mediastinal area could be appreciated. The visual appearance at thoracoscopy was disheartening; heaps and mounds of mesothelioma invading the diaphragm, mediastinal pleura, and parietal pleura, with invasion of the visceral pleura, could be easily delineated. Biopsies confirmed diffuse mixed mesothelioma, which was obviously unresectable and incurable. Chemotherapy and irradiation were started concurrently. An x-ray film 3 months later revealed unabated growth of the tumor (Fig. 10–3*B*).

PATHOGENESIS, SYMPTOMS, AND HISTOLOGY

Mesothelioma arises most commonly from the pleura, although it can develop in the pericardium, peritoneum, and tunica vaginalis. This malignant tumor usually appears 20 or more years following inhalation of asbestos fibers. The mechanical properties of the asbestos fibers, rather than their chemical composition, seem to incite the tissue change. Fibers less than 2.5 μ in diameter and 10 to 80 μ in length can penetrate deeply into the lung.

Approximately 99% of asbestos fibers are filtered via the nasopharyngeal area. The small number entering the lung are phagocytized by macrophages, after which proteinaceous material and hemosiderin are absorbed, forming a ferruginous body. It is believed this process contributes to asbestosis. Fragmented asbestos fibers are not as readily cleared by the upper airway and pass through the alveoli and then out to the dependent portions of the parietal pleura. Typically, after 20 to 40 years of continuous irritation, malignant changes can occur.

Although clinical symptoms and roentgenographic findings are usually minimal, the disease may be widespread and unresectable when the first subtle symptoms occur. Visualization by thoracoscopy consistently reveals the process to be much more advanced than suggested by x-ray or physical findings. The lesion usually arises from many areas of the parietal pleura but is most advanced in the dependent portions of the thorax. Very rigid adhesions can be seen obliterating the lower pleural cavity, whereas firm deposits of tumor, not clearly delineated on conventional chest x-ray examination, can be found in the apex of the thorax. In fact, it is discouraging to view directly this vast amount of tumor invading organs throughout the thorax. Early in its course, mesothelioma appears to be multicentric in origin, involving large but separate areas of the pleura and diaphragm. Frequently the mediastinal pleura is fixed and has a woodlike consistency. In some cases, a hemorrhagic mucoid material is diffusely and irregularly distributed over a normal-appearing parietal pleura. Elsewhere, only erythema and edema

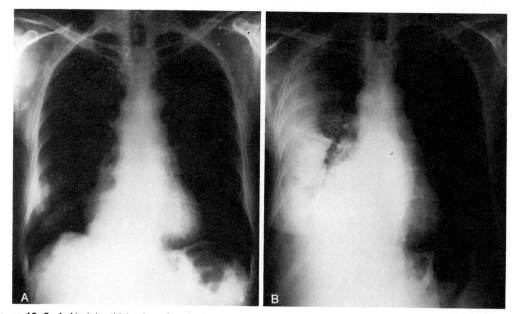

Figure 10–3. *A*, Nodular thickening of parietal pleura on right. *B*, Progressive growth of tumor despite radiation and chemotherapy.

may be seen, or there may be multiple nodules or masses, which coalesce to form loculated cystic spaces.

Initially, involvement of diaphragmatic and costophrenic areas by neoplasm corresponds to gravitational deposition of asbestos fibers. In some patients with minimal gross findings, a blind biopsy from the costophrenic area will frequently return tumor. As the disease progresses, tumor excrescences and invasive adhesions are found posteriorly and laterally. Pleural effusion can occur early, but later reabsorption of fluid and tumor coalescence will obliterate the thoracic cavity. At this stage of the disease, severe compression of organs begins to occur.

Mesothelioma invades lung, chest wall muscles, diaphragm, and mediastinal structures, eliminating any possibility for developing a clean plane of resection free of tumor. Terminally, the neoplasm debilitates the patient by compression, envelopment, and strangulation of organs. In our experience, a complete resection or even a substantial debulking procedure is not possible in over 95% of our carefully evaluated patients.

In general, diffuse mixed mesothelioma has a variable histologic appearance. Portions of the tumor have an intermix of cuboidal and spindle cells, usually with obvious transitions from one cell type to the other. The cuboidal cells appear mainly in small groups, forming glandlike spaces or cores, whereas the adjacent spindle cells produce sheets and, rarely, distinct fascicles. In other areas, either the epithelial (tubulopapillary) or the sarcomatous (fibrosarcomatous) type can predominate, occasionally side by side, without obvious blending. In these areas there is generally a considerable uniformity of cell morphology, but in the mixed areas there may be considerable pleomorphism. All of our patients had the mixed type of mesothelioma, and all were exposed to amosite, crocidolite, and chrysotile fibers.

RESULTS: RESECTION VERSUS NONOPERATIVE MANAGEMENT

In our series of 62 patients, those undergoing resection survived an average of only 6.8 months before dying of massive recurrence involving both pleural cavities and the peritoneal cavity. One patient lived 15 months following resection but had a prolonged period of progressive painful deterioration before dying of recurrent disease. Of the patients managed nonoperatively, those receiving chemotherapy or radiation therapy, or both, following the diagnosis of mesothelioma survived slightly more than 9 months; those untreated also survived more than 9 months on the average. Clearly, in the nonoperative group, survival did not differ significantly for the treated and untreated patients.

Even though chemotherapy and irradiation were used as a last resort, the overall survival period of the nonoperative group was still better than that of patients undergoing resection. Even patients receiving no treatment survived longer than did those whose tumor was surgically treated. Paradoxically, the shortest duration of survival was in the resection group—in those patients who clinically appeared to have the least amount of tumor when first seen. We suggest that the intact pleura may present a barrier to the growth of the tumor, since mesothelioma has been found to grow through needle aspiration tracts and thoracoscopy sites where the pleura has been disrupted, and that pleural resection may potentiate spread. In support of our experience, a review of the literature has failed to reveal a single substantial series with satisfactory survival statistics following resection for mesothelioma.

A report by Butchart and colleagues[5] in 1976 was based on experience with 29 patients whose tumor was treated by pleuropneumonectomy. Their reported complication rate was 43%, and the hospital mortality, 31%. Only three of their patients survived 2 years. These authors suggested that if resection was contemplated, only patients with epithelial lesions should undergo operation.

Churg[6] believes that a major problem with mesothelioma is establishing a correct histopathologic diagnosis. Carcinoma and sarcoma—which can metastasize to the pleura and peritoneum, mimicking mesothelioma—must be excluded. It must be remembered that bronchogenic carcinoma occurs much more commonly in asbestos workers than does mesothelioma.

DeLaria and coworkers[7] performed extrapleural pneumonectomy in their patients with malignant mesothelioma. Although their series revealed a significantly lessened operative mortality, the rapid demise or recurrence of disease in seven of their last nine reported patients suggests that the natural course of the disease rather than operative intervention may explain the occasional long-term survivor. Their patients differed from those in our series in several ways: Few of their patients had a history of asbestos exposure, whereas all of our patients had confirmed exposure. Most of their patients, especially the longer survivors, had epithelial mesothelioma; however, all of ours had mixed mesothelioma. We suspect that the lesion in at least a few of their patients was infiltrating adenocarcinoma. Their patients frequently had distant metastases, whereas even at autopsy, distant metastases were found very infrequently in our series. At the time of resection, these workers frequently left a rim of diaphragm; yet in our patients, a blind biopsy in the costophrenic area returned evidence of disease in many cases. Shortness of breath was relieved following resection in their patients. In our series, however, since 60% of the patients had concurrent asbestosis, shortness of breath was increased with resection. In their series, pleural effusion occurred late, and thoracentesis was never positive for malignant cells; in contrast, we found that pleural effusion occurred early and was commonly positive for malignant cells. So many dissimilarities suggest that their patients and ours did not have the same disease process.

Finally, Jensik has described malignant mesothelioma as "essentially an incurable disease irrespective of the therapeutic approach."[8] Elms and Simpson[9] support this viewpoint in their report of a study of 300 patients in the British Isles. In fact, they maintain that surgery, chemotherapy, and radiation encouraged spread of the tumor and that conservative management apparently offers the best quality of life. Because all tissue types were invariably present on histologic examination, the mesotheliomas in their series were considered to be of the mixed variety.

The report by Wanebo and colleagues[10] at Memorial Sloan-Kettering Cancer Center described results with partial resection followed by external irradiation and systemic chemotherapy. Best results in this study were also in patients with the epithelial type of lesion. Wanebo's group did not have confirmation of asbestos exposure in all patients and frequently did not have confirmation of mesothelioma at autopsy. Interestingly, they did describe metastases to cervical nodes, whereas we have seen metastases only very infrequently and very late in advanced disease. Patients as young as 13 years of age were included in their series. Since the lesion is thought to develop over 20 to 40 years following exposure, the accuracy of the diagnosis in a 13-year-old must be questioned. Many children in our area had exposure to asbestos, but none developed mesothelioma until late in the third decade of life.

Once again we find serious disparities between this series and ours.

Legha and Muggia[11] maintain that an adequate specimen obtained by open biopsy is usually necessary for diagnosis. Tumors having a propensity for serosal spread, such as ovarian carcinoma, appendiceal mucocele, adenocarcinoma, and bronchoalveolar carcinoma, must be carefully excluded. These workers have found no therapeutic modality that suggests improvement in survival of patients with mesothelioma in the last 20 years. Since their review of the literature has produced only rare cases surviving 5 years, they believe that "the 25% mortality rate for pleuropneumonectomy found in some series makes this procedure even more unjustifiable."[11]

Gaensler believes that mesothelioma "is not now nor likely ever will be a surgical disease."[8] In his series of 65 patients, none underwent surgical resection and few received chemotherapy. Yet there were two 3-year survivors and one 4-year survivor. He suggests that any invasive procedure, even for diagnosis, is meddlesome.

It is difficult to rationalize scientifically how incomplete removal of bits and pieces of firm, fibrous, diffusely invasive tumor could benefit any patient. Moreover, in many of our patients, extrapleural pneumonectomy was not feasible because of advanced pulmonary fibrosis due to heavy industrial exposure on the contralateral side. In the entire literature, only a small number of patients have survived 5 years following resection. We reemphasize that prolongation of life may be attributed to patient selection and to the timing of intervention in the course of the disease rather than the specific form of therapy employed.

Despite an acute awareness of this lesion and early tissue diagnosis, resection has never been curative. Furthermore, we question whether resection has any place at all in the management of patients with this tumor. These concerns are substantiated by the following findings:

1. Cigarette smokers exposed to asbestos have an unusually high incidence of pulmonary carcinoma. Possibly in some of the reported 2-, 3-, and 4-year survivors, the lesion that was resected, irradiated, and treated with chemotherapeutic agents was carcinoma of the lung rather than the so-called epithelial variant of mesothelioma. On occasion, carcinoma of the lung invading the pleura is extremely difficult to differentiate from mesothelioma; significantly, most good results reported in the literature have been found in that group of

patients with epithelial mesothelioma. The lesion in several of our patients was initially diagnosed as mesothelioma by biopsy; yet at autopsy it was found to be carcinoma of the lung.

2. At autopsy, we occasionally see involvement of all three cavities, so at least in some patients, the disease is not localized to one thoracic cavity. Unilateral pleurectomy would be of little benefit in these patients. Recently CT scans of the chest have demonstrated bilateral involvement, not appreciated in conventional chest films.

3. In our experience, the disease becomes more virulent and aggressive following disruption of the parietal pleura. This has been demonstrated by the rapid demise of our patients undergoing resection and also by the growth of tumor through thoracoscopy sites and needle tracts.

4. In the autopsy room, our attempts to delineate a clean plane of resection in areas of minimal involvement have been unsuccessful, so we are skeptical that a clean plane of resection can be found in the operating room. In fact, microscopic sections have shown invasion of intercostal muscles by tumor, obviating the possibility of a curative resection.

5. Survival with nonoperative management in our series and others was notably longer than that following surgery. Perhaps preservation of an intact parietal pleura is more important to prolongation of life than is debulking of tumor mass.

In conclusion, the futility of attempting a curative resection quickly becomes apparent as the clinician gains experience with this intractable disease process. Moreover, no evidence is available to substantiate the idea that a massive radical incomplete resection prolongs life in a patient with diffuse, mixed malignant pleural mesothelioma.

References

1. Borow M, Constan A, Livornese L, Shalet N: Mesothelioma following exposure to asbestos: A review of 72 cases. Chest 64:641, 1973.
2. Selikoff I, Cheng J, Hammond E: Relation between exposure to asbestos and mesothelioma. N Engl J Med 272:560, 1965.
3. Aisner J, Wiernik PH: Malignant mesothelioma: Current status and future prospects. Chest 74:438, 1978.
4. Lewis RJ, Kunderman PF, Sisler GE, Mackenzie JW: Direct diagnostic thoracoscopy. Ann Thorac Surg 21:536, 1976.
5. Butchart EG, Ashcroft T, Barnsley WC, Holden MP: Pleuro-pneumonectomy in the management of diffuse malignant mesothelioma of the pleura: Experience with 29 patients. Thorax 31:15, 1976.
6. Churg A: Current issues in the pathologic and mineralogic diagnosis of asbestos-induced disease. Chest 84:275, 1983.
7. DeLaria GA, Jensik R, Faber LP, Kittle CF: Surgical management of malignant mesothelioma. Ann Thorac Surg 26:375, 1978.
8. Lewis RJ, Sisler GE, Mackenzie JW: Diffuse mixed malignant pleural mesothelioma. Ann Thorac Surg 31:53, 1981.
9. Elmes PC, Simpson MJC: The clinical aspects of mesothelioma. Q J Med 45:427, 1976.
10. Wanebo H, Martini N, Melamed M, et al: Pleural mesothelioma. Cancer 38:2481, 1976.
11. Legha S, Muggia F: Therapeutic approaches in malignant mesothelioma. Cancer Treat Rev 4:13, 1977.

11

Malignant Pleural Mesothelioma: A Combined Modality Approach

Karen H. Antman, M.D.
Richard J. Shemin, M.D.
Joseph M. Corson, M.D.

Malignant mesotheliomas arise most frequently from the pleura and peritoneum, and occur rarely in the pericardium[5, 6] and the tunica vaginalis propria.[3, 22] Because these tissues are of mesodermal embryologic origin, mesotheliomas are classified as soft tissue sarcomas.[52, 54, 56] Only pleural malignant mesotheliomas are considered in this discussion.

At the Dana-Farber Cancer Institute (DFCI), we are currently evaluating a multimodality investigational approach to malignant mesothelioma. Because the diagnosis of malignant mesothelioma is plagued by both false positives (up to one third of cases)[40] and false negatives, an expert pathologist is an essential member of the treatment team. Since virtually all patients die of their disease, experienced supportive and palliative care is a key in improving the quality and perhaps also the duration of survival.

The treatment of mesothelioma remains unsatisfactory. Although some authors have advocated supportive care alone because current treatments have not demonstrated increased survival, occasional patients have remained disease-free for periods in excess of 5 years after intensive multimodality treatment.[6, 16, 23, 59] The premise that mesothelioma is untreatable is clearly untenable, since palliation from radiotherapy and chemotherapy with response rates from various chemotherapeutic regimens of up to 30% has been reported by a number of investigators.[1] We believe patients with mesothelioma should be offered investigational therapy. Three points deserve emphasis:

1. The median survival for a chemotherapy-treated group will not be prolonged until the response rate of a given regimen reaches 50%. Despite a substantial survival advantage for responders, the median survival is not affected if less than 50% respond.

2. Intensive individualized treatment exposes the patient to complications of surgery, chemotherapy, and radiotherapy with no certainty of benefit and no opportunity for identifying a better treatment. Thus, nonstandard treatment should not be undertaken in other than a research setting.

3. Advocating "supportive care alone" ensures that no new therapy is evaluated and therefore that no promising regimen can be found. A similar conservative philosophy was advocated in the past for Hodgkin's disease, advanced testicular cancer, and childhood leukemia—all of which are now curable diseases.

EPIDEMIOLOGY

Recognizing the Patient at High Risk

The most important etiologic factor is exposure to asbestos, although chronic severe pulmonary disease [13] including tuberculosis and lipoid aspiration pneumonia,[44] radiation,[7] and zeolite contact[9, 57] have been associated with the development of malignant mesothelioma. About half of all patients with malignant pleural mesothelioma will eventually recall a clear history of asbestos exposure.[5] (In various series from different institutions the percentage of patients with a history of asbestos contact varies considerably, ranging from zero[14] to almost 80%.[5, 6])

Patients whose history apparently includes none of these factors may have had a long-forgotten, cryptic, or trivial asbestos exposure. (Asbestos bodies, fiber cores coated by hemosiderin and glycoprotein, can be identified in most urban dwellers at autopsy.[39, 58])

Table 11–1. Staging of Malignant
Mesothelioma

Stage	Structures Involved by Tumor
I	Ipsilateral pleura and lung
II	Chest wall, mediastinum, pericardium, or contralateral pleura
III	Thorax and abdomen, or lymph nodes outside the chest
IV	Distant hematogenous metastases

Modified from Butchart EG et al: Pleuropneumonectomy in the management of diffuse malignant mesothelioma of the pleura: experience with 29 patients. Thorax 31:15–24, 1976.

An increased risk of mesothelioma can be identified 20 years after first asbestos exposure; however, the incidence of the disease continues to rise after 35 to 45 years.[55] The cumulative lifetime risk of developing mesothelioma increases as a constant times the third or fourth power of time since first exposure,[49, 50] i.e., risk = K (time since first exposure)$^{3.5}$. Dose and duration of exposure are reflected in the constant part of the equation.[49, 50] Thus, the lower the age at first exposure, the higher the cumulative lifetime risk. Obviously then, significant levels of exposure in schools may be particularly hazardous.

Asbestos is virtually indestructible; thus, once particles have settled in the body, "exposure" continues for the remainder of the patient's lifetime.

Other Asbestos-related Malignancies

Unless either the classic mixed form or the sarcomatoid variants of mesothelioma are identified (see section on Pathology), the differential diagnosis must always include pleural metastases from an occult primary adenocarcinoma. Asbestos workers who smoke have a significantly higher-than-expected risk of lung cancer and perhaps head and neck malignancies as well.[48, 55] The risk of lung cancer appears to be synergic rather than merely additive. Compared with nonsmoking unexposed persons, nonsmoking asbestos workers have an increased risk of lung cancer of only one- to fivefold. However, asbestos workers who smoke have approximately a 90-fold increased risk[55] (Table 11–1). In asbestos workers, the lifetime risk of bronchogenic carcinoma (approximately 1 in 4) substantially exceeds that of mesothelioma (1 in 10). Although exposed persons should avoid smoking to decrease the substantial risk of bronchogenic cancer, the incidence of mesothelioma is similar in both smokers and nonsmokers.

PRESENTATION AND SUPPORTIVE CARE

Patients with malignant pleural mesothelioma first seek medical attention for dyspnea, chest pain, or both.[4–6] Most patients have a large unilateral pleural effusion on the chest x-ray film. (Bilateral involvement at presentation occurs in fewer than 5%.) Rarely, patients are asymptomatic, with effusion an incidental finding on routine chest x-ray film. A scoliosis with contracture of the ipsilateral hemithorax is a relatively late finding on the chest film, but decreased lung volume is frequently seen on computed tomography (CT) scan at presentation.[2, 21, 31, 38, 45] Fluid may become loculated or disappear with advancing disease.

Although pleural plaques or characteristic interstitial fibrosis are visible on the chest x-ray film in only 20% of cases, small pleural calcifications can be seen on CT scan in 50%.[31]

Diagnosis and Staging

Pleural fluid cytology or needle biopsy specimens will confirm the presence of a malignancy and may occasionally suggest mesothelioma; however, they frequently yield a misleading diagnosis of "metastatic adenocarcinoma."[7] Sputum cytology and bronchoscopy should be considered to rule out a bronchogenic adenocarcinoma in asbestos-exposed smokers since the risk of lung cancer in this group is two and a half times that of mesothelioma.[55] Open thoracotomy has been generally required to obtain adequate biopsy tissue for definitive diagnosis. However, the ability to diagnose mesothelioma from needle biopsy samples has improved somewhat with the use of supplemental methods, especially immunoperoxidase studies and electron microscopy. Because open biopsy may compromise any later attempt at surgical resection (due to tumor growth through the operative scar involving the intercostal space and the surrounding musculature), invasive diagnostic procedures should be undertaken at the institution where definitive surgery would be performed if indicated. To avoid diagnostic thoracotomy, investigational approaches include electron microscopy of tissue from needle biopsies or of cytocentrifuged specimens from pleural fluid.

Alternatively, an adequate sample for biopsy may be obtained under direct visualization via pleuroscopy.[10, 11]

The Butchart staging system[16] is simple and predicts survival with statistical significance[51] (Table 11–1). A CT scan to assess the extent of thoracic disease is indicated for staging or if treatment is contemplated.[31] Other radioisotopic scans are appropriate only if symptoms or laboratory values suggest metastases, since brain, bone, and abdominal involvement including liver metastases is uncommon at presentation. X-ray films and scans may be indicated, however, to rule out an occult primary adenocarcinoma in cases where the pathologic findings are less than definitive. The sites and extent of known tumor involvement may make a diagnosis of metastatic adenocarcinoma unlikely. Conversely, x-ray films and CT scans may identify an occult primary tumor, or may identify tumor in locations that are rarely involved by malignant mesothelioma. A markedly elevated serum carcinoembryonic antigen (CEA) suggests a diagnosis of adenocarcinoma.

GROSS PATHOLOGY

Discrete nodules of firm, grayish tumor stud the pleura early in the disease. Parietal and visceral surfaces subsequently become adherent, forming a thick rind. Tumor encases and constricts but only superficially invades the lung, frequently extending into major fissures. Invasion of the chest wall, pericardium, and diaphragm may occur early.[34, 42]

Lymphatic and hematogenous spread are usually late manifestations. At autopsy, thoracic regional lymph node metastases are present in up to 67% of cases.[36] Hematogenous metastases are found in 33% to 67%,[26, 36] chiefly to liver, lung, kidney, adrenal, and bone, and are often small and clinically unsuspected.

MICROSCOPIC PATHOLOGY

Malignant mesothelioma may be epithelial, sarcomatoid or mixed histologically.[34, 60] From 50% to 60% are epithelial, with a predominantly tubular, papillary, solid, or vacuolated pattern. Tumor cells of the sarcomatoid variant are ovoid to spindle-shaped, with cellularity and hyperchromatism similar to that of a fibrosarcoma. Both epithelial and sarcomatoid patterns are present in the mixed type. The percentage of mixed lesions appears to increase with the amount of tissue examined; extensive

sampling may be required to demonstrate the minor component.

Differential Diagnosis

Inflammatory or reactive processes and other malignant tumors may mimic mesothelioma.[34–36] The lack of cytologic atypia and hyperchromatism, and the absence of invasion should distinguish mesothelial hyperplasia resulting from underlying infection or inflammation of serosal membranes. Metastatic adenocarcinoma of the pleura may be extremely difficult to distinguish from the considerably rarer epithelial variant of mesothelioma. "Pseudomesothelioma," a small peripheral pulmonary adenocarcinoma with widely generalized pleural involvement, has been described.[32] Breast, ovarian, gastric, renal, or prostatic adenocarcinomas may metastasize to the pleura. Sarcomatoid mesothelioma must be distinguished from primary fibrosarcoma, malignant fibrous histiocytoma, malignant schwannoma, hemangiopericytoma, synovial sarcoma, and carcinosarcomas (which have a similar mixed histologic pattern but generally form a pulmonary parenchymal mass rather than involve the pleura).

Specimens obtained by open biopsy and by pleurectomy or pneumonectomy should be extensively sampled. A small piece of tissue should be processed in glutaraldehyde for electron microscopy, and a sample of uninvolved lung should be submitted for counting of asbestos fibers.[20, 53] (Asbestos counts, including those obtained at autopsy, have legal as well as diagnostic and epidemiologic value.)

Unless an unequivocal mixed pattern is pathognomonic of mesothelioma, we currently require characteristic findings in at least two of three supplemental methods—histochemical, immunoperoxidase, and electron microscopy—for a definitive diagnosis of mesothelioma.

Supportive Care

Shortness of breath and chest pain can initially be controlled by repeated thoracenteses and minor narcotics; however, pleural fluid eventually becomes loculated and difficult to drain or disappears as the tumor obliterates the pleural space.[26] Pleurodesis renders any subsequent surgical resection technically difficult and is frequently unsuccessful owing to rapid fluid accumulation.

A painful chest wall mass develops in more than 10% of patients[9, 26] growing through sites of repeated thoracentesis or chest tube drainage or thoracotomy scars. High doses of radiotherapy delivered to a small port encompassing a chest wall lesion may relieve pain; radiation therapy should be considered when such a mass is detected, because irradiating larger lesions is frequently ineffective.[30] We recommend evaluation of nonconventional fractionation such as hyperfractionation twice a day, or a large fraction once a day over a shorter total treatment duration, since the tumor is usually not radioresponsive.[30]

After a median survival of 6 to 14 months (ranging from a few weeks to 16 years), patients generally die of respiratory infections.[5, 6] Small bowel obstruction resulting from extension through an involved diaphragm develops in about one third. A few die of pericardial or myocardial involvement.[6] Direct extension to ribs, esophagus, venous structures, and vertebrae causes pain, dysphagia, vena cava syndromes, and rarely cord compression, respectively.

Physicians should be aware that *rare* patients with a well-differentiated variant of mesothelioma may survive for periods of years after diagnosis.[28, 29, 37, 46]

Daily fevers with no identified source of infection are common and poorly tolerated, accompanied by significant weight loss, poor performance, and early death. Disseminated intravascular coagulation, thromboses of extremities, thrombophlebitis, pulmonary emboli, and Coombs'-positive hemolytic anemia have been observed in up to one fifth of patients.[8]

THERAPY

Surgery

Although virtually all authors agree on the necessity of open thoracotomy for adequate biopsy of most pleural mesotheliomas, the efficacy of tumor excision remains disputed.

Surgeons advocate at least three different strategies in the management of patients with pleural mesothelioma:

1. **Supportive care alone after definitive biopsy**: Since reported cures with any treatment remain anecdotal, and prolonged survival from treatment is difficult to document, some physicians believe that any surgical procedure other than that required to establish accurately the diagnosis is contraindicated. We feel that all patients should be offered investigational therapy; no effective management will ever be identified by pursuing the option of supportive care only.

2. **Pleurectomy alone**: The Chest Surgery Group at Memorial Sloan-Kettering Cancer Center has advocated pleurectomy performed when feasible at the time of thoracotomy for diagnosis.[13, 43, 59] Pleurectomy ensures adequate tissue for diagnosis, retains maximum lung volume and pulmonary function, and eliminates recurrent pleural effusions. If histologic examination proves the lesion to be other than mesothelioma, the procedure is equally palliative. Although pleurectomy is time-consuming and technically demanding, operative mortality and morbidity are very low in experienced hands.

In 1974, Worn in Germany reported a series of 248 patients with malignant mesothelioma treated by either radical extrapleural pneumonectomy or merely pleurectomy.[61] The fact that 9% to 10% of patients survived for 5 years in both groups is frequently cited as evidence for the superiority of the less radical procedure. However, certain difficulties exist with this study. Neither the number of patients surviving disease-free nor the operative mortality was specified. It is also unclear whether the histology of the mesotheliomas was pathologically reviewed (particularly that of the long-term survivors).

3. **Radical extrapleural pneumonectomy**: This procedure, advocated by authors at institutions in Boston, England, and Chicago[15, 16, 23, 47] is most likely to remove the entire lesion. Because perioperative deaths occurred in 31% of their initially reported series, Butchart and colleagues recommended careful selection of surgical candidates.[15] Although this high mortality rate is frequently cited by noninterventionists, recent reports from institutions with a significant surgical experience with the disease have observed an operative mortality of less than 3%.

Either pleurectomy or pneumonectomy yields considerable palliation of chest pain and prevents recurrent pleural effusions.[41] Because it would be virtually impossible to do a randomized trial of resection versus medical therapy, and because selection biases are otherwise difficult to avoid, the impact of surgery on survival is difficult to evaluate.

Chemotherapy

Prior to the availability of CT scanning to assess disease extent,[2, 21, 31, 38, 45] chemotherapy was difficult to evaluate in mesothelioma.

Table 11–2. Clinical Studies of Effectiveness of Chemotherapeutic
Agents in Malignant Mesothelioma

Study[a]	No of Patients	Number of Patients Responding CR	PR	RR(%)	Dose (mg/m^2) Doxorubicin	Cyclophosphamide	Other
Review[1] (single agent)	36		16	44	Variable		
DFCI[51]	48	1	14	31	≥60	600	
MDA[24]	20	0	5	25	≥60	≥600	DTIC
Mt. Sinai[19]	36	3	5	22	75	Azacytidine	
	16	1	2	19	90	Radiotherapy	
ECOG[40]	66	2	5	11	45–70	DTIC	

[a]DFCI: Dana-Farber Cancer Institute, Boston, Mass; MDA: M. D. Anderson Hospital, Houston, Texas; Mt. Sinai Hospital, New York; ECOG: Eastern Cooperative Oncology Group.
CR: complete response; PR: partial response; RR: overall response (CR + PR).

Pleural and peritoneal effusions on chest x-ray film are neither evaluable nor measurable by classical criteria because their volume depends on many variables (e.g., hydration); moreover, effusions frequently disappear as the pleural space is obliterated by advancing disease. In addition, at any one institution, a given regimen was used in only a few patients.

Response rates with regimens containing doxorubicin (Adriamycin) have varied considerably (11–44%) in various studies.[1, 6, 8, 40] The use of doxorubicin combinations has been reported to prolong survival.[62] Observed differences may result from a steep dose-response curve for doxorubicin or from biases introduced by patient selection (Table 11–2).

Alkylating agents have response rates in the range of 20% to 30%. Other alkylating agents, such as 5-azacytidine, 5-fluorouracil, and methotrexate with rescue,[25] may also have significant activity.[1]

Although intravenous cisplatin initially appeared to lack single-agent activity in mesothelioma (response in only 3 of 31 patients in one review),[1] several recent studies have demonstrated synergism when cisplatin has been combined with a number of other chemotherapeutic agents in certain in vitro experimental systems and in clinical trials in other tumors. In a very small pilot study of a combination of doxorubicin and cisplatin, each given in a dose of 50 mg per square meter of body surface, four of six patients responded (one complete and three partial responses),[63] with response durations of 5 to 17 months. The observed response rate may be an effect of small numbers, or the addition of doxorubicin to cisplatin may be synergistic in mesothelioma. Dose may also be a factor; in another study, large doses of cisplatin delivered intraperitoneally resulted in objective responses in a few cases.[33]

The efficacy of most other chemotherapeutic agents remains largely unknown. A regimen of mitomycin (10 mg/m^2) and cisplatin (50 mg/m^2) given every 4 weeks was designed at Mt. Sinai Hospital in New York, based on the results of screening of many single agents in an experimental model of two human malignant mesotheliomas serially transplanted in nude mice.[17, 18] Preliminary results showed objective responses in 4 of 12 patients (one partial response in 5 previously treated patients and one complete and two partial responses among 7 previously untreated patients).[18]

Radiotherapy

Several radiotherapists have defined techniques intended to deliver high doses of radiotherapy to the pleura without compromising central lung function.[12, 30] These include the following:

1. Utilizing anterior to posterior (AP) and posterior to anterior (PA) ports with protection of the midportion of the lung by lead blocks. Electrons are then delivered to the previously blocked areas. Maximum electron penetration into normal lung tissue is determined by CT scan to include only the pleura.
2. Rotating a radiation source about the patient's chest to treat the peripheral lung, in combination with AP and PA mediastinal ports for the mediastinum.
3. Tangentially irradiating peripheral pleura in combination with AP and PA mediastinal ports.

If radiotherapy results in a de facto radiation pneumonectomy, or is complicated by radiation pneumonitis, surgical pneumonectomy may be preferred. (Six to 12 months after radiotherapy, when fibrosis ensues or tumor progresses, pulmonary arterial blood perfusing the involved lung will remain relatively hypoxic, whereas after surgical pneumonectomy, all pulmonary blood will be oxygenated in the contralateral normal lung.)

Palliation of pain by radiotherapy in our series at DFCI was complete or substantial in only 5 of 29 courses, moderately effective in 6, and inadequate in 18.[30] Adequate palliation strongly correlated with doses of 4000 rad or more over 4 weeks. In the series at the Memorial Sloan-Kettering Cancer Center, the median survival of patients receiving radiotherapy after surgery was 13 months, compared with 15 months for patients undergoing surgery alone.[13, 43, 59] However, patients with incompletely resectable disease received both modalities, whereas many patients with completely resected tumor were spared radiotherapy. Prolonged survival and diminished pain have been reported by French investigators after a median of 4500 rad delivered to the hemithorax.[27] The study group survived a median of 13 months, compared with 9.8 months for nonrandomized controls receiving conventional radiotherapy. Thus, of the three available treatment modalities, radiotherapy appears to offer the least in terms of either survival or palliation. This is believed to be due to the poor radioresponsiveness of the tumor in addition to the very large tumor volume. If treatment of the entire pleural surface by radiotherapy is attempted, normal tissue tolerance prevents delivery of an effective safe dose.

Combined Modality

An intensive combined modality approach is under investigation at a number of cancer centers in an effort to prolong survival and ultimately to increase the number of long-term disease-free survivors.[4, 12, 24] Patients able to tolerate intensive treatment are obviously selected to some extent. The actuarial survival from time of diagnosis for 23 patients (DFCI) treated with a combined modality protocol between 1978 and 1982 was 46% at 2.5 years, compared with 19% for the 23 patients treated on protocol with chemotherapy alone.[51] Of 20 patients entered into a study at the M. D. Anderson Hospital in Houston, Texas,[24] five patients who achieved a partial response to cyclophosphamide, doxorubicin, and dacarbazine (DTIC) underwent "surgical debulking." These patients survived for 59, 33+, 65+, 83+, and 104+ weeks, respectively. The median survival for nonresponders was 36 weeks.

Thus, the median survival of intensively treated patients appears longer than that of patients receiving supportive or palliative therapy or that of historical controls.[24, 51, 62]

The rate of long-term disease-free survival ("cure") is woefully small after surgery alone—however radical the procedure. This might have been anticipated by the diffuse nature of the pleural involvement. Clearly, the need at this time is to identify active drugs and then to compare combinations of such agents in randomized phase III trials in patients with advanced measurable disease. Finally, the most effective combination would be administered prior to or following optimal surgical resection.

Clearly, much work remains to be done in determining the optimal treatment of mesothelioma. Because this is not a common tumor, multi-institutional, multimodality cooperation becomes key in making a significant impact on this disease, which appears destined to increase in incidence.

References

1. Aisner J, Wiernik PH: Chemotherapy in the treatment of malignant mesothelioma. Semin Oncol 8:335–343, 1981.
2. Alexander E, Clark RA, Colley DP, et al: CT of malignant pleural mesothelioma. Am J Radiol 137:287–291, 1981.
3. Antman K, Cohn S, Green M: Malignant mesothelioma of the tunica vaginalis testis. J Clin Oncol 2:447–451, 1984.
4. Antman KH: Malignant mesothelioma. N Engl J Med 303:200–202, 1980.
5. Antman KH: Clinical presentation and natural history of benign and malignant mesothelioma. Semin Oncol 8:313–320, 1981.
6. Antman KH, Blum RH, Greenberger JS, et al: Multimodality therapy for malignant mesothelioma based on a study of natural history. Am J Med 68:356–362, 1980.
7. Antman KH, Corson JM, Li FP, et al: Malignant mesothelioma following radiation exposure. J Clin Oncol 1:695–700, 1983.
8. Antman KH, Pomfret EA, Aisner J, et al: Peritoneal mesothelioma: natural history and response to chemotherapy. J Clin Oncol 1:386–391, 1983.
9. Artvinli M, Baris YI: Malignant mesothelioma in a small village in the Anatolian region of Turkey: an epidemiologic study. J Natl Cancer Inst 63:17–22, 1979.
10. Boutin C, Farisse P, Choux R, et al: Intérêt de la pleuroscopie dans le diagnostic des mésothéliomes malins diffus. Revue française des Maladies respiratoires 4:972–974, 1976.
11. Boutin, C, Viallat JR, Cargnino P: La biopsie sous thoracoscopie dans le diagnostic des pleurésies. Le Concours Medical 23:4213–4218, 1979.
12. Brady LW: Mesothelioma—the role for radiation therapy. Semin Oncol. 8:329–334, 1981.
13. Brenner J, Sordillo PP, Magill GB, et al: Malignant

mesothelioma of the pleura: review of 123 patients. Cancer 49:2431–2435, 1982.

14. Brenner J, Sordillo PP, Magill GB, et al: Malignant peritoneal mesothelioma: review of 25 patients. Am J Gastroenterol 75:311–313, 1981.

15. Butchart EG, Ashcroft T, Barnsley WC, et al: The role of surgery in diffuse malignant mesothelioma of the pleura. Semin Oncol 8:321–328, 1981.

16. Butchart EG, Ashcroft T, Barnsley WC, et al: Pleuropneumonectomy in the management of diffuse malignant mesothelioma of the pleura: experience with 29 patients. Thorax 31:15–24, 1976.

17. Chahinian AP, Beranek JT, Suzuki Y, et al: Transplantation of human malignant mesothelioma into nude mice. Cancer Res 40:181–185, 1980.

18. Chahinian AP, Norton L, Szrajer L, et al: Mitomycin C and cisplatin in human malignant mesothelioma xenografts in nude mice: clinical correlation. Proc Am Assoc Cancer Res 24:151(597), 1983.

19. Chahinian AP, Pajak TF, Holland JF, et al: Diffuse malignant mesothelioma: prospective evaluation of 69 patients. Ann Intern Med 96:746–755, 1982.

20. Churg A: Fiber counting and analysis in the diagnosis of asbestos-related disease. Hum Pathol 13:381–392, 1982.

21. Cohen BA, Efremidis A, Chahinian AP, et al: Computed tomography of the chest in diffuse malignant pleural mesothelioma. Am Rev Resp Dis 123:131, 1981.

22. DeKlerk DP, Nime F: Adenomatoid tumors (mesothelioma) of testicular and paratesticular tissue. Urology VI:635–641, 1975.

23. DeLaria GA, Jensik R, Faber LP, et al: Surgical management of malignant mesothelioma. Ann Thorac Surg 26:375–382, 1978.

24. Dhingra H, Valdivieso M, Tannir N, et al: Combined modality treatment for mesothelioma with Cytoxan (CTX), Adriamycin (ADR), and DTIC (CYADIC) and adjuvant surgery. Proc Am Soc Clin Oncol 2:205(C-800), 1983.

25. Dimitrov NV, Egner J, Balcueva E, et al: High-dose methotrexate with citrovorum factor and vincristine in the treatment of malignant mesothelioma. Cancer 50:1245–1247, 1982.

26. Elmes PC, Simpson MJC: Insulation workers in Belfast. 3. Mortality 1940–66. Brit J Industr Med 28:226–236, 1971.

27. Eschwege F, Schlienger M: La radiothérapie des mésothéliomes pleuraux malins: A propos de 14 cas irradiés a doses élevées. J Radiol Electrol 54:255–259, 1973.

28. Fischbein A, Suzuki Y, Selikoff IJ, et al: Unexpected longevity of a patient with malignant pleural mesothelioma. Cancer 42:1999–2004, 1978.

29. Foyle A, Al-Jabi M, McCaughey WTE: Papillary peritoneal tumors in women. Am J Surg Pathol 5:241–249, 1981.

30. Gordon W, Antman KH, Greenberger JS, et al: Radiation therapy in the management of patients with mesothelioma. Int J Rad Oncol Biol Phys 8:19–25, 1982.

31. Grant DC, Seltzer SE, Antman KH, et al: Computed tomography of malignant pleural mesothelioma. J Comp Assist Tomog 7:626–632, 1983.

32. Harwood TR, Grecey DR, Yokoo H: Pseudomesotheliomatous carcinoma of the lung. A variant of peripheral lung carcinoma. Am J Clin Pathol 65:159–167, 1976.

33. Howell SB, Pfeifle CL, Wung WE, et al: Intraperitoneal cisplatin with systemic thiosulfate protection. Ann Intern Med 97:845–851, 1982.

34. Kannerstein M, Churg C, McCaughey WTE: Asbestos and mesothelioma: a review. Pathol Annu 13:81–130, 1978.

35. Kannerstein M, Churg J: Peritoneal mesothelioma. Hum Pathol 8:83–94, 1977.

36. Kannerstein M, McCaughey WTE, Churg J, et al: A critique of the criteria for the diagnosis of diffuse malignant mesothelioma. Mt Sinai J Med 44:485–494, 1977.

37. Katsube Y, Mukai K, Silverberg SG: Cystic mesothelioma of the peritoneum: a report of five cases and review of the literature. Cancer 50:1615–1622, 1982.

38. Kreel L: Computed tomography in mesothelioma. Semin Oncol 8:302–312, 1981.

39. Langer AM, Selikoff IJ, Sastre A: Chrysotile asbestos in the lungs of persons in New York City. Arch Environ Health 22:348–361, 1971.

40. Lerner H, Amato D, Shiraki M, et al: A prospective study of Adriamycin programs in malignant mesothelioma. Proc Am Soc Clin Oncol 2:230(C-901), 1983.

41. Martini N, Manjit SB, Beattie EJ: Indications for pleurectomy in malignant effusion. Cancer 35:734–738, 1975.

42. McCaughey WTE: Criteria for diagnosis of diffuse mesothelial tumors. Ann NY Acad Sci 132:603–613, 1965.

43. McCormack P, Nagasaki F, Hilaris BS, et al: Surgical treatment of pleural mesothelioma. J Thorac Cardiovasc Surg 84:834–842, 1982.

44. Meyniard O, Boissonnas A, Laisne MJ, et al: Pneumopathie chronique a l'huile de paraffine et modifications pleurales. Rev Fr Mal Resp 8:259–264, 1980.

45. Mirvis S, Dutcher JP, Haney PJ, et al: CT of malignant pleural mesothelioma. Am J Radiol 140:665–670, 1983.

46. Moore JH, Crum CP, Chandler JG, et al: Benign cystic mesothelioma. Cancer 45:2395–2399, 1980.

47. Nauta RJ, Osteen RT, Antman KH, et al: Clinical staging and the tendency of malignant pleural mesotheliomas to remain localized. Ann Thorac Surg 34:66–70, 1982.

48. Newhouse M: Epidemiology of asbestos-related tumors. Semin Oncol 8:250–257, 1981.

49. Peto J, Henderson BE, Pike MC: Trends in mesothelioma incidence in the United States and the forecast epidemic due to asbestos exposure during World War II. In Peto R, Schniderman M (eds): Quantification of Occupational Cancer. Banbury Report. Vol 9. New York, Cold Spring Harbor Laboratory, 1981, pp 51–69.

50. Peto J, Seidman H, Selikoff IJ: Mesothelioma mortality in asbestos workers: implications for models of carcinogenesis and risk assessment. Brit J Cancer 44:001–012, 1981.

51. Pomfret E, Antman K, Corson J, et al: Intensive treatment of patients (pts) with malignant mesothelioma (MM). Proc Am Assoc Cancer Res 24:156(619), 1984.

52. Robbins SL, Cotran RS: Pathologic Basis of Disease, 2d ed. Philadelphia, WB Saunders, 1979, p 144.

53. Roggli VL, McGavran MH, Subach J, et al: Pulmonary asbestos body counts and electron probe analysis of asbestos body cores in patients with mesothelioma. Cancer 50:2423–2432, 1982.

54. Russell WO, Cohen J, Enzinger F, et al: A clinical and pathological staging system for soft tissue sarcomas. Cancer 40:1562–1570, 1977.

55. Selikoff IJ: Cancer Risk of Asbestos Exposure. In Hiatt HH, Watson, JD, and Winsten, JA (eds.):

Origins of Human Cancer. New York, Cold Spring Harbor Laboratory, 1977, pp 1765–1784.

56. Stout AP, Lattes R: Tumors of the soft tissues. In Atlas of Tumor Pathology. Washington DC, Armed Forces Institute of Pathology, 1967, pp 176–177.
57. Suzuki Y: Malignant mesothelioma induced by asbestos and zeolite in the mouse peritoneum. Proc. Am Assoc Cancer Res 24:61(240), 1983.
58. Thomson JG, Kaschula ROC, MacDonald RR: Asbestos as a modern urban hazard. South Afr Med J 37:77–81, 1963.
59. Wanebo HJ, Martini N, Melamed MR, et al: Pleural mesothelioma. Cancer 38:2481–2488, 1976.
60. Winslow DJ, Taylor HB: Malignant peritoneal mesotheliomas. Cancer 13:127–136, 1960.
61. Worn H: Moglichkeiten und Ergebnisse der chirurgischen Behandlung des malignen Pleuramesothelioms. Thoraxchirurgie 22:391–393, 1974.
62. Yap B, Benjamin RS, Burgess A, et al: The value of Adriamycin in the treatment of diffuse malignant pleural mesothelioma. Cancer 42:1692–1696, 1978.
63. Zidar B, Pugh R, Schiffer L, et al: Treatment of six cases of mesothelioma with doxorubicin and cisplatinum. Proc Am Soc Clin Oncol 2:225(C-880), 1983.

12

Malignant Pleural Mesothelioma: Operative Treatment by Pleurectomy

Patricia M. McCormack, M.D.
Nael Martini, M.D.

According to American Cancer Society statistics, 2000 new cases of malignant mesothelioma were diagnosed in 1982. This ranks it far below the leading cancer killer—lung cancer. However, malignant mesothelioma is gaining prominence because of its link etiologically to industrial carcinogens, mainly asbestos. Plumbers, welders, painters, naval yard workers, and asbestos factory workers carry an increased risk of developing this cancer. Selikoff and others[1-4] have also proved that family members who have been exposed to the asbestos fibers carried home on clothing have a 300-fold increased risk of developing mesothelioma.

A two- to three-decade lag period between exposure and onset of disease means that the peak incidence of this disease is just now approaching. Since cures of this malignancy are anecdotal, treatment is challenging.

HISTOLOGY AND DIAGNOSIS

Histologically, malignant mesotheliomas present as two separate entities. **Fibrosarcomatous** mesotheliomas are like soft tissue sarcomas elsewhere in the body. They grow as masses and invade contiguous structures. If the tumor is localized, complete surgical excision is usually possible[5, 6] (Fig. 12–1). **Epithelial** mesotheliomas are more common and

more lethal.[7] These tumors grow in sheets involving the parietal pleura first and then the visceral pleura. Continued growth patterns are outward into chest wall and inward into lung parenchyma. More diffuse tumors are those with direct extension into major structures such as vena cava, diaphragm, heart, or esophagus, or with extension beyond the hemithorax.

From 1939 to 1981, 149 patients received treatment for malignant mesothelioma at the Memorial Sloan-Kettering Cancer Center. Of these, 47 had fibrosarcomatous tumors. Results of surgical excision of all tumor and contiguous tissues have been published.[8, 9] Pleura is resected in these tumors where direct invasion exists; a pleurectomy per se, however, is not indicated.

The remaining 102 patients had epithelial mesotheliomas involving most of the parietal or visceral pleura, or both, within one hemithorax. The youngest of these patients was 13 years of age, the oldest 79. The male-to-female ratio was 3.5:1.

In 89% of the patients, major symptoms initiated the diagnostic chest x-ray film (Table 12–1. The presence of pleural effusion is generally characteristic of epithelial mesothelioma[10, 11] (Fig. 12–2). Chest pain, usually pleuritic in nature, is unique in that in most other diseases affecting the parietal pleura, effusion developing a space between the pleural layers

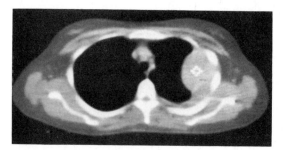

Figure 12–1. CT scan showing localized fibrosarcomatous mesothelioma.

Table 12–1. Major Symptoms of Malignant Epithelial Mesothelioma

Symptoms	No. of Patients
Dyspnea	61
Pain	54
Weight loss	38
Cough	33
Other	29
Total	91

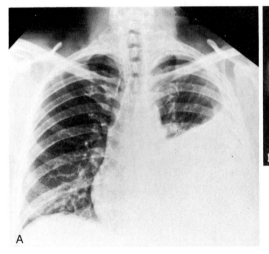

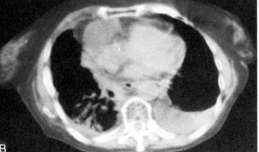

Figure 12–2. Pleural effusion on chest x-ray film *(A)* and CT scan *(B)*.

usually effects pain relief. This does not happen with malignant mesothelioma. The tumor invades directly into chest wall tissues, and the pain increases in intensity (Fig. 12–3).

Diagnosis of malignant epithelial mesothelioma can be very difficult (Table 12–2). Differentiation from metastatic adenocarcinoma to pleura is paramount. Adenocarcinomas of the lung and bronchoalveolar carcinomas are frequently mistaken for mesotheliomas on cytologic specimen alone.[12] Bronchoscopy is needed in every case to rule out endobronchial pathology. We have never obtained a diagnosis of malignant mesothelioma from a bronchial biopsy or aspirate.

The diagnosis of malignant epithelial mesothelioma carries such a grave prognostic implication that an unequivocal tissue diagnosis is mandatory. In most cases, an open pleural biopsy is necessary.

TREATMENT

Since no single method of treatment has yielded success in this group of patients, we have tried various combinations of the three basic modalities over the years. Prior to 1977, the median survival in our clinical experience was 14 months.[9]

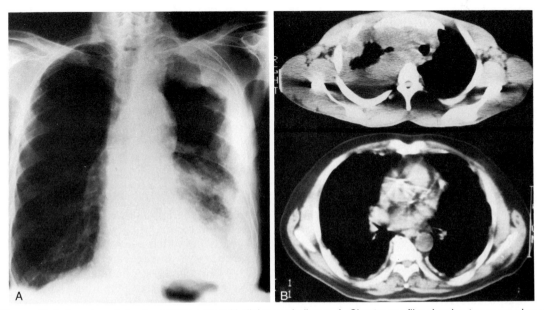

Figure 12–3. Invasion of chest wall tissue by epithelial mesothelioma. *A,* Chest x-ray film showing tumor growing as infiltrating pleural masses. *B,* CT scan illustrating tissue invasion by tumor in early *(top)* and late *(bottom)* stages.

In 1977 we began a new protocol, combining surgery, radiation therapy, and chemotherapy. Surgical exploration is done to establish a definitive tissue diagnosis and determine the extent of the intrathoracic spread of disease. A parietal pleurectomy is then carried out as completely as possible, including the pericardium if necessary.

In three areas it is especially difficult to strip the parietal pleura: superior mediastinum, pericardium, and diaphragm. Because of this, these areas show the most frequent tumor recurrence. In our patients, therefore, they receive special attention at the time of operation. Internal radiation therapy is then delivered by the most appropriate methods. Radioactive iodine-125 sources are placed in bulky nonresectable tumor masses. In areas of residual microscopic tumor rather than bulky disease, special Silastic catheters (4 mm × 15 cm) are secured about 2 cm apart and brought through and anchored to the skin. On about the third postoperative day, radioactive iridium-192 sources are inserted through the catheters into the predetermined area. Iridium sources and catheters are removed 3 to 4 days later.

Phosphorus-32 is instilled into the pleural cavity via a 14-gauge catheter placed intraoperatively. This is delayed until all other tube sites are healed following removal of tubes to prevent contamination from leakage.

These three forms of internal radiation therapy do not prolong hospitalization, and the discharge is routinely between the seventh and tenth postoperative day.

In our patients, external radiation therapy is given 4 to 6 weeks postoperatively. The lung is shielded, and both superficial electron beam and deep photon irradiation are used.

Upon completion of the radiation treatment, the patients are placed on systemic chemotherapy.[13-15]

RESULTS

From 1977 to 1981, 33 patients with malignant epithelial mesothelioma have been treated using this new protocol. Ages ranged from 34 to 74 years, with a median of 58. Of the 33 patients, 28 were men and 5 were women. Eight patients gave no history of exposure to asbestos or cigarette smoking prior to their illness. The remaining 25 patients were exposed to both.

All patients were symptomatic. Dyspnea, pain, and cough occurred in two thirds in

Table 12–2. Results of Diagnostic Studies in 33 Patients with Malignant Epithelial Mesothelioma

Study	Findings		
	Negative	Cancer	Meso-thelioma
Pleural fluid cytology	19	5	0
Closed pleural biopsy	9	1	5
Open biopsy	0	0	28

varying combinations. Rarer symptoms included fever, dysphagia, hemoptysis, and anorexia.

All chest x-ray films were abnormal. Findings were pleural effusion or pleural thickening in 22 patients, effusion as well as a mass in 10, and mass alone in 1.

Since a positive diagnosis is essential to treatment, multiple diagnostic tests were performed. According to our experience, open pleural biopsy is usually necessary; this is followed immediately by pleurectomy if mesothelioma is confirmed in those cases presenting with localized disease and negative findings on bronchoscopy.

Malignant epithelial mesotheliomas fall into two subgroups at the time of clinical presentation: Localized tumors are those whose limited extent permits resection of all gross disease. Advanced tumors have already invaded major structures such as diaphragm, esophagus or vena cava or are already metastatic beyond the hemithorax.

There were no operative deaths in this group of patients. Postoperative complications occurred in four patients: In one patient, a ruptured bleb required operative closure; two patients had subcutaneous emphysema; and in the fourth, prolonged chest tube drainage was necessary.

In our series, 20 patients died of their disease at 5 to 28 months after treatment, for a median survival of 21 months. Thirteen patients are still alive from 10 to 53 months after treatment.

Recommendations for treatment of this disease vary widely. Reputable medical centers in the United States have advocated the following: no treatment, chemotherapy alone, radiation therapy alone, or an extrapleural pneumonectomy.[16-21]

We believe that a combination of all effective methods is necessary. We have not observed benefit from pneumonectomy and now take pains to preserve the lung.[22]

Survival rates justify our recommended approach for now, but a true cure for this disease must still be sought.

References

1. Selikoff IJ, Hammond EC, Churg J: Asbestos exposure, smoking and neoplasia. JAMA 204:106–112, 1968.
2. Selikoff IJ, Churg J, Hammond EC: Relation between exposure to asbestos and mesothelioma. N Engl J Med 272:560–565, 1965.
3. Whitwell F, Rawcliffe RM: Diffuse malignant pleural mesothelioma and asbestos exposure. Thorax 26:6–22, 1971.
4. Legha SS, Muggia FM: Pleural mesothelioma. Clinical features and therapeutic implications. Ann Intern Med 87:613–621, 1977.
5. McDonald AD, McDonald JC: Malignant mesothelioma in North America. Cancer 46:1650–1656, 1980.
6. McCormack P, Bains MS, Beattie EJ Jr, Martini N: New trends in skeletal reconstruction after resection of chest wall tumors. Ann Thorac Surg 31:45–52, 1981.
7. Oels HC, Harrison EG, Carr DT, Bernatz PE: Diffuse malignant mesothelioma of the pleura. A review of 37 cases. Chest 60:564–579, 1971.
8. Ratzer ER, Pool JL, Melamed MR: Pleural mesothelioma. Clinical experiences with thirty-seven patients. Am J Radiol 99:863–880, 1967.
9. Wanebo HJ, Martini N, Melamed MR, et al: Pleural mesotheliomas. Cancer 38:2481–2488, 1976.
10. Taryle DA, Lakshminarayan S, Sahn SA: Pleural mesotheliomas. An analysis of 18 cases and review of the literature. Medicine 55:153–162, 1976.
11. Shearin JC, Jackson D: Malignant pleural mesothelioma. Report of 19 cases. J Thorac Cardiovasc Surg 71:621–627, 1976.
12. Roberts GH, Campbell GM: Exfoliative cytology of diffuse mesothelioma. J Clin Pathol 25:577–582, 1972.
13. Yap BS, Benjamin RS, Burgess MA, Bodey GP: The value of Adriamycin in the treatment of diffuse malignant pleural mesothelioma. Cancer 42:1692–1696, 1978.
14. Antman KH: Malignant mesothelioma. N Engl J Med 303:200–202, 1980.
15. Aisner J, Wiernik PH: Malignant mesothelioma. Current status and future prospects. Chest 74:438–444, 1978.
16. Shabanah FH, Sayegh SF: Solitary (localized) pleural mesothelioma. Report of two cases and review of the literature. Chest 60:558–563, 1971.
17. Chahinian AP, Suzuki Y, Mandel EM, Holland JF: Diffuse pulmonary malignant mesothelioma. Response to doxorubicin and 5-azacytidine. Cancer 42:1687–1691, 1978.
18. Butchart EG, Ashcroft T, Barnsley WC, Holden MP: Pleuropneumonectomy in the management of diffuse malignant mesothelioma of the pleura. Experience with 29 patients. Thorax 31:15–24, 1976.
19. DeLaria GA, Jensik RA, Faber LP, Kittle CF: Surgical management of malignant mesothelioma. Ann Thorac Surg 26:375–382, 1978.
20. Antman, KH, Blum RH, Greenberger JS, et al: Multimodality therapy for malignant mesothelioma based on a study of natural history. Am J Med 68:356–362, 1980.
21. Legha SS, Muggia FM: Therapeutic approaches in malignant mesothelioma. Cancer Treat Rev 4:13–23, 1977.
22. Martini N, Bains MS, Beattie EJ Jr: Indications for pleurectomy in malignant effusion. Cancer 35:734–738. 1975.

13

Malignant Pleural Mesothelioma: Operative Treatment by Extrapleural Pneumonectomy

L. Penfield Faber, M.D.

Malignant mesothelioma is a tumor characterized by relentless growth causing compression of the mediastinum with severe pain, pulmonary compromise, and, ultimately, death. Control of pain usually requires increasing amounts of narcotics, and the invariably terminal course of the disease is difficult for all.

Various forms of therapy have been recommended for this malignancy, but none has been successful in terms of cure.[1] Radiotherapy and chemotherapy have been only minimally effective in lengthening the time of survival. The surgical forms of treatment have offered some palliative benefit; these include pleurectomy and extrapleural pneumonectomy, usually with adjunctive chemotherapy and irradiation. Nevertheless, the use of any of these forms of therapy remains controversial. The aggressive nature of the tumor has led some clinicians to recommend supportive measures alone.[7]

Malignant mesothelioma frequently starts in the dependent portion of the thoracic cavity. Because of their proximity, the diaphragm and the pericardium are commonly deeply invaded by tumor. In the early stages of disease, however, the tumor is localized to the ipsilateral thoracic cavity and can be approached surgically. *Pleurectomy* involves removal of the parietal pleura in conjunction with the pericardium if tumor has spread to that structure, but invasion of the lung, when present, makes it difficult to separate tumor and pleura from the pulmonary parenchyma. No attempt is made to remove tumor invading the diaphragm and the mediastinum or to dissect tumor adherent to the surface of the lung. Consequently, pleurectomy leaves a significant amount of residual tumor, which is then treated with internal and external irradiation and chemotherapy.

It is impossible to strip tumor or pleura from the diaphragmatic surface; therefore, removal of the diaphragm along with the tumor mass seems appropriate. *Extrapleural pneumonectomy* is a radical procedure that entails removal en bloc of the parietal pleura, lung, pericardium, and diaphragm (Fig. 13–1). Minimal, if any, residual tumor remains following this procedure. Extrapleural pneumonectomy has been demonstrated to offer significant palliation and occasional long-term survival and therefore is worth considering in properly selected patients.

STAGING

Butchart and colleagues have recommended a simplified staging system that is used to identify surgical candidates[5] (Table 13–1). In general, Stage I patients are considered for resection, but positive mediastinal lymph nodes do not contraindicate extrapleural pneumonectomy.

The three histologic types of malignant mesothelioma are epithelial, fibrosarcomatous, and mixed. The epithelial type has been reported to carry a more favorable prognosis when surgical therapy is carried out, but in most series, histologic type has not been used as an indication for or contraindication to extrapleural pneumonectomy. Histologic differentiation of malignant mesothelioma from metastatic adenocarcinoma is difficult, so a

Table 13–1. Pathologic Staging of Diffuse Malignant Mesothelioma of the Pleura[5]

Stage	Degree of Involvement
I	Tumor confined within capsule of parietal pleura, i.e., involving only ipsilateral pleura, lung, pericardium, and diaphragm
II	Tumor invading chest wall or involving mediastinal structures, e.g., esophagus, heart; lymph node involvement inside chest
III	Tumor penetrating diaphragm to involve peritoneum; involvement of opposite pleura; lymph node involvement outside chest
IV	Distant blood-borne metastases

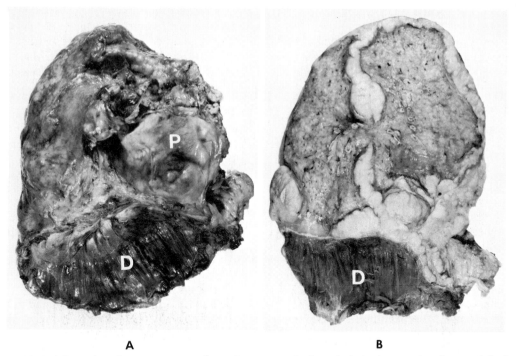

A   **B**

Figure 13–1. *A,* Extrapleural pneumonectomy for malignant mesothelioma includes lung, pericardium, and diaphragm. *B,* The mesothelioma invades the major fissure and diaphragm.

careful evaluation for a primary carcinoma elsewhere is always warranted when the diagnosis of malignant mesothelioma is considered.

Computed tomography (CT) is the best radiologic technique for staging the extent of the tumor. CT scans should include the chest and abdomen in order to evaluate the opposite pleura, mediastinum, and peritoneum (Fig. 13–2A). If invasion of the heart, esophagus, or abdominal organs is suspected, further selective studies are indicated. Routine radionuclide scans of the bones and brain are not warranted because the mesothelioma patient rarely presents with distant metastases. Mediastinoscopy is not used as a staging procedure; any involved lymph nodes can be removed with the lung, and such involvement does not contraindicate surgery.

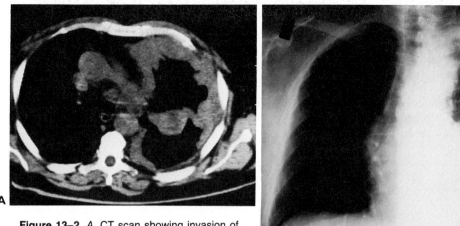

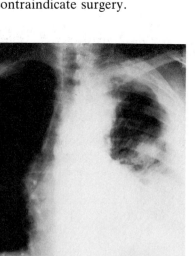

Figure 13–2. *A,* CT scan showing invasion of the major fissure. *B,* Typical chest x-ray appearance of a malignant mesothelioma. Note the decreased size of the involved thorax.

DIAGNOSIS

The most frequent symptoms associated with malignant mesothelioma are cough, chest pain, and weight loss. Although exposure to asbestos fibers has long been reported to be an etiologic factor in the development of malignant mesothelioma, approximately 30% of patients do not recall an instance of possible exposure.

Any physician who treats chest disease should be familiar with the radiologic appearance of malignant mesothelioma (Fig. 13–2B). The diaphragm is obliterated, the pleura is thickened, and the irregular, rounded tumor is easily identified. Despite the large amount of tumor and fluid present in the chest cavity, the involved thorax is diminished in size when compared with the opposite side. If the patient has a history of asbestos exposure, the diagnosis can be made from interpretation of the x-ray film. A proper diagnosis is essential so that unnecessary thoracentesis, needle biopsies, and diagnostic studies can be avoided.

Cytologic examination of the pleural fluid and needle biopsy specimens of the pleura generally does not establish the correct histologic diagnosis. Although malignant cells may be identified, there is not enough material in such small specimens to allow determination of cell type. The correct diagnosis usually requires an open pleural biopsy, accomplished at either thoracoscopy or thoracotomy. However, all these procedures run the risk of seeding of the biopsy site with tumor.[8] If nonsurgical therapy is contemplated, thoracoscopy is recommended for the biopsy procedure.[7] If the patient is a candidate for surgery, the diagnosis should be made at the time of one-stage biopsy and resection, thereby avoiding a second procedure with the attendant operative risk and minimizing the chance of biopsy site seeding. Many patients evaluated for resection at 2 to 3 months after biopsy have been found to have tumor growing in the biopsy site.[8]

The pathologist must be alerted to the possibility of mesothelioma because, as noted, it is frequently difficult to differentiate this tumor · from adenocarcinoma. Proper correlation of the gross appearance of the tumor with its frozen-section histologic characteristics then permits selection of the definitive surgical procedure.

INDICATIONS FOR EXTRAPLEURAL PNEUMONECTOMY

Extrapleural pneumonectomy is recommended only in patients in good general condition who do not have major systemic disease and who are able to withstand the physiologic insult associated with radical resection. Age is only a relative contraindication, but patients over the age of 65 years are generally not suitable candidates. Pulmonary function should be adequate to tolerate pneumonectomy. Clinically, the involved lung has little function, and quantitative ventilation-perfusion lung scans usually identify a significant deficit.

Extrapleural pneumonectomy should be reserved for Stage I patients in whom the tumor is localized to one side of the chest. However, positive mediastinal nodes do not contraindicate resection. If the tumor is growing through the chest wall at a previous open biopsy site, the extrapleural plane is usually obliterated; in such cases, the procedure is technically difficult and therapeutically unrewarding.

Butchart and colleagues recommend that a pure epithelial type of tumor is "more deserving of a radical surgical approach."[5] However, histology is generally not used as a criterion for extrapleural pneumonectomy.

The patient and family must be aware of the risks of the procedure and understand that an aggressive attempt at palliation is being attempted and that cure or long-term survival is unlikely.

OPERATIVE TECHNIQUE

Extrapleural pneumonectomy is best accomplished by posterolateral thoracotomy through the sixth intercostal space. If the diagnosis has not been previously established, initially a small incision is made to obtain an appropriate piece of pleura for biopsy. The surgeon must also plan for additional exposure if necessary in order to resect the diaphragm. With retraction of the chest wall muscles inferiorly, this can be accomplished through a second intercostal incision between the ninth and tenth rib. The use of a thoracoabdominal incision through the sixth intercostal space provides excellent exposure for diaphragmatic resection and extrapleural pneumonectomy.

Dissection is started in the extrapleural plane and is carried as far as possible. Bleeding may be persistent until the lung has been removed, and transfusion is frequently necessary. Because the large bulk of the tumor limits lung mobility, exposure of the hilum in the usual manner is difficult. In order to maximize hilar exposure, one-lung anesthesia using a long single-lumen tube or a double-lumen endotracheal tube, with deflation of the operated lung, can be employed.

It is frequently necessary to approach the bronchus and pulmonary artery posteriorly. Once the pleura has been removed from the vertebral bodies and aorta, the hilar structures are mobilized. It may be necessary to transect the bronchus first; stapling techniques are helpful in this regard. The pulmonary artery can also be approached posteriorly and then stapled or ligated as desired. The pericardium can be entered anteriorly or posteriorly and is resected from the surrounding chest wall and inferior pericardium.

On the left side, care must be taken to avoid injury to the vagus and recurrent laryngeal nerves, but tumor invasion may preclude their preservation. If the esophagus is involved by tumor, the lateral muscle wall must be carefully freed. A prosthetic patch is used to reconstruct the diaphragm. The patch must be water-tight to prevent passage of fluid from the pleural space into the peritoneal cavity, and it must be stable enough to retain the abdominal organs in the peritoneal cavity. Dacron velour meets these criteria and is available in sizes large enough to replace the resected diaphragm. The diaphragm is also replaced by a prosthetic patch on the right side, despite the presence of the liver.

When the pericardium is resected on the right side, the defect must be closed with a prosthetic patch. If the defect is not repaired, the heart will herniate to the right side, creating torsion of the superior and inferior vena cavae, with a resultant significant decrease in cardiac output. Pericardial reconstruction is not necessary on the left side because the heart cannot herniate if the *entire* pericardium has been removed, and it will continue to function quite well.

A chest tube is left in the pleural cavity to help position the mediastinum after surgery and to provide drainage if postoperative bleeding is a problem. The tube remains clamped unless drainage becomes necessary and is removed at 4 or 5 days postoperatively.

RESULTS

Worn in Germany has had the best results with extrapleural pneumonectomy for malignant mesothelioma.[10] In his series, the 2-year survival rate was 37%, and the 5-year survival, 10%. No details concerning pathologic stage or histologic type are presented in his report. In a similar group of patients with mesothelioma treated symptomatically, only 12.5% were alive at 1 year, and none were alive at 2 years.

Butchart and coworkers have reported a 10% 2-year survival and a 3.5% 5-year survival in 29 patients following pleural pneumonectomy.[4] Results were best in Stage I patients with the pure epithelial histologic type. However, in this series, the operative mortality was 31%, and the complication rate was a significant 43%. These figures indicate the need for both meticulous postoperative care and stringent criteria for patient selection in order to obtain optimal results. Butchart's group concluded that this operative procedure is appropriate in patients less than 60 years of age without major systemic disease, whose tumors are of the epithelial type.

Bamler and Maassen have reported a 35% 2-year survival rate for their group of 17 patients.[3] The operative mortality in this series was 23%.

In our current series of 32 patients (25 males and 7 females), there were three operative deaths for a mortality of 9.4%. Of the 32 procedures, 17 were performed on the left side and 15 on the right. Although a careful history regarding asbestos exposure was obtained in each case, only 16 patients (50%) could recall contact with asbestos. Pathologic study revealed that 21 tumors were epithelial, 9 were of the mixed type, and 2 were sarcomatous.

The procedure afforded good palliation in eight patients (25%). Good palliation was defined as survival for 24 months or longer, with a return to fairly normal activities. Five patients survived for at least 36 months, and one patient expired at 82 months postoperatively from recurrent disease. Another patient remained free of disease at 39 months following surgery. The 3-year survival was 15%, and the median survival time for the entire group was 13.25 months.

Serious complications occurred in eight patients (25%). One patient had a persistent recurrent right pleural effusion following left extrapleural pneumonectomy that required right pleurectomy 3 weeks after the initial procedure. Cause of the persistent effusion was not determined, but extensive mediastinal dissection was required at the time of the original operation. This patient expired 6 months after the first operation. Two other patients developed a bronchopleural fistula and empyema, which were managed successfully by open drainage; although there were no other complications specifically involving the prosthetic patches in these cases, the patches obviously remained a nidus for infection. Left vocal cord paralysis occurred in two patients as a result of resection of the vagus nerve but was satisfactorily managed by Teflon injection of the vocal cord. In another patient, a chylothorax developed after a right extra-pleural pneumonectomy; this problem required reoperation for thoracic duct ligation. Retention of secretions requiring tracheostomy and refractory cardiac arrhythmia were the remaining two complications. One other patient developed ascites from the pleural space as a result of reconstruction of the diaphragm with unreinforced Marlex; however, the ascites eventually resolved spontaneously.

The majority of patients received postoperative adjunctive therapy, which consisted of adriamycin alone or in combination with other agents and radiation therapy to any area of gross residual disease. Radiation therapy was also given at the first sign of local recurrence. As there has been no prospective study to evaluate surgery alone, it is difficult to determine whether adjunctive therapy has been of significant benefit. However, we continue to use such measures following extrapleural pneumonectomy.[6]

CONCLUSIONS

Difficulties encountered with the surgical management of malignant mesothelioma include local recurrence in the incision, a sometimes shortened life span, and the morbidity and mortality associated with the operation. Radiation therapy or chemotherapy alone has had minimal effect on the course of the disease, but neither has the associated mortality of extrapleural pneumonectomy.[2] However, extrapleural pneumonectomy can offer significant palliation in selected patients and occasionally can provide long-term survival.[6]

Currently we manage our patients with malignant mesothelioma in the following manner. When the tumor is suspected on clinical and radiologic evaluations, proper staging is accomplished by means of CT scans of the chest and abdomen and further evaluation for metastases if symptoms warrant. Stage I patients are considered to be surgical candidates, and in our practice the histologic type of tumor is not a criterion for selection of patients. A one-stage biopsy and resection operation is accomplished following all necessary preparations for pleurectomy or extrapleural pneumonectomy; upon cytologic confirmation of the diagnosis of malignant mesothelioma, either pleurectomy or extrapleural pneumonectomy, as indicated, is accomplished.

If the tumor is not adherent to the lung, then complete parietal pleurectomy is done. As much tumor as possible is removed from the diaphragm, and the pericardium is excised

if necessary. This procedure carries less morbidity and mortality than reported for extrapleural pneumonectomy, and Wanebo and colleagues have shown a 21-month mean survival with pleurectomy alone.[9]

Frequently, however, the tumor mass has invaded the lung parenchyma, and a large tumor is identified on the CT scan. In such cases, parietal pleurectomy is not technically feasible, and extrapleural pneumonectomy is the procedure of choice. With proper technique, morbidity and mortality are within acceptable limits, and little residual disease remains. Palliation is achieved in 25% of patients, and there is an occasional long-term survivor. Adjunctive therapy consisting of irradiation or chemotherapy may further extend the length of survival.

Malignant mesothelioma compresses the involved lung, pushes the mediastinum to the opposite side, and restricts function of the contralateral lung. Extrapleural pneumonectomy can alleviate the symptoms and physiologic abnormalities caused by this tumor with a small operative risk, even though prospects of cure are small.

References

1. Aisner J, Wiernik PH: Malignant mesothelioma—current status and future prospects. Chest 74:4, 1978.
2. Antman KH, Blum RH, Greenerger JS, et al: Multimodality therapy for malignant mesothelioma based on a study of natural history. Am J Med 68:156–162, 1980.
3. Bamler KJ, Maassen W: Uber die Verteilung der benignen und malignen Pleuratumoren in Krankengut einer lungenchirurgischen Klinik mit besonderer Berukichtigung des malignen Pleuramesothelioms und seiner radikalen Behandlung einschliesslich der ergebnisse des Zwerchfellersatzes mit konservieter Dura Mater. Thoraxchirurgie 22:386–391, 1974.
4. Butchart EG, Ashcroft A, Barnsley WC, et al: Pleuropneumonectomy in the management of diffuse malignant mesothelioma of the pleura. Thorax 31:15, 1976.
5. Butchart EG, Ashcroft T, Barnsley WC, Holden MP: The role of surgery in diffuse malignant mesothelioma of the pleura. Semin Oncol 8:321–328, 1981.
6. DeLaria GA, Jensik RJ, Faber LP, Kittle CF: Surgical management of malignant mesothelioma. Ann Thorac Surg 36:4, 1978.
7. Lewis RJ, Sisler GE, MacKenzie JW: Diffuse, mixed malignant pleural mesothelioma. Ann Thorac Surg 31:53–60, 1981.
8. Shearin JC Jr, Jackson D: Malignant pleural mesothelioma: Report of 19 cases. J Thorac Cardiovasc Surg 71:621–627, 1976.
9. Wanebo HJ, Martini N, Melamed MR, et al: Pleural mesothelioma. Cancer 38:2481, 1976.
10. Worn H: Moglichkeiten und Ergebnisse der chirurgischen Behandlung des malignen Pleuramesothelioms. Thoraxchirurgie 22:391–393, 1974.

IV

Needle Biopsy for the Diagnosis of Intrathoracic Lesions

Attention to needle biopsy began in Berlin at the November 1882 meeting of the Society of Internal Medicine. Only ten days previously, Leyden (1883) told the audience he had used this procedure to obtain tissue and identify organisms from the lung of a patient with pneumonia. His claim was short-lived, however, because the first discussant, Günther, rose to state that he had done the same thing, but six months earlier! A few years later (1886), Ménétrier described a patient in whom he had diagnosed a primary bronchogenic carcinoma by needle biopsy. These reports deserve a good deal of credit because they were done prior to the invention of x-rays (1895).

Needle aspiration was then used in the diagnosis of infectious disease problems. Widespread interest in this technique was aroused by Greig and Gray (1904), who demonstrated by needle aspiration that enlarged lymphatic glands in patients with sleeping sickness contained trypanosomes, not streptococci, as had previously been claimed. It was also possible to identify spirochetes by lymph gland aspiration (White and Pröscher, 1907).

The early reports of lung needle aspiration, although enthusiastic about obtaining specimens, were soon dimmed by accounts of complications and even death from hemorrhage, usually when large trocars were used in an attempt to secure more tissue.

In 1914 Ward conjectured that the examination of cells obtained by needle aspiration might aid in the diagnosis of various lymphomas; this was re-enforced by the investigations of Guthrie (1921). He was able to diagnose Hodgkin's disease, leukemia, metastatic tumor, and various types of adenitis. Similar findings in lymph nodes were obtained by Forkner (1927) using a small dental broach inserted through a 17- or 18-gauge needle.

Needle puncture and aspiration became established with the report of Martin and Ellis (1930) in their series of 65 patients, two of whom had carcinoma of the lung. These authors showed the reliability and safety of this technique and advised that "The indications for biopsy by needle puncture and aspiration are tumor masses which lie below the surface of normal tissue where surgical exposure is deemed contraindicated for any reason." Their article demonstrated the value of this procedure for neoplastic diseases and popularized *aspiration biopsy*. In 1936 Sappington and Favorite collected more than 2,000 instances in which needle aspiration for bacteriologic sampling had been done.

Craver and Binkley (1938) reviewed aspiration biopsy of the lung, particularly in 92 patients with bronchogenic carcinoma. They stated: "Aspiration biopsy is used as a method of choice in that group of cases in which the roentgenographic evidence indicates that the tumor is not accessible by bronchoscopy," thus stressing its value and low morbidity.

Despite these favorable reports and technical improvements, many surgeons did not endorse this method, fearing the risks of tumor cell implantation, tumor cell spread into the bloodstream, air embolism, or life-threatening pneumothorax.

Recently needle biopsy through the rigid bronchoscope (Versteegh and Swierenga, 1963) and through the flexible scope (Kato et al., 1978) has been developed to biopsy extrabronchial tumors or tracheobronchial lymph nodes.

The questions of diagnostic reliability and procedural safety are answered, but the question of when the procedure should be used still remains.

85

14

Needle Biopsy for the Diagnosis of Intrathoracic Lesions: Transthoracic Needle Biopsy

Willard A. Fry, M.D.

Transthoracic needle biopsy of focal pulmonary lesions by fine-needle aspiration has finally gained acceptance by the thoracic surgical community in the United States, long after its acceptance in other countries.[1] Its accuracy in tumor diagnosis is in the range of 80% to 90%, and it has become recognized as the single most accurate diagnostic procedure for detection of peripheral lung lesions short of thoracotomy. Nevertheless, there are still many areas of controversy concerning transthoracic needle biopsy, ranging from nomenclature to indications.

The concept of needle aspiration biopsy of lung lesions dates over 50 years from the early reports by Hayes Martin at Memorial Hospital in New York.[2] The basic concept remains that of procurement of a specimen by needle aspiration, which is smeared on a slide, stained, and interpreted by a cytopathologist. Other terms for the procedure include *aspiration lung biopsy, fine needle aspiration, fine needle aspiration biopsy, percutaneous lung biopsy,* and *skinny needle biopsy;* we have fixed on *transthoracic needle biopsy* (TTNB), because our interest in the procedure was stimulated mainly by the work of Dahlgren and Nordenstrom—specifically, their book *Transthoracic Needle Biopsy.*[3] They have described the technique in detail. Several other investigators have also described various maneuvers in performing TTNB.[4]

PROCEDURE

We do our TTNB with a standard image intensifier in the radiology department. If the lesion cannot be localized fluoroscopically, usually because of small size (< 1 cm in diameter) then TTNB cannot be performed. Some groups use computed tomography (CT) to facilitate needle placement. This will certainly work but increases the time as well as the cost of the procedure considerably and, in our opinion, represents an overuse of new technology; therefore, we do not recommend CT-guided TTNB.

Instrumentation

At our institution we generally use a 6-inch, 22-gauge needle. A syringe pistol is very helpful in TTNB, though not essential. Syringe pistols available include the following:

1. ASPIR-GUN by Everest Company, 5 Sherman Street, Linden, New Jersey 07036.
2. Cameco Pistol by Precision Dynamics Corp., 3031 Thornton Avenue, Burbank, California 91504.
3. The 22-gauge needle that we use is #1-0374-T-462LNR from Becton Dickinson Corp., Cardiovascular and Special Instruments Division, Rutherford, New Jersey 07070.

Technique

A study of standard chest radiographs, and of tomograms when appropriate, will usually define the selected approach, whether anterior, posterior, or lateral, and the approximate depth of the lesion. The area is localized fluoroscopically (we have not found biplane fluoroscopy necessary), and a mark is made on the skin. The puncture site is swabbed with an antiseptic. Gloves are not necessary, and we have yet to see a septic complication of TTNB. A small wheal is raised with a local anesthetic, and the deeper tissues are then anesthetized.

An 18-gauge needle is inserted through the skin and superficial chest wall tissues to help direct the finer 22-gauge needle and to keep it from being bent by the skin. Under fluoroscopic control the needle is manipulated down to the lesion by a clamp (Fig. 14–2). The patient can be gently moved from side to side

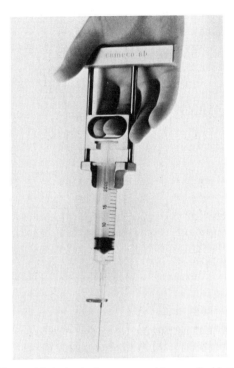

Figure 14–1. Aspiration gun used for needle biopsies. Made by Precision Dynamics Corp. (Cameco), 3031 Thornton Ave., Burbank, Calif. 91504.

to check that the tip of the needle is in the mass; smaller lesions can be seen to "dance around" when they have been pierced by the needle and the clamp is wiggled. The needle is twisted a bit, the obturator is removed, and a 20-cc syringe is attached. With suction applied, several short jabbing movements are made. Suction is released, and the needle is removed (Fig. 14–3). The syringe is disconnected, filled with air, and reattached to the needle.

The specimen, which is contained in the needle and is rarely present in the syringe itself, is blown onto a glass slide; smears are prepared; and the slide is immediately placed in 90% alcohol and then stained by the Papanicolaou technique. One smear can be air-dried and stained by Giemsa or Wright's stain, or Dif-Quik if desired. If the material is bloody, initial immersion of the slide in Carnoy's solution is recommended. The needle and syringe are rinsed in 50% alcohol, and then another preparation is obtained from the needle wash specimen from its passage through a Millipore filter.

A chest film is taken 30 to 60 minutes after the procedure to ascertain the presence or absence of pneumothorax; as a general rule, if a pneumothorax of significance is to occur, it

will be apparent by that time. A small pneumothorax with the lung apex separated off the chest wall for only 2 to 3 cm usually presents no problem. Collapse of over 30% is probably best managed by placement of a small intrapleural chest tube.

Many of our TTNB procedures are performed on an outpatient basis.[5] Outpatients are informed in advance that they should come prepared to stay overnight if a significant pneumothorax develops. Transient hemoptysis occurs in about one fifth of cases. The patient should be informed of this possibility preoperatively, and reassured that if bleeding does occur, it will stop spontaneously.

Who should perform TTNB? This is less a matter of controversy and more a matter of interest, experience, and skill. The invasive radiologist is probably the physician most commonly called upon to perform TTNB. In some centers the pulmonary physician is the preferred operator.[6] In our hospital TTNB is performed on the thoracic surgical service. At other institutions it is performed by the cytopathologist.[7] Whoever does the TTNB should either be able to insert a chest tube or have someone immediately available who can;[5] this is an important aspect of patient care that cannot be a subject of "turf" or other controversy.

Every bit as important as the proper procurement of TTNB specimens is the competence, interest, and experience of the cytopathologist who will be reading the slides. If diagnostic accuracy of TTNBs performed is not in the 80% range, an outside audit of the collection and interpretation of TTNB specimens is recommended.

COMPLICATIONS

Pneumothorax has occurred in 28% of our patients, but less than one third of these (26%, representing 7% of all TTNBs performed) have required placement of a chest tube. If there is any question, we feel that the safest course is assured by use of a small chest tube. We tell all our TTNB patients in advance that they have a 10% chance of "getting a chest tube."

Needle size has been a subject of some controversy. Berquist and colleagues at the Mayo Clinic feel that their pneumothorax incidence of 36% should limit the use of TTNB.[8] However, most of their procedures were done with an 18-gauge needle. Zavala and Schoell

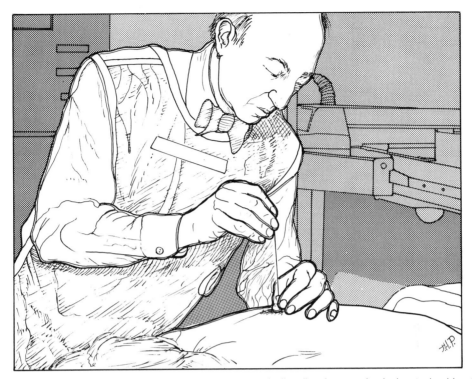

Figure 14–2. The site of skin puncture is chosen fluoroscopically, directly over the lesion to be biopsied. After infiltration of the skin with a local anesthetic, an 18-gauge, 2-inch needle is passed through the skin and superficial fascia. A 22-gauge, 6-inch needle is then passed through the 18-gauge needle. With a hemostat, it is maneuvered to the lesion in the lung under fluoroscopic control.

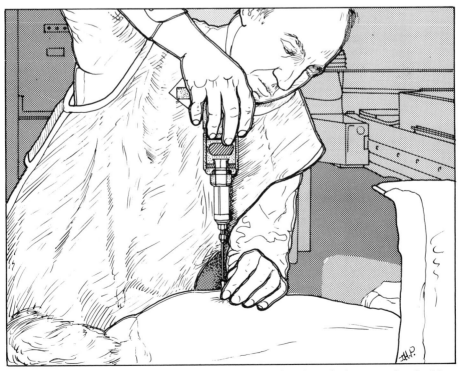

Figure 14–3. When the tip of the long 22-gauge needle is in the lesion, the stylet is removed and a 20-cc disposable plastic syringe fitted to a syringe pistol is attached. Suction is applied, followed by several short, vertical jabbing movements. Suction is released before the needle is removed.

have described an "ultrathin" TTNB technique using a 25-gauge needle with a very low incidence of pneumothorax.[9]

The earlier controversy over whether or not seeding of the needle tract by tumor cells occurs with TTNB was particularly marked in the United States. It is hard to document the genesis of that argument; apparently, however, the thoracic surgeons who opposed TTNB on these grounds for so many years were extrapolating from experiences with Cope and Abrams pleural biopsy needles in the biopsy of malignant pleural effusions, in which there is in fact occasional growth of cancer along the needle tract. This even led to some rather heated exchange in the surgical literature.[10] It is fair to state that seeding the needle tract with tumor cells by TTNB does not occur when fine (20-gauge or smaller) needles are used.[11] It is generally agreed that this argument is over.

There is difference of opinion over how many times needle aspiration should be done during the procedure. Although pneumothorax has occurred after a single needle pass in an easy case, the incidence of pneumothorax increases not only with the size of the needle but also with the number of passes.[8] Our experience has led us to limit the number of passes as much as possible. If the needle tip is on target and if there is enough specimen to prepare a slide, a single aspiration is satisfactory and is preferred whenever possible. Some groups have a cytotechnologist present to perform a rapid stain and assess the adequacy of the material. We do not consider this necessary, however, and it certainly prolongs the procedure.[5] Sagel's group at Washington University repeats the examination later in the day if the initial TTNB is nondiagnostic.[1]

INDICATIONS AND CONTRAINDICATIONS

Two major areas of controversy over TTNB involve when it should be done and what are the real contraindications. The procedure's area of greatest usefulness is in tumor diagnosis. If there is a reasonable chance that the suspect lung lesion can be visualized by flexible fiberoptic bronchoscopy, or that at fiberoptic bronchoscopy there is a strong likelihood that a brush or biopsy forceps can be guided to the lesion, then we prefer bronchoscopy over TTNB to confirm the diagnosis. Our preference for bronchoscopy is strengthened if the

patient appears to be a candidate for thoracotomy, as bronchoscopy would have to be performed under any circumstance prior to thoracotomy when malignancy is under consideration. That attitude is strengthened also by the incidence of pneumothorax.

There are very few contraindications to TTNB. Absolute contraindications include inability of the patient to cooperate or the presence of a hemorrhagic diathesis or a pulmonary lesion suspected to be a hydatid cyst. The depth of the lesion does not present a problem when fine (22-gauge) needles are used, and we have successfully performed TTNB on azygous lymph nodes. The incidence of pneumothorax is increased in patients with advanced chronic obstructive pulmonary disease, particularly when emphysematous cysts or bullae are present; we categorize such cases as presenting a relative contraindication to TTNB.

Since there is a false-negative rate of about 16% in TTNB for tumor diagnosis, we would not do TTNB for a small peripheral lung lesion that has a high risk of being malignant, because if the diagnosis is positive on TTNB, the patient will obviously undergo surgery.[12] But if the TTNB is negative for tumor and tumor remains a significant possibility, the patient should be operated upon regardless, because the 16% false-negative rate becomes unacceptable in a good-risk patient with a radiographically suspect peripheral lesion. To counter by saying that TTNB will pick up small peripheral small cell lung cancers is unrealistic, as such a presentation is truly rare for these lesions.[13]

We consider the most suitable candidates for TTNB to be (1) the marginal-risk patient with a lesion suspected of being cancer, in whom sputum cytologic studies and bronchoscopy have yielded negative results, but in whom the increased operative risk is acceptable if lung cancer is found, and (2) the obviously inoperable patient for whom the quickest diagnosis of a lesion beyond the immediate

Table 14–1. Various Benign Lesions Diagnosed by TTNB

Lesion	No. Of Cases
Lung abscess	5
Mediastinal cyst	4
Coccidioidomycosis	3
Tuberculoma	3
Mediastinal neurofibroma	1
Hamartoma	1

Table 14–2. Accuracy of TTNB in 236
Patients with Malignancy

Finding	% or No. of Patients
Positive	84%
Negative	16% (false-negatives)
False-positive	1 patient (tuberculoma mistaken for adenocarcinoma)

reach of the bronchoscope is necessary. Confirmation of cell type in each case is essential, for even the palliative treatment will vary according to cell type of the primary lung lesion.

TTNB is not particularly useful in diagnosis of diffuse lung disorders such as sarcoid and interstitial pneumonitis. It has been used in the past to diagnose some opportunistic infections such as *Pneumocystis carinii* pneumonia, but in such cases, transbronchial brushing and lung biopsy have since been shown to be preferable.[14, 15]

In our experience, TTNB has been diagnostic in several cases of tuberculoma, mediastinal cyst, coccidioidomycosis granuloma, and lung abscess (Table 14–1). Although most cases for TTNB center on tumor diagnosis, facilities for microbiology studies should always be readily available. Extra smears can be made for special staining, and minute amounts of TTNB specimen material can be blown onto a blood agar plate, a Lowenstein slant, or a Sabouraud plate for culture.

RESULTS

In our experience of 350 TTNBs done over a 15-year period, there has been no mortality associated with the procedure. None of our patients experienced air embolism, and we know of no seeding of the needle tract by tumor. Our incidence of pneumothorax is 28% overall, and of those requiring a chest tube, 7% overall. Of 236 patients who were ultimately proved to have cancer, TTNB was positive in 84% of the cases (Table 14–2). Our false-negative rate is, therefore, 16%. We have had only one false-positive case, in which a coin lesion that was identified as adenocarci-

noma on TTNB turned out to be a tuberculoma at the time of thoracotomy.

ACKNOWLEDGMENT

The author wishes to express appreciation to three colleagues in cytopathology who have made this work meaningful and possible: Pacita Manalo, Miriam Christ, and William J. Frable.

References

1. Sagel SS, Ferguson TB, Forrest JV, et al: Percutaneous transthoracic needle aspiration biopsy. Ann Thorac Surg 26:399, 1978.
2. Martin HE, Ellis EB: Biopsy by needle puncture and aspiration. Ann Thorac Surg 92:169, 1930.
3. Dahlgren S, Nordenstrom B: Transthoracic Needle Biopsy. Chicago, Year Book Medical Publishers, 1966.
4. Zajicek J: Aspiration biopsy cytology. Monographs in Clinical Cytology, vol 4. New York, S. Karger, 1974.
5. Stevens GM, Jackman RJ: Outpatient needle biopsy of the lung: its safety and utility. Radiology 151:301, 1984.
6. Gilney RT, Man GC, King EG, LeRiche J: Aspiration biopsy in the diagnosis of pulmonary disease. Chest 80:300, 1981.
7. Johnston WW, Frable WJ: Diagnostic Respiratory Cytology. Masson Publishing USA, Inc., 1979.
8. Berquist TH, Bailey PB, Cortese DA, Miller WE: Transthoracic needle biopsy. Mayo Clin Proc 55:475, 1980.
9. Zavala DC, Schoell JE: Ultrathin needle aspiration of the lung in the infectious and malignant disease. Am Rev Resp Dis 123:125, 1981.
10. Naylor B: Dissemination of cancer cells after needle biopsy of lung. J Thorac Cardiovasc Surg 64:324, 1972.
11. Nordenstrom B, Bjork VO: Dissemination of cancer cells by needle biopsy of the lung. J Thorac Cardiovasc Surg 65:671, 1973.
12. Baker RR: The role of percutaneous needle biopsy in the management of patients with peripheral pulmonary nodules. J Thorac Cardiovasc Surg 79:161, 1980.
13. Todd TR, Weisbrod G, Tao LC, et al: Aspiration needle biopsy of thoracic lesions. Ann Thorac Surg 32:154, 1981.
14. Repscher LH, Schroter G, Hammond WS: Diagnosis of *Pneumocystis carinii* pneumonitis by means of endobronchial brush biopsy. N Engl J Med 287:340, 1972.
15. Poe RH, Utell MJ, Israel RH, Eshleman JD: Sensitivity and specificity of the nonspecific transbronchial lung biopsy. Am Rev Resp Dis 119:25, 1979.

15

Needle Biopsy for the Diagnosis of Intrathoracic Lesions: Transbronchial Needle Biopsy

Ko Pen Wang, M.D.

Bronchoscopic techniques have permitted the evaluation of a variety of extrabronchial mediastinal abnormalities. Transbronchial needle puncture of the aorta, pulmonary artery, and left atrium was performed safely in hemodynamic studies even before the availability of current angiographic techniques.[1] Methods for needle aspiration of cytologic and other biopsy specimens from the subcarinal area have also been developed for use with the rigid bronchoscope.[2-8] At our institution transbronchial needle aspiration (TBNA) through the rigid bronchoscope was first performed in selected patients with right paratracheal neoplasms.[9] The technical feasibility and safety of obtaining specimens from other mediastinal sites have been confirmed in a more extensive series.[10] Development of a flexible needle for use in fiberoptic bronchoscopy has permitted further evaluation of TBNA.[11-13] Its initial diagnostic applications[11] and potential value in staging bronchogenic carcinoma[11-13] have been reported previously. This discussion presents an update of these experiences, with emphasis on available instruments, related anatomy, technical factors, and the value of TBNA in staging of bronchogenic carcinoma.

INSTRUMENTATION

Two types of TBNA needles are available. The *Type I single-lumen fixed* needle is 120 cm long and consists of two parts: an inner steel stylet and an outer semitranslucent (Teflon) sheath tipped with a 1.3-cm-long 22-gauge needle (Fig. 15–1). The stylet protrudes beyond the tip of the needle and is rounded to protect the bronchoscope from laceration when the needle is passed through the channel. A side channel for the aspiration of the cytopathologic specimen has been added to the proximal end of the catheter. Thus, only par-

tial removal of the flexible stylet is necessary for the aspiration of specimens.[28]

The *Type II double-lumen* retractable needle (Fig. 15–2) consists of three parts: an inner catheter tipped with a 1.3 cm-long 22-gauge needle; an outer catheter tipped with a smooth metal hub that functions to protect the bronchoscope from laceration when the needle is inserted through the channel; and a flexible stylet which provides the rigidity necessary for securing a specimen.

RELATED ANATOMY

Performance of TBNA demands familiarity with endobronchial landmarks and their relationship to extrabronchial mediastinum structures (Fig. 15–3). We have used the following guidelines in our approach to specific locations.

Aspiration of *subcarinal nodal* sites is achieved most easily. Although neoplastic infiltrate or rock-hard tumor may not permit puncture occasionally, the membranous posterior tracheal wall usually provides less resistance to the needle at this area, and satisfactory angulation of the bronchoscope is not as difficult to maintain as at paratracheal locations. Specimens should be obtained from the right side of the carina either anteriorly or posteriorly.

For *right paratracheal nodal* aspiration a site is selected 2 cm (or 2 to 4 tracheal rings) proximal to the carina, anterolaterally—a level at which the azygous arch will usually be avoided. The use of this anterolateral approach rather than a lateral approach effectively avoids puncture of the azygous arch and also avoids the mediastinal parietal pleura adjacent to the lateral tracheal wall, thereby minimizing the likelihood of pneumothorax. The 1.3-cm needle usually cannot reach the superior vena cava, so that bleeding complications can also be avoided.

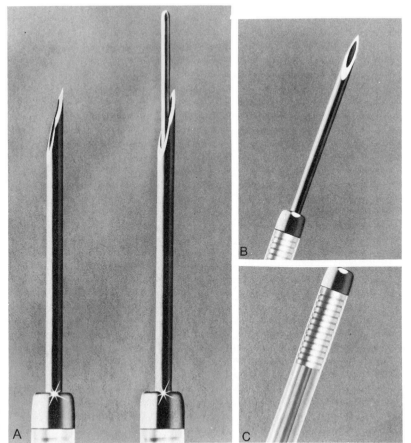

Figure 15–1. Type I needle, single-lumen fixed. (Courtesy of Mill-Rose Laboratories, Inc., Mentor, Ohio.)

The *aortic pulmonary window node* is approached at the level of the carina. An imaginary perpendicular line is extended from the carina to the lateral wall of the left main-stem bronchus, and aspiration is performed from the anterolateral aspect of the airway wall at this level.

TBNA specimens may sometimes be required at other locations; the puncture site varies with the anatomic distribution of a given lesion. Puncture of the bronchus intermedius is permissible, but its anterior wall should be avoided because of the proximity of the main right pulmonary artery. Aspiration specimens may be taken from the lateral and posterior walls of the bronchus at the orifice of the middle lobe bronchus. Similarly, because the truncus anterior branch of the right pulmonary artery passes anterior to the right upper lobe bronchus, aspiration from the right upper lobe spur requires direct caudal or posterior orientation of the needle. In the approach to the spur between the left upper and lower lobe, the needle is passed directly into the spur in a caudal direction or into the lateral wall of the lower lobe bronchus at its origin. Aspiration specimens are otherwise not obtained from the left main-stem bronchus because of its relationship to major vessels: the descending aorta lies posteriorly, the left superior pulmonary vein passes anteriorly at the orifice of the left upper lobe, and the left pulmonary artery courses superior and lateral to this spur.

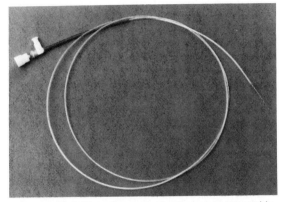

Figure 15–2. Type II needle, double-lumen retractable. (Courtesy of Mill-Rose Laboratories, Inc., Mentor, Ohio.)

In most patients, these guidelines have been

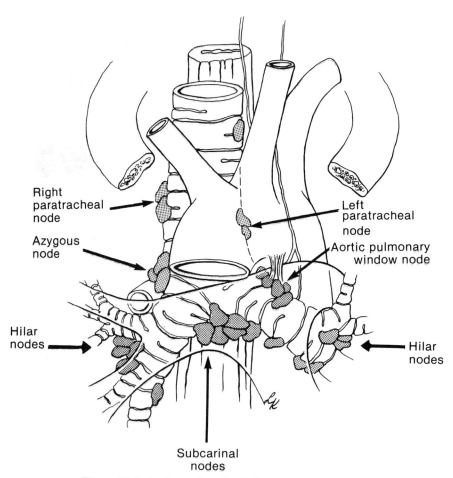

Right
paratracheal
node

Azygous
node

Hilar
nodes

Left
paratracheal
node

Aortic pulmonary
window node

Hilar
nodes

Subcarinal
nodes

Figure 15–3. Anatomy of mediastinal and hilar lymph nodes.

sufficient for safe airway puncture, but the potential distortion of normal anatomic relationships by mediastinal disease requires cautious planning of each procedure. Potentially safe high-yield sites for TBNA have been demonstrated using a variety of imaging procedures. Preoperative computed tomography (CT) with contrast enhancement has proved valuable, and such scans are obtained in most patients.[14] Angiography occasionally has provided additional useful information. These studies may guide aspiration from otherwise hazardous locations in some patients. However, in spite of all precautions, occasionally the bronchoscopist will aspirate pure blood into the catheter, indicating that the needle tip has punctured a large vessel; in this event, the needle is simply withdrawn, and another site is chosen to obtain specimens. There is no relationship of intrabronchial hemorrhage to large vessel puncture. It seems that intrabronchial bleeding following TBNA is related to puncture of intramural vessels.

TECHNIQUE

The bronchoscope used at our institution is the regular 5-mm flexible bronchoscope with a 2-mm working channel. The procedure is generally done using local anesthesia. The bronchoscope is passed either nasally or orally, and is positioned in the airway with the area of the carina or trachea to be punctured in full view.

With the Type I instrument (single-lumen fixed needle), the needle is passed through the bronchoscope channel with the stylet protruding beyond the needle tip, while the bronchoscope tip is in the trachea without any angulation. When the needle tip is seen in the viewing field, the stylet is partially withdrawn by pulling on the head of the stylet. The stylet is withdrawn minimally so that its tip is within the hollow part of the needle. This is essential to give the needle and sheath sufficient rigidity to permit puncture of the bronchial or tracheal wall. The bronchial or tracheal wall is next punctured with a quick thrust of the needle.

The stylet is then withdrawn partially so that its tip is outside the hollow part of the needle and inside the Teflon catheter. The space surrounding the flexible stylet provides enough space for aspiration. An aspiration syringe filled partially with 3 to 5 cc of normal saline is attached to the proximal end of the catheter, and suction is supplied by an assistant to draw the specimen into the partially translucent sheath. Once the sample is obtained, the needle is withdrawn from the channel, and the specimen is flushed into a container and processed for cytologic examination.

With the Type II instrument (double-lumen retractable needle), the needle is withdrawn into the metal hub of the outer catheter during its insertion through the biopsy channel of the bronchoscope.[15] Under direct vision the needle is advanced by pushing and locking the inner catheter to the outer catheter from its proximal end. The tracheobronchial wall is then punctured using a technique similar to that described for the Type I needle. The guidewire is removed completely, and a 20- to 50-cc syringe that has been preloaded with 2 to 5 cc of normal saline is attached to the inner catheter. Suction is applied while gently advancing and withdrawing the needle within the lesion. The entire system is then removed, and the specimen is collected for cytologic examination.

The type of needle used is a personal preference. We have found the Type I needle more convenient to use and easier to clean. The Type II needle seems to provide better protection of the small airway, making it particularly useful in biopsy of peripheral coin lesions; however, complete removal of the guidewire is necessary, making the procedure more complicated when this needle is used in biopsy of central lesions. Two or three punctures are made in each anatomic site; a different needle is not necessary to aspirate each site. Needle aspiration for staging always precedes brushing or biopsy of an airway distal to the trachea or to the main-stem bronchus.

TBNA may appear to be an easily accomplished procedure for the experienced bronchoscopist, but thorough training is mandatory to ensure its safe application. At our institution, instruction in the procedure prior to its use in patients includes detailed review of mediastinal anatomy and supervised practice sessions in which the needle is used both in the lung model and in the anesthetized dog.

The training experience has identified several potential errors in technique that can decrease the yield of the procedure and increase its risk; some of these are illustrated in Figure 15–4. The target site for aspiration should be approached as closely as possible, with the bronchoscope tip near the mucosal surface and with a minimum of needle tip exposed. When the needle extends far beyond the tip of the bronchoscope so that a long segment of Teflon catheter is within the viewing field, several problems may occur: first, the target site may be missed altogether because of decreased control of the needle tip; second, when excess catheter protrudes beyond the instruments, some of the force for puncture will be dissipated when the catheter bends despite its internal support by the stylet, so that the airway wall may not be completely penetrated. Furthermore, viewing the distal needle from a distance along the long shaft of exposed catheter may suggest that the needle has completely pierced the airway, even though only its tip is partially imbedded within the wall. After airway puncture, all of the needle should have pierced the airway wall. The needle should be advanced to its metal hub, with only the hub and the Teflon catheter visible. The bronchoscope should be advanced over the catheter close to the hub to confirm this needle position prior to aspiration. The

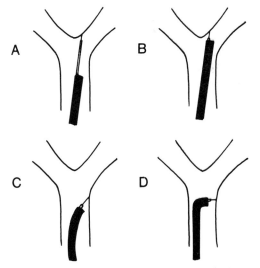

Figure 15–4. Transbronchial needle aspiration approaches: *A* and *B,* Subcarinal areas. *C* and *D,* Right paratracheal areas. Diminished yield may be associated with the procedure when excess catheter is exposed, as in *A,* or when the airway wall is approached obliquely, as in *C.* Ideally, the target site should be approached as closely as possible, with a minimum of needle tip protruding beyond the bronchoscope, as seen in *B,* and with as perpendicular an orientation as possible to the airway wall, as seen in *D.*

1.3-cm needle will not reach vascular structures at the usual carefully identified puncture site.

Another common technical error relates to the unique problem of aspirating through the paratracheal area with a flexible instrument. The airway wall should be approached with the needle in as perpendicular an orientation as possible. This approach will assure that puncture is made in the membranous intercartilaginous area, thereby permitting more complete transmission of force across the shortest distance of airway wall. If an oblique approach is taken, puncture becomes more difficult. The needle may completely miss the target and it must cross a greater distance. Although the apparent puncture site may be in the intercartilaginous space, the needle tip can become lodged in the lower tracheal ring bounding this space. Thus, it is possible to imbed the needle within the airway wall without obtaining an extrabronchial specimen.

Although the airway can ordinarily be punctured with a quick thrusting motion of the needle alone, when necessary the entire bronchoscope can be advanced toward the airway wall in order to aid puncture. It is useful for the proximal end of the bronchoscope to be secured in its position at the nose, mouth, or endotracheal tube by the bronchoscopy assistant to avoid recoil of the instrument during the puncture.

TBNA requires the same general principles of careful patient selection that are used in the identification of candidates for other bronchoscopy procedures. In particular, patients with coagulopathies or any anatomic variant that might increase the likelihood of hemorrhage or pneumothorax should not be subjected to this procedure.

STRATEGIES IN STAGING OF BRONCHOGENIC CARCINOMA

Clinical strategies used in preoperative diagnosis and staging[16-23] must combine knowledge of the histologic and biologic characteristics of the neoplasm (which determine the likelihood of mediastinal involvement at the time of evaluation) with an appreciation of the anatomic site of origin, recognized patterns of lymphatic drainage, and the accessibility of specific nodal sites to staging procedures, as well as the yield, safety, and limitations of these procedures. An extensive array of tests that provide information about the mediastinum is available.

TBNA provides safe access to many metastatic sites within the mediastinum. The availability of specimens from the inferior tracheobronchial nodes with this technique is of particular importance because of the central role of the subcarinal area in pulmonary lymphatic drainage and its position as an intermediary station in the contralateral spread of disease. Splaying of the main-stem bronchi or carinal blunting consistent with subcarinal disease can elude detection on the plain chest film, but the recognition of the involvement of this N_2 location may prove to have unique prognostic value.[24, 25] Naruke and coworkers[24] performed pulmonary resection with complete mediastinal lymph node dissection in 270 patients. Among their 64 patients with mediastinal metastasis, those with subcarinal lymph node involvement had a significantly reduced 5-year survival (9.1%) compared to that of N_2 patients without subcarinal metastasis (29%). These workers noted no significant differences in survival related to metastasis to other carefully identified N_2 nodal sites. Versteegh and Swierenga correlated the results of subcarinal aspiration with surgical outcome: 14 patients in whom the aspirate represented the only recognized site of metastasis underwent thoracotomy, and none of them had a curative resection.[26]

Increasing experience with needle aspiration has confirmed the safety of this technique and extended its application to use with the fiberoptic bronchoscope, suggesting that staging of bronchogenic carcinoma with respect to mediastinal nodal involvement (N status), as well as by standard criteria regarding the extent of endobronchial disease (T status), could be carried out routinely at diagnostic bronchoscopy. At institutions where TBNA for cytopathologic investigation is available, more invasive surgical procedures that are associated with higher risk and the need for general anesthesia could be avoided.

The ultimate place of TBNA in staging awaits further evaluation of its sensitivity in the varied clinical presentations of bronchogenic carcinoma. A potential role in patient evaluation is outlined in Figure 15–5. Patients with a radiologically abnormal mediastinum (on either standard chest roentgenogram or CT scan) or with clinical factors that are correlated with mediastinal metastasis (central primary tumor, mass exceeding 3 cm in size, unfavorable histologic findings) might benefit from the procedure. If cytopathologic findings are negative in these settings, the more inva-

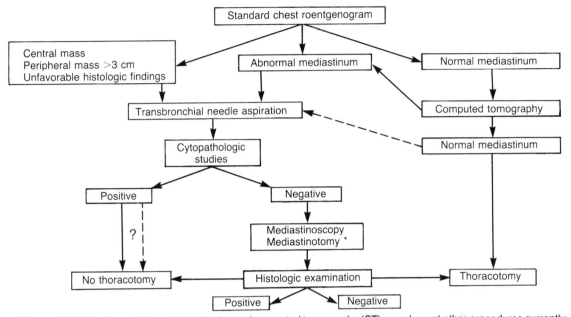

Figure 15–5. Transbronchial needle aspiration and computed tomography (CT) complement other procedures currently used in the diagnosis and staging of bronchogenic carcinoma. CT scanning may detect otherwise inapparent mediastinal disease, and transbronchial puncture may establish tissue diagnosis in patients at increased risk for mediastinal involvement, obviating the need for more invasive studies. Choice of procedure at the asterisk depends upon the location of nodal involvement. (Modified from Haponik EF, Wang KP: New methods for diagnosis and staging of mediastinal disease. *In* Aisner J (ed): Lung Cancer. New York, Churchill Livingstone, 1983.)

sive but complementary procedure of mediastinoscopy or mediastinotomy may be required, depending upon the most likely site of mediastinal involvement.

We currently believe that patients with roentgenographically demonstrable mediastinal lymphadenopathy and positive transbronchial needle aspiration from N_2 sites are not candidates for curative resection. The significance of positive findings following needle aspiration in the absence of radiographic evidence of mediastinal disease is unclear. It is unknown whether TBNA identifies patients with micrometastases confined within the node.

INDICATIONS AND COMPLICATIONS

At our institution, TBNA has been used successfully for diagnosing lymphoma, sarcoidosis,[27] and metastatic tumors in the mediastinum and hilar area;[28] for aspiration of mediastinal abscesses, thymic cysts, and, in one patient, an esophageal cyst;[14] and for ^{125}I seed implantation. However, the major value of TBNA is in diagnosis and staging of bronchogenic carcinoma. In extraluminal lesions with a normal overlying mucosa, with or without slight extrinsic compression, an 80% diagnostic yield was reached using either rigid bronchoscopy or flexible bronchoscopy.[11, 13] In staging of bronchogenic carcinoma, a prospective study showed positive findings in specimens obtained by TBNA in 50% of patients judged to be surgical candidates. In those patients with negative findings following TBNA, more invasive staging procedures, such as mediastinoscopy and mediastinotomy, yielded positive findings in only an additional 15%.

In more than 300 patients undergoing TBNA, only two complications have been observed: pneumothorax requiring chest tube placement in one patient and asymptomatic pneumomediastinum in another. Neither significant bleeding into the airway nor infection in the mediastinum occurred, and there have been no deaths. Although the procedure of TBNA appears to carry significant risk, experience has proved it much safer than transbronchial forceps lung biopsy. Pneumothorax can be virtually prevented by avoiding the lateral wall of the trachea in patients without obvious lymphadenopathy. The needle should be placed anterolaterally to avoid mediastinal reflection of the pleura; in a normal-looking carina, the needle should be placed so that it points vertically downward rather than posteriorly.

In conclusion, our experience suggests that with TBNA, the diagnostic yield should be of more concern than the risk. Both optimal yield and minimal risk are associated with a high degree of technical skill and familiarity with the instrument used. It should also be emphasized that the expertise of cytology laboratory personnel is critical in this regard; without proper handling and processing of biopsy specimens and interpretation of cytopathologic findings, the aim of TBNA, even when done with faultless technique, will be lost.

References

1. Crymes TP, Fish RG, Smith DE, et al: Complications of transbronchial left atrial puncture. Am Heart J 58:46, 1959.
2. Schieppati E: Mediastinal lymph node puncture through the tracheal carina. Surg Gynecol Obstet 110:243, 1958.
3. Versteegh RM, Swierenga J: Bronchoscopic evaluation of the operability of pulmonary carcinoma. Acta Otolaryngol (Stockh) 56:603–611 1963.
4. Fox RT, Lees WM, Shields TW: Transcarinal bronchoscopic needle biopsy. Ann Thorac Surg 1:92–96, 1965.
5. Simecek C: Cytological investigation of intrathoracic lymph nodes in carcinoma of the lung. Thorax 21:369–371, 1966.
6. Bridgman AH, Duffield GD, Takaro T: An appraisal of newer diagnostic methods for intrathoracic lesions. Dis Chest 53:321–327, 1968.
7. Atay Z, Brandt JH: Die Bedeutung der Zytodiagnostik der Perbronchialen Feinnadelpunktion von Mediastinalen oder Hilaren Tumoren. Dtsch Med Wochenschr 102:345–348, 1977.
8. Lemer J, Malberger E, Konig-Nativ R: Transbronchial fine needle aspiration. Thorax 37:270–274, 1982.
9. Wang KP, Terry P, Marsh B: Bronchoscopic needle aspiration biopsy of paratracheal tumors. Am Rev Respir Dis 118:17–21, 1978.
10. Wang KP, Marsh BR, Summer WR, et al: Transbronchial needle aspiration for diagnosis of lung cancer. Chest 80:48–50, 1981.
11. Wang KP, Terry PB: Transbronchial needle aspiration in the diagnosis and staging of bronchogenic carcinoma. Am Rev Respir Dis 127:344–347, 1983.
12. Haponik EF, Wang KP: New methods for diagnosis and staging of mediastinal disease. In Aisner J (ed): Lung Cancer. New York, Churchill Livingstone, 1983.
13. Wang KP, Brower R, Haponik EF, Siegelman S: Flexible transbronchial needle aspiration for staging of bronchogenic carcinoma. Chest 84:571–576, 1983.
14. Wang KP, Nelson S, Scatarige J, Siegelman S: Transbronchial needle aspiration of a mediastinal mass: therapeutic implications. Thorax 38:556–557, 1983.
15. Wang KP, Haponik EF, Britt EJ, et al: Transbronchial needle apsiration of peripheral pulmonary nodules. Chest 86:819–823, 1984.
16. Benfield JR, Juillard GJF, Pilch YH, et al: Current and future concepts of lung cancer. Ann Intern Med 83:93, 1975.
17. Cohen MH: Diagnosis, staging and therapy. In Harris CC (ed): Pathogenesis and Therapy of Lung Cancer. New York, Marcel Dekker, 1979.
18. Mittman C, Bruderman I: Lung cancer: to operate or not? Am Rev Respir Dis 116:477, 1977.
19. Paulson DL, Urschel HC: Selectivity in the surgical treatment of bronchogenic carcinoma. J Thorac Cardiovasc Surg 62:554, 1971.
20. Straus MJ: Lung Cancer. Clinical Diagnosis and Treatment. New York, Grune & Stratton, 1977.
21. Mountain CF: Assessment of the role of surgery for control of lung cancer. Ann Thorac Surg 24:365, 1977.
22. Baker RR, Stitik FP, Marsh BR: The clinical assessment of selected patients with bronchogenic carcinoma. Ann Thorac Surg 20:520, 1975.
23. Guinn GA, Tomm KE, North L, et al: Clinical staging of primary lung cancer. Chest 64:51, 1973.
24. Naruke T, Seumasu K, Ishikawa S: Lymph node mapping and curability at various levels of metastasis in resected lung cancer. J Thorac Cardiovasc Surg 76:832, 1978.
25. Kirsh MM, Sloan H: Mediastinal metastases in bronchogenic carcinoma: influence of postoperative irradiation, cell type, and location. Ann Thorac Surg 33:459, 1982.
26. Versteegh RM, Swierenga J: Bronchoscopic evaluation of the operability of pulmonary carcinoma. Acta Otolaryngol (Stockh) 56:603, 1963.
27. Wang KP, Britt EJ, Haponik EF, et al: A rigid transbronchial needle aspiration biopsy for histological specimens. Ann Otol Rhinol Laryngol (in press).
28. Wang KP, Gupta PK, Haponik EF, Erozan YS: Flexible transbronchial needle aspiration: technical considerations. Ann Otol Rhinol Laryngol 93:233, 1984.

V

Thoracoscopy

Genitourinary diseases were primarily responsible for the development of the technique of thoracoscopy. For many centuries the demands of stone, stricture, and urinary retention were such an important part of the physician's daily routine that some device had to be made to inspect and treat the bladder and its problems. The development of endoscopy was a challenge and is a tribute to the ingenuity and perseverance of scientists.

In 1806 Bozzini, a German physician, demonstrated before a medical meeting in Vienna his new apparatus, the *Lichtleiter,* or light conductor, for the inspection of various body cavities (Fig. 1). The *Lichtleiter* was a vase-shaped structure containing a candle in a round window that was divided vertically into two parts. One side was for the candle, the light source, and the other side was a viewing port. The *Lichtleiter* was used by fitting the open end of a speculum to the window. The apparatus was ingenious and clever, but it was not a success because the idea was counter to the conservatism of many German physicians, the device was painful and difficult to use, and the light was too dim.

Ségalas (1826) and Fisher (1827) made further attempts at performing endoscopy with reflected light, but cumbersome instrumentation and insufficient lighting prevented any enthusiasm for their equipment. The breakthrough for endoscopy began with Desormeaux (1853), "the father of cystoscopy," with his *gazogene* lamp that burned a mixture of alcohol and turpentine and produced a bright light. His apparatus was the first to be accepted widely; it provided great impetus to further development of endoscopy.

Until 1867, illumination in these early endoscopes came from a source outside the patient's body. At that time Brück, a dentist, developed an instrument called the diaphanoscope, with the light source (in this instance an electrically heated platinum loop) placed inside the patient.

Nitze, working first with an optician, Beneche, and later with a skilled instrument maker, Leiter, produced the first cystoscope,

with the dual features of a lens system and an electrical source of illumination close to the field to be inspected (1879). An exposed incandescent platinum loop was used for light. A cooling system for the loop had been designed, but this was cumbersome, and burns of the bladder wall were not infrequent. However, a few years later the Edison lamp (1880) appeared, and soon the *mignon* light was incorporated into the cystoscope (Newman, 1883; Leiter, 1886).

Kelling reportedly first examined the pleural cavity in dogs using a cystoscope (Unverricht, 1922), but it remained for the Swedish physician Jacobeus to develop a serious interest in thoracoscopy. He pioneered its use, initially for the diagnosis of tuberculous effusions (1910) and subsequently for cauterizing and lysing intrapleural adhesions (1916, 1922). In-

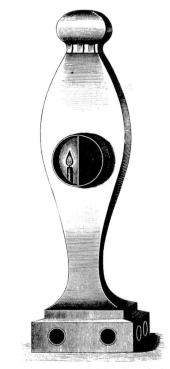

Figure 16–1. Bozzini's Lichtleiter (1807). A more cumbersome and ineffective instrument can scarcely be imagined, but it was a start. The original is in the Museum of the American College of Surgeons, Chicago.

terest in this operative approach was stimulated by many phthisiologists in treating tuberculosis and inducing pneumothorax that when complete resulted in a cure rate of approximately 70% as compared with about 33% or less when the pneumothorax was incomplete because of adhesions.

Intrapleural pneumolysis or the Jacobeus procedure was widely used, particularly in Europe, where artificial pneumothorax constituted the main treatment for tuberculosis. Bloomberg (1978) in the United States utilized this procedure in about 2000 instances between 1936 and 1950.

Gradually, as pneumothorax was replaced by thoracoplasty and, in turn, thoracoplasty was pushed aside by antimicrobials, the Jacobeus operation was abandoned. However, many European surgeons continued use of the thoracoscope for diagnosis and biopsy of many intrathoracic diseases. Interest in needle biopsy of the pleura began and rapidly found application. References to thoracoscopy between 1950 and 1965 are rare, particularly in the United States, but there has been a general renewal of interest in this procedure, culminating in the *Atlas* by Brandt, Loddenkemper, and Mai (1983).

16

Thoracoscopy: An Old Procedure Revisited

Paul Thomas, M.D.

An accurate diagnosis in patients with obscure intrathoracic lesions generally requires the recovery of representative tissue for examination. Many such patients are not candidates for surgical treatment. Therefore, thoracoscopy has been reintroduced to avoid diagnostic thoracotomy in selected patients. In recent years, thoracoscopy has been heralded by enthusiasts and derided by the uninspired, although its use was first suggested and reported by Jacobeus as long ago as 1910.[1] The procedure was widely used as an adjunct to pneumothorax therapy for lysis of adhesions between the lung and chest wall in patients with pulmonary tuberculosis prior to the discovery of effective antituberculous chemotherapy. The potential diagnostic application was also recognized; however, the procedure fell into disuse with the evolution of the direct surgical approach to intrathoracic diseases.

The terms *thoracoscopy* and *pleuroscopy* are used interchangeably in the literature. Weissberg and colleagues[2] prefer pleuroscopy for clarity, suggesting that it is the more specific term. Their objection to thoracoscopy is the connotation of a more general endoscopic examination. A thoracoscope is an instrument for examining the pleural cavity that is inserted through an intercostal space. Therefore, thoracoscopy is direct examination of the pleural cavity and its contents by means of an endoscope. Thoracoscopy implies a capability to examine and recover tissue samples from the chest wall and lung, which would seem to be a preferred definition of the procedure.

Interest in thoracoscopy has been stimulated by both the increasing requirement for diagnostic accuracy and the coincidental technical advances in instrumentation. There are increasing numbers of patients with unusual or difficult-to-diagnose pleural and pulmonary diseases. These include a large population of immunosuppressed individuals for which a wide variety of chemotherapeutic agents with specific activity are available. Therefore, etiologic diagnosis is essential for successful treatment.

INSTRUMENTATION

A variety of instruments have been used, some adapted to the procedure and some specifically designed. Preexisting instruments such as the mediastinoscope, bronchoscope, and laparoscope have been adapted to thoracoscopy.[2–4] Boushy and coworkers[5] reported using a needle scope developed for arthroscopy. Some investigators designed an introducer to allow passage of a flexible fiberoptic bronchoscope.[4,6] Several groups used available instruments and were obliged to make a second opening into the pleural space to insert biopsy forceps independent of the telescopic instrument.[7] Specific instruments designed for thoracoscopy include an introducer, instrument sheath with a valve to maintain a closed pleural space, an optical system, a light source, and biopsy forceps. The instrument system we have used and found quite satisfactory is illustrated in Figure 16–1. Although this is a rigid system, it has interchangeable accessories and additional access ports for aspiration and for coagulation.

PROCEDURE AND LIMITATIONS

Thoracoscopy can be done under either local or general anesthesia.[8,9] Having used both, we prefer to do the procedure under general anesthesia with ventilatory control, which provides for a more complete and satisfactory examination. Entry into the pleural space is made through a small intercostal incision; a hemostat is used to open the intercostal muscles and to puncture the pleura, as for chest tube inser-

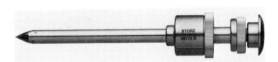

Figure 16–1A. Trocar and cannula with valve (either 9-mm or 11-mm). (Courtesy of Karl Storz, Endoscopy-America, Inc.)

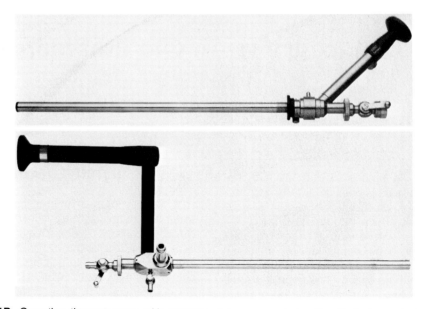

Figure 16–1B. Operating thoracoscopes with operating telescope and sheath with instrument channel for rigid operating instruments. *Top,* An 11-mm scope. *Bottom,* A 9-mm scope. (Courtesy of Karl Storz, Endoscopy-America, Inc.)

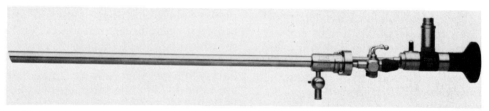

Figure 16–1C. Biopsy thoracoscope with forward-oblique telescope and fiberoptic light system and sheath for instruments. (Courtesy of Karl Storz, Endoscopy-America, Inc.)

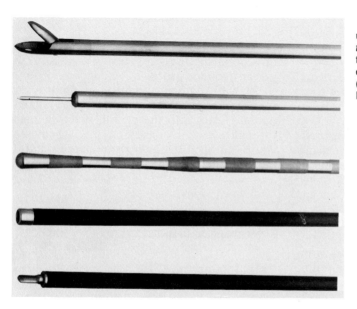

Figure 16–1D. Operating instruments for use with operating thoracoscope. *Top to bottom,* Biopsy forceps, injection needle, palpation probe, insulated cannula for suction and coagulation, and coagulating electrode. (Courtesy of Karl Storz, Endoscopy-America, Inc.)

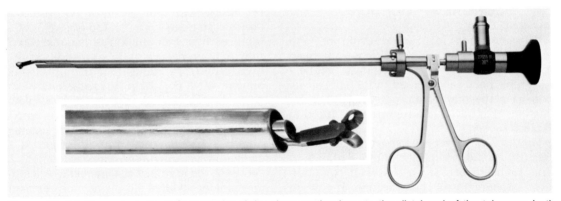

Figure 16–1E. Biopsy forceps. Note proximity of the sharp cutting jaws to the distal end of the telescope in the detailed view *(bottom)*. (Courtesy of Karl Storz, Endoscopy-America, Inc.)

tion. Although the instrument used is provided with a trocar for insertion, we discourage its use to avoid damage to the underlying lung. The optical system is introduced through the sheath into the pleural cavity, and air is insufflated through the access port to create a pneumothorax space. Thoracoscopy examination is limited or impossible if the lung is adherent to the chest wall at the site selected for insertion of the instrument. On several such occasions we have used alternative insertion sites. Airway management with a divided lumen endotracheal tube is an advantage but is not essential. However, it is important that the soft tissues of the intercostal space be sealed around the sheath to prevent loss of the pneumothorax during the procedure.

On completion of inspection, tissue sampling sites are selected and biopsy specimens se-

cured. The number of specimens taken varies with the diagnostic probabilities in each patient. However, we have found that in immunosuppressed patients, four tissue samples are sufficient for the requirements of light and electron microscopy, bacterial and viral studies, and fungal and parasitic examinations. A cautery device for coagulation hemostasis should be available as well as an aspirator, although these are seldom needed. On withdrawal of the instrument, a chest tube is inserted through the same incision for aspiration of the pleural space. In selected patients the tube is left in place for pleural space drainage, particularly if the indication for thoracoscopy was pleural effusion. However, the chest tube has been removed in the operating room in most of our patients undergoing lung biopsy without subsequent pneumothorax.

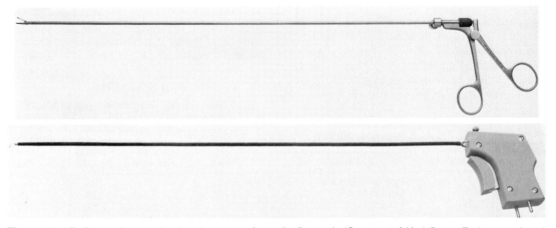

Figure 16–1F. Biopsy forceps *(top)* and cautery electrode *(bottom)*. (Courtesy of Karl Storz, Endoscopy-America, Inc.)

CLINICAL APPLICATIONS

Thoracoscopy is in a state of evolution, and indications for the procedure have not been defined with finality. The diagnostic applications have been investigated more extensively than have the therapeutic potentials. The indications that have been reported are listed in Table 16–1.[1–18]

Thoracoscopy has been used most frequently either to establish a specific etiology of pleural effusion or to exclude a treatable condition such as tuberculosis. The procedure is advised in lieu of thoracotomy after thoracentesis and percutaneous needle biopsy have not yielded satisfactory diagnostic information. Thoracoscopic lung biopsy to define the nature of pulmonary infiltrates has been frequently employed to avoid thoracotomy and open lung biopsy. Our interest in the procedure resulted from the increasing number of immunosuppressed patients presenting with pulmonary infiltrates of equivocal origin.

Since 1978, thoracoscopy has been used selectively as a diagnostic procedure in our patients who would otherwise require thoracotomy. In a consecutive series of 39 patients, two conclusions were reached: first, biopsy specimens removed via thoracoscopy were representative of the lesion; and second, sufficient tissue could be recovered for all required laboratory studies.

RESULTS

More than 600 patients have undergone thoracoscopy as reported in the literature cited. The majority of thoracoscopies were done for diagnosis of pleural or pulmonary parenchymal diseases or both. However, the procedure was used in a number of patients for different reasons. Review and analysis of this accumulated experience, including our series of patients, to determine exactly the probability of accurate diagnosis and the potential for false-negative or false-positive results are difficult. In many patients, the objective of the thoracoscopic examination is diagnostic exclusion. The procedure may be considered "positive"—that is, yielding definitive results—in a patient with persistent or recurrent pleural effusion if metastatic malignancy or pleural tuberculosis is excluded. Similarly, a lung biopsy may be recorded as a positive examination if *Pneumocystis carinii* infection is excluded in an immunosuppressed patient. In addition, the accuracy of diagnostic conclusion may not be evident until postmortem tissues are examined, viral cultures are reported, or the course of illness is resolved. The most important correlation would be an evaluation, retrospectively, of patient management decisions based on the diagnostic conclusion established via thoracoscopy. Data are not available to make such an analysis. However, it is possible to arrive at a preliminary estimate of the usefulness and accuracy of thoracoscopy by considering its application in patients with pleural effusion and patients with diffuse lung disease.

Thoracoscopy for diagnosis of pleural effusion provides an optimal result for a clinical decision in an estimated 94% of patients examined. The results reported by four groups of investigators with large series of patients studied are given in Table 16–2. Unsatisfactory diagnoses and failed diagnoses occurred as a result of technical difficulties and tissue sampling errors. In our series, for example, we were unable to enter the pleural space after multiple attempts in one patient with undiagnosed pleural effusion. However, a diagnostic yield of 94% is comparable to that achieved by direct thoracotomy. The results in our series of patients undergoing thoracoscopy for pleural effusion were as follows: malignant pleural effusion established, 40%; malignant pleural effusion excluded but with a finding of

Table 16–1. Indications for Thoracoscopy

Diagnostic	Therapeutic
Pleural effusion	Lysis of adhesions
Chest wall mass	Hemothorax
Diffuse lung infiltrate	Pleurodesis
Focal lung infiltrate	Foreign body removal
Pneumothorax	Sympathectomy
Hemothorax	Pulmonary cyst drainage
	Cancer staging

Table 16–2. Diagnostic Accuracy of Thoracoscopy for Pleural Effusion

Series	No. of Patients	Positive Results	Diagnostic Yield (%)
Weissberg et al[2]	113	107	96
DeCamp et al[7]	121	114	94
Oldenburg and Newhouse[8]	32	28	88
Canto et al[14]	172	164	95
Totals	438	413	94

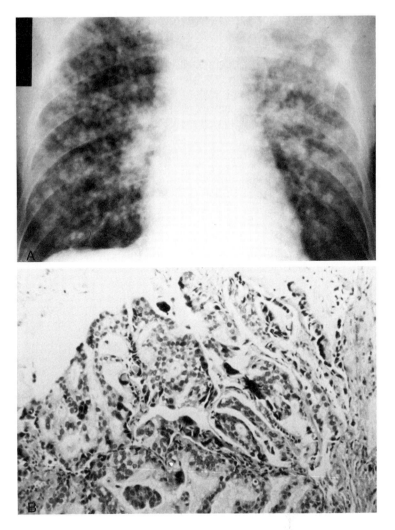

Figure 16–2. Thoracoscopy permitted definitive diagnosis in a patient whose chest roentgenogram, postero-anterior projection, demonstrated bilateral, diffusely distributed nodular disease *(A)*. Microscopic examination of tissue obtained at thoracoscopy revealed adenocarcinoma *(B)*.

nonspecific pleuritis, 20%; and tuberculous pleural effusion excluded with a finding of nonspecific pleuritis, 30%.

Diagnostic thoracoscopy has been used to avoid thoracotomy in both immunocompetent and immunosuppressed patients with diffuse pulmonary disease (Fig. 16–2). The results in several reported series of patients are given in Table 16–3. It must be emphasized that the interpretation of a positive result is determined by the investigators. The 100% diagnostic yield reported by one group, for instance, was based on a diagnosis of *Pneumocystis carinii* infection in 20 of 34 patients suspected and exclusion of the infection in the remaining 14 patients.[4] However, thoracotomy was obviated by thoracoscopy in these patients.

We have used thoracoscopic lung biopsy in selected patients to diagnose masses, diffuse nodules, and focal and diffuse infiltrates in both immunocompetent and immunosup-

pressed individuals. A satisfactory diagnosis, either specific or by exclusion, was achieved in 94% of these patients. This experience included the unusual findings of pulmonary calcinosis in a renal transplant recipient and of refractile foreign bodies in the infiltrate of a lymphoma patient following therapy. Diagnosis of *Pneumocystis carinii* was established in a patient with acquired immune deficiency

Table 16–3. Diagnostic Accuracy of Thoracoscopy for Diffuse Lung Disease

Series	No. of Patients	Positive Results	Diagnostic Yield (%)
Rodgers and Talbert[4]	46	46	100
Boutin et al[10]	20	20	100
Dijkman et al[11]	91	84	92
Totals	157	150	96

syndrome; the organism was subsequently re-demonstrated on repeat thoracoscopic lung biopsy during a clinical relapse.

Thoracoscopy has been employed in a smaller number of patients for diagnosis of intrathoracic tumors and pulmonary nodules and for staging of bronchogenic carcinoma. Although a pre-resection diagnosis of a mass may provide information if surgical removal is contemplated, this is not critical as a method of obviating thoracotomy. There may be objections to biopsy of potentially resectable neoplasms of the chest wall or lung relative to possible dissemination of tumor cells. Staging the extent of disease in patients with bronchogenic carcinoma may be advantageous in selected patients, but limitations must be recognized. Obviously, the mediastinal lymph node drainage area is not within the field of inspection of the thoracoscope. Areas of adherence between the lung and parietal pleura of the chest wall, mediastinum, or diaphragm may be inflammatory at the site of biopsy and therefore histologically misleading.

The therapeutic applications for thoracoscopy have been tentatively explored but as yet have not been widely accepted. Instillation of a wide variety of irritating materials into the pleural space to produce pleurodesis in patients with either pleural effusion or pneumothorax has been studied repeatedly. Therefore, it is not surprising that the use of such irritants in the pleural space at the time of thoracoscopy is increasing.[2, 4, 10, 17] Patients with traumatic hemothorax have benefited from thoracoscopy to determine the source and extent of bleeding into the pleural space and to control the site by cautery treatment in order to avoid thoracotomy.[15, 16] At the present time it is impossible to determine the usefulness of thoracoscopy in a patient with threatening hemothorax who needs urgent surgery for resuscitation. A most intriguing procedure accomplished via thoracoscopy is upper thoracic sympathectomy.[16, 18] Endoscopic removal of iatrogenically deposited foreign bodies from the pleural space has also been accomplished.[17]

COMPLICATIONS

The complications of thoracoscopy thus far reported have been minor. Bleeding has been observed in immunosuppressed patients with preoperative thrombocytopenia; transfusion was required, but the bleeding stopped spontaneously without thoracotomy.[12] Transient hemoptysis may occur after lung biopsy.[10]

Pneumothorax has been the most troublesome problem. Some investigators, including ourselves, have not routinely placed a chest tube after thoracoscopic lung biopsy and have observed postoperative pneumothorax as a complication. Others have reported pneumothorax as a complication in patients who have post-thoracoscopy pleural space drainage.

References

1. Jacobeus HC: The cauterization of adhesions in artificial pneumothorax treatment of pulmonary tuberculosis under thoracoscopic control. Proc R Soc Med 16:45–62, 1923.
2. Weissberg D, Kaufman M, Zurkowski Z: Pleuroscopy in patients with pleural effusions and pleural masses. Ann Thorac Surg 29:205–208, 1980.
3. Gwin E, Pierce G, Boggan M, et al: Pleuroscopy and pleural biopsy with the flexible bronchoscope. Chest 67:527–531, 1975.
4. Rodgers BM, Talbert JL: Thoracoscopy for diagnosis of intra-thoracic lesions in children. J Pediatr Surg 11:703–708, 1976.
5. Boushy SF, North LB, Helgason AH: Thoracoscopy: Technique and results in eighteen patients with pleural effusion. Chest 74:386–389, 1978.
6. Ben-Isaac FE, Simmons DH: Flexible fiberoptic pleuroscopy: Pleural and lung biopsy. Chest 67:573–576, 1975.
7. DeCamp PT, Moseley PW, Scott ML, Hatch HB Jr: Diagnostic thoracoscopy. Ann Thorac Surg 16:79–84, 1973.
8. Oldenburg FA, Newhouse MT: Thoracoscopy: A safe, accurate diagnostic procedure using the rigid thoracoscope and local anesthesia. Chest 75:45–50, 1979.
9. Miller JI, Hatcher CR: Thoracoscopy: A useful tool in the diagnosis of thoracic disease. Ann Thorac Surg 26:68–72, 1978.
10. Boutin C, Viallat JR, Cargnino P, Rey F: Thoracoscopic lung biopsy. Chest 82:44–48, 1982.
11. Dijkman JH, van der Meer JWM, Bakker W, et al.: Transpleural lung biopsy by the thoracoscopic route in patients with diffuse interstitial pulmonary disease. Chest 82:76–83, 1982.
12. Rodgers BM, Moazam F, Talbert JL: Thoracoscopy in children. Ann Surg 189:176–180, 1979.
13. Rodgers BM, Ryckman FC, Moazam F, Talbert JL: Thoracoscopy for intrathoracic tumors. Ann Thorac Surg 31:414–420, 1981.
14. Canto A, Blasco E, Casillas M, et al: Thoracoscopy in the diagnosis of pleural effusion. Thorax 32:550–554, 1977.
15. Ratliff JL, Johnson N, Clever JA: Pleuroscopy and cautery control of intrathoracic hemorrhage with a flexible fiberoptic bronchoscope. Chest 71:216–217, 1977.
16. Radigan LR, Glover JL: Thoracoscopy. Surgery 82:425–428, 1977.
17. Oakes DD, Sherck JP, Brodsky JB, Mark JBD: Therapeutic thoracoscopy. J Thorac Cardiovasc Surg 87:269–273, 1984.
18. Kux M: Thoracic endoscopic sympathectomy in palmar and axillary hyperhidrosis. Arch Surg 113:264–266, 1978.

17

Thoracoscopy: A Clinical Perspective

David H. Martin, M.D.
Michael T. Newhouse, M.D.

Thoracoscopy is an important, although in North America underutilized, adjunct to procedures for diagnosis of pleural and parenchymal lung disease. In recent years there has been renewed interest in this technique by thoracic surgeons and respirologists because thoracoscopy usually provides a reliable diagnosis in the 30% of cases that remain undiagnosed after thoracentesis and blind pleural biopsy.

Recently, promising applications have been developed, including pleuroscopic lung biopsy and cyanoacrylic glue pleurodesis.

HISTORICAL BACKGROUND

Jacobaeus introduced thoracoscopy in 1910 as a therapeutic procedure,[1] which was initially performed with a cystoscope to lyse pleural adhesions to aid induction of artificial pneumothorax for the treatment of tuberculosis. In 1921, he described the use of thoracoscopy for diagnosis of lung carcinoma.[2] In 1953 Lloyd recognized the value of thoracoscopy in undiagnosed pleural effusions.[3] Heine, in 1957, first reported the use of thoracoscopic lung biopsy for diagnosis of diffuse interstitial disease.[4]

In Europe, thoracoscopy has long been widely and effectively used, and numerous articles have been published in the literature there. Brandt and colleagues, reported a series of 1130 diagnostic thoracoscopies with biopsy for pleural effusions, with only 2.5% of pleural effusions remaining undiagnosed.[5] This group has also recently published a comprehensive atlas of thoracoscopy that details methodology and results.[6]

Despite the utility of thoracoscopy, well demonstrated in the European literature, this procedure is available in relatively few centers in North America, and most patients continue to be subjected unnecessarily to general anesthesia and open thoracotomy.

ADVANTAGES OVER OTHER DIAGNOSTIC TECHNIQUES

Thoracoscopy can be performed safely under local anesthesia even in relatively ill patients, requires only a very small incision, and usually results in a a definitive diagnosis or excludes a specific diagnosis. In contrast, thoracentesis, alone or combined with blind needle biopsy, fails to yield a diagnosis in up to 30% of cases of pleural effusion.[7-11] Thoracoscopy avoids most of the risks of open thoracotomy while achieving a comparable diagnostic and, in selected cases, therapeutic yield.

In various forms of diffuse pulmonary parenchymal disease, lung biopsy via the thoracoscope has also been very successful in providing a definitive diagnosis, with results similar to those with open lung biopsy, although no direct comparison has been made.[12-14]

INDICATIONS

The majority of thoracoscopies are done for exudative or persistent pleural effusions when thoracentesis and pleural biopsy are nondiagnostic; most patients will previously have undergone bronchoscopy. Occasionally, thoracoscopy has been used for investigation and therapy of pneumothorax. In some patients with established diagnoses, we have successfully used thoracoscopy to produce pleurodesis or to obtain tissue for breast cancer hormone receptor studies.[14a] The procedure has also been used for exploration of penetrating chest injuries[15, 16] and for retrieval of foreign bodies.[17]

CONTRAINDICATIONS

Relative contraindications to thoracoscopy include the presence of transudative pleural fluid or of major adhesions or an inadequate pleural cavity. The procedure obviously carries increased risk in the patient with coagulopathy or unstable cardiorespiratory status. Inability of the patient to cooperate (e.g., in a semiconscious state owing to extreme illness) or the necessity of mechanical ventilation may preclude the safe and effective use of the thoracoscope.

PROCEDURE

The instrumentation for thoracoscopy, the Storz set, is shown and described in Figure 16–1.

Preparation of the Patient

The risk of bleeding or the possibility of the need for prolonged chest tube drainage is carefully explained to the patient, and informed written consent is obtained.

We obtain a chest radiograph with decubitus views, a pleural sonogram if loculated fluid is suspected, and an electrocardiogram; if indicated, arterial blood gas analysis and spirometric studies are also performed. The patient is cross-matched for 2 units of packed red cells and instructed to take nothing by mouth after midnight the evening before the procedure. Thirty minutes prior to instrumentation, an intravenous line is established, and the patient is premedicated with 50 mg of meperidine intramuscularly and, provided the patient does not have glaucoma, with 0.6 mg of atropine subcutaneously.

Technique

For the performance of thoracoscopy in our unit, administration of supplemental oxygen by nasal catheter at 2 to 4 L/min and cardiac monitoring are routinely employed in the operating room.

The technique of thoracoscopy is simple. After the patient is placed with the involved side facing upward in the lateral decubitus position, the appropriate incision site is marked; this is usually the third intercostal space in the anterior axillary line or the fifth intercostal space in the posterior axillary line, or as indicated by sonography if sufficient fluid is loculated. Under sterile conditions, the Storz instruments are thoroughly inspected for cor-

rect assembly and operation. After standard skin preparation the selected intercostal space is anesthetized, as well as the two adjacent intercostal nerve bundles, with 2% lidocaine with epinephrine, using a total of not more than 5 mg/kg of lidocaine.

A 1.5-cm incision is made parallel and immediately adjacent to the upper border of the chosen rib to avoid the neurovascular bundle. The subcutaneous and intercostal tissue layers are bluntly dissected with curved forceps until the pleural space is entered. Blind exploration with a gloved fifth finger will assure that the pleural space is patent and that the lung is not adherent to the site of introduction of the trocar.

The trocar and cannula are introduced, and when the cannula has barely entered the pleural space, the trocar is removed and the cannula advanced. The thoracoscope is then carefully introduced under direct vision, and room air is allowed to enter the chest to deflate the lung and allow visualization. Any fluid is aspirated with a maximum suction of 30 cm H_2O applied to the side port channel. Excessive suction pressure may result in severe chest pain, respiratory and cardiovascular distress, and local lung trauma. A controlled pneumothorax is maintained by opening the lateral suction channel to air as needed.

The pleural space is systematically examined for abnormalities of the parietal or visceral pleura including the region of the apex, mediastinum, pericardium, and diaphragm. If desired, the parietal pleura at the site of insertion can be examined by replacing the thoracoscope with a gas-sterilized fiberoptic bronchoscope, which can be retroflexed to view the site of insertion. The bronchoscope can also be used for photography, or a special 35-mm camera adapted for the thoracoscope can be used. However, the flexible fiberoptic bronchoscope should not be used for thoracoscopy because it is clearly inferior to the rigid thoracoscope in both optical quality and in ability to obtain suitable biopsy material.

Lesions should first be palpated with the probe to evaluate pulsatile structures and to distinguish bone or cartilage from cystic and fleshy or granulation tissue. A long needle can be introduced under direct vision to avoid a biopsy of a vascular lesion or to inject lidocaine onto the parietal pleura prior to biopsy. For parietal pleura biopsies, the needle should be directed to areas over a rib to avoid the intercostal neurovascular bundle.

Rarely, excessive bleeding may occur; this can be controlled by electrocautery, instillation of vasopressin, or lung reexpansion. Adequate specimens for histopathologic and microbiologic studies and special staining procedures should be obtained.

Upon termination of the procedure, a rubber catheter is used to evacuate air as fully as possible if no thoracostomy tube is to be left in place. Alternatively, a large Argyle chest tube is inserted and attached to an underwater drainage tube and secured with purse-string and retention sutures and tape; the chest tube is left in place if metastatic carcinoma is to be treated with chemotherapy instillation or if a lung biopsy has been performed. Following lung biopsy, subcutaneous emphysema may be marked, particularly if the patient coughs, unless the chest tube completely fills the chest wall incision or the purse-string suture pulls the intercostal muscles tightly around the thoracostomy tube.

A chest radiograph is obtained after the procedure to evaluate lung expansion, and vital signs are monitored for 1 to 2 hours.

COMPLICATIONS

Potential complications of thoracoscopy include hemothorax; empyema; hypoxemia and arrhythmias; and cough and local pain. Recurrence of tumor at the thoracoscopy site is a rare possibility. Bronchopleural fistula and subcutaneous emphysema are other uncommon sequelae.

RESULTS

Over a 10-year period starting in 1973, 69 rigid thoracoscopies were performed in our unit: 58 by two respirologists and 11 by the surgical service. In the first 5-year period, as reported by Oldenburg and Newhouse,[18] diagnostic yield for the flexible bronchoscope used as a thoracoscope was only 56%, compared with 88% for the rigid (Storz) thoracoscope (see Table 17–1). Thus, thoracoscopy should be performed only with a rigid thoracoscope.

In our group of patients, no arrhythmias were detected by cardiac and ear oximetry monitoring, and the mean oxyhemoglobin saturation following controlled pneumothorax using room air was 93%. The mean fall in Sa_{O_2} was 1.4%; the lowest recorded saturation, associated with severe coughing during insertion of the thoracoscope, was 83%. Faurschou and

Table 17–1. Diagnostic Accuracy of Fiberoptic Bronchoscope Versus Rigid Thoracoscope

Instrument	Total Cases in Series	Cases Undiagnosed*	Correct Diagnosis
Fiberoptic bronchoscope			
All lesions†	9	7	5 (56%)
Neoplasms	3	2	1 (33%)
Rigid (Storz) thoracoscope			
All lesions†	32	25	28 (88%)
Neoplasms	10	7	8 (80%)

*Results of number of cases undiagnosed at previous needle biopsy.
†Lesions included nonspecific pleuritis, carcinoma, sarcoma, neurofibroma, tuberculosis, systemic lupus erythematosus, and pancreatitis.

coworkers have confirmed these observations.[19]

Histologic diagnosis following thoracoscopic biopsy compared with findings at follow-up is shown in Table 17–2. The most common histologic diagnosis was nonspecific pleuritis, made in 37 patients (54%). During a follow-up period of up to 2 years, a subsequent specific diagnosis was achieved in only six of these patients (8.7%) (Table 17–3). In this group of patients, therefore, the diagnostic accuracy of thoracoscopic biopsy was 80%. There are several possible reasons for the false-negative or inconclusive results in the remaining 20% of patients; for example, a carcinoma may block the lymphatics at a distant site, causing local pleural fluid accumulation without local invasion or pleural metastasis. In this example a genuinely negative result would be classified as false-negative at follow-up. Of course, false-negative results will occur where

Table 17–2. Histologic Diagnosis at Biopsy Versus Findings at Follow-Up in 69 Patients

Lesion	Diagnosis Histologic	Follow-up
Nonspecific pleuritis	37	31
Carcinoma		
Undifferentiated	6	7
Adenocarcinoma	12	12
Squamous	2	3
Small cell	—	1
Mesothelioma	1	1
Osteogenic sarcoma	1	1
Neurofibroma	1	1
Tuberculosis	1	4
Systemic lupus erythematosus	1	1
Pancreatitis	—	1

Table 17–3. Specific Diagnoses* in 6 Patients Following False-negative Thoracoscopy

Patient	Lesion Demonstrated at Follow-up	Diagnostic Method or Parameter
1	Tuberculosis	Gastric fluid culture
2	Tuberculosis	Clinical response
3	Tuberculosis	Clinical response
4	Small cell carcinoma	Biopsy
5	Squamous cell carcinoma	Hilar node biopsy
6	Undifferentiated carcinoma	Biopsy

*Made by clinical follow-up.

the involved pleura is not biopsied. Failure to obtain representative pleura is unlikely at thoracoscopy but may occur if the inflammatory reaction has produced a large amount of reactive granulation tissue or fibrin deposition.

Of the three cases of tuberculosis not diagnosed by thoracoscopy, only one was proved by culture of gastric fluid; the remaining two were presumed to be tuberculosis because of highly suggestive signs and symptoms despite the negative thoracoscopic biopsy and, subsequently, on the basis of the clinical response to antituberculosis therapy.

Specific diagnoses were made in 25 patients (41%), of whom 23 (37%) had neoplasia; of the remaining 2 patients, one had tuberculosis and the other, systemic lupus erythematosus. The negative predictive value of the histologic diagnosis was 84%. The overall diagnostic accuracy was 90% (Table 17–4).

In 19 of the 58 medical-service patients, the presence or absence of carcinoma was confirmed on thoracoscopic visual appearance alone; the results are illustrated in Table 17–5. The positive predictive value of visual appearance in diagnosis of malignancy was 67%; the corresponding negative predictive value was 71%. The overall diagnostic accuracy of visual appearance alone was 68%.

In the medical-service group of 58 patients, there were only four minor complications: subcutaneous emphysema following lung biopsy, pneumothorax, ventricular ectopic activity and acute dyspnea and chest pain related to excessive pleural suction. The only potentially serious complication was a hemothorax (400 mL) following biopsy of nodular granulation tissue; fortunately, the bleeding ceased spontaneously. In the surgical-service group of 11 patients, there was one instance of post-thoracoscopy empyema and one of intraoperative cardiac arrest, resulting in death 10 days later. These data, though collectively too small a base for statistical interpretation, suggest that a minimal complication rate is related to careful attention to patient selection, technique, and postoperative management, making the procedure suitable for performance by internists in centers where surgical support is available.

The largest reported follow-up series, composed of 51 patients, describing results of thoracotomy for undiagnosed pleural effusion comes from the Mayo Clinic.[20] In 61% of these patients, no specific diagnosis could be made in the follow-up period even after thoracotomy. Of the remaining patients in whom a specific diagnosis was made, the majority (72%) proved to have a malignancy. The rest of the patients had collagen vascular disease (17%), and there was one case of mitral stenosis and one of "yellow nail syndrome."Although the two methods have not been directly compared, these results suggest that thoracotomy with open pleural biopsy is no more likely to provide a diagnosis than is thoracoscopy.

Transthoracoscopic lung biopsy has been effectively applied in the diagnosis of diffuse pulmonary infiltrates, particularly in the immunocompromised patient. In a series of 49 thoracoscopies in 45 patients aged 8 months to 68 years, the overall diagnostic accuracy was 92%.[21] In another series of 65 thoracoscopies in 57 children, 34 of whom were immunocompromised, a diagnostic accuracy of 100% was achieved in 20 cases of infection by *Pneumocystis carinii*.[22]

A recent study suggests that the problem of

Table 17–4. Predictive Value of Thoracoscopic Biopsy Results Determined by Follow-up Findings in 62 Patients

Thoracoscopic Biopsy Results	Follow-Up Findings		
	Diagnostic	*Nondiagnostic*	
Diagnostic	25	0	(positive predictive value = 100%)
Nondiagnostic	6	31	(negative predictive value = 84%)

Sensitivity = 80%, specificity = 100%, diagnostic accuracy $(25 + 31)/62 = 90\%$.

Table 17–5. Predictive Value of Thoracoscopic Visual Appearance in Carcinoma (CA) Determined by Histologic Diagnosis in 19 Patients

Thoracoscopic Visual Appearance	Histologic Diagnosis		
	CA Present	CA Absent	
CA present	8	4	(positive predictive value = 67%)
CA absent	2	5	(negative predictive value = 71%)

Sensitivity = 80%, specificity = 56%, diagnostic accuracy = 68%.

prolonged bronchopleural air leak following lung biopsy may be minimized by *not* applying suction after connecting the chest tube to underwater drainage. In a series of 28 thoracoscopic lung biopsies managed postoperatively by drainage alone, only 4 patients had a persistent pneumothorax, with a mean duration of chest drainage of 4.4 days (range 1–21 days) for the entire group.[23]

It is evident that thoracoscopy with pleural or lung biopsy is a useful diagnostic tool whose success rate equals that of open pleura or lung biopsy.[24] Further technical advances, such as the use of tissue glue,[25–27] have extended the value of thoracoscopy to make it a useful therapeutic tool in spontaneous pneumothorax and bronchopleural fistula.

Thoracoscopy with pleural biopsy is far superior to thoracentesis alone, even with blind pleural biopsy, because the diagnostic results are similar to those of open biopsy; moreover, as with blind pleural biopsy, general anesthesia is not needed, and postoperative morbidity is low. Furthermore, transthoracoscopic pleural and lung biopsy may supplant open surgical procedures for these selected diagnostic and therapeutic purposes,[28] including therapy of persistent or recurrent pneumothorax. In the future, Nd:YAG laser systems, which can readily be utilized through the thoracoscope, promise to make these instruments even more useful. It is not clear why, in North America, this relatively benign and simple procedure is available in so few centers. We hope that this technique will be rediscovered by the current-generation respirologists and thoracic surgeons, thus facilitating the diagnosis and therapy of lesions of the lungs and pleura while reducing morbidity and the related costs of hospital care to a minimum.

ACKNOWLEDGEMENTS

The authors thank Drs. N. Jones, L. Kahana, J. Morse, and S. Puksa for their constructive criticism and Josephine Garstin for preparation of the manuscript.

References

1. Jacobaeus H: Ueber die Moglichkeit die Zystoskopie bei Untersuchung Seroser Hohlungen Anzuwenden. Munch Med Wschr 57:2090–2092, 1910.
2. Jacobaeus H, Key H: Some experiences of intrathoracic tumors, their diagnosis and their operative treatment. Acta Chir Scand 53:573, 1921.
3. Lloyd MS: Thoracoscopy and biopsy in the diagnosis of pleurisy with effusion. Q Bull Sea View Hosp 14:12–33, 1953.
4. Heine F: Die Probeexcision aus Veranderungen im Thoraxraum und lung unter thoracoskopischer sicht. Beitr Klin Tuberk 116:615–627, 1957.
5. Brandt H-J, Mai J: Differential diagnosis of pleural effusion using thoracoscopy. Pneumonologie 145:192–203, 1971.
6. Brandt H-J, Loddenkemper R, Mai J: Atlas der Diagnostischen Thorakoskopie [Atlas of Diagnostic Thoracoscopy]. Stuttgart, Georg Thieme Verlag, 1983. (English edition in press. Thieme-Stratton, New York.)
7. Black LF: Pleural effusions (editorial). Mayo Clin Proc 56:201–202, 1981.
8. Enk B, Viskum K: Diagnostic thoracoscopy. Eur J Respir Dis 62:344–351, 1981.
9. Rao NV, Jones PO, Greenberg SD, et al: Needle biopsy of parietal pleura in 124 cases. Arch Intern Med 115:34–41, 1965.
10. Storey DD, Dines DE, Coles DT: Pleural effusion: a diagnostic dilemma. JAMA 236:2183–2186, 1976.
11. Scerbo J, Keltz H, Stone DJ: A prospective study of closed pleural biopsies. JAMA 218:377–380, 1971.
12. Boutin C, Viallat JR, Cargnino P, Rey F: Thoracoscopic lung biopsy. Experimental and clinical preliminary study. Chest 82:44–48, 1982.
13. Janik JS, Nagarcy HS, Groff DB: Thoracoscopic evaluation of intrathoracic lesions in children. J Thorac Cardiovasc Surg 83:408–413, 1982.
14. Rogers BM, Moazam F, Talbert JL: Thoracoscopy. Early diagnosis of interstitial pneumonitis in the immunologically suppressed child. Chest 75:126–130, 1979.
14a. Levine MN, Young JEM, Ryan E, Newhouse MT: Pleural effusion in breast cancer. Thoracoscopy for hormone receptor determination (submitted to Cancer).
15. Branco JMC: Thoracoscopy as a method of exploration in penetrating injuries of the thorax. (Preliminary report.) Dis Chest 12:330–335, 1946.
16. Jones JW, Ditahama A, Webb WR, McSwain N: Emergency thoracoscopy: a logical approach to chest trauma management. J Trauma 21:280–284, 1981.
17. Brodsky JB, Welti RS, Mark JB: Thoracoscopy for retrieval of intrathoracic foreign bodies (letter). Anesthesiology 54:91–92, 1981.

18. Oldenburg FA, Newhouse MT: Thoracoscopy. A safe, accurate diagnostic procedure using the rigid thoracoscope and local anesthesia. Chest 75:45–50, 1979.

19. Faurschou P, Madsen F, Viskum K: Thoracoscopy: influence of the procedure on some respiratory and cardiac values. Thorax 38:341–343, 1983.

20. Ryan CJ, Rogers RF, Unni KK, Hepper NG: The outcome of patients with pleural effusion of indeterminate cause at thoracotomy. Mayo Clin Proc 56:145–149, 1981.

21. Rogers BM, Ryckman FC, Moazam F, Talbert JL: Thoracoscopy for intrathoracic tumors. Ann Thorac Surg 31:414–420, 1981.

22. Rodgers BM, Moazam F, Talbert JL: Thoracoscopy in children. Ann Surg 189:176–180, 1978.

23. Dijkman JH, van der Meer JWM, Bakker W, et al: Transpleural lung biopsy by the thoracoscopic route in patients with diffuse interstitial pulmonary disease. Chest 82:76–83, 1982.

24. Gaensler EA, Carrington CB: Open biopsy for chronic diffuse infiltrative lung disease: clinical, roentgenographic and physiological correlations in 502 patients. Ann Thorac Surg 30:411–426, 1980.

25. Hatakenaka R, Ikeda S, Hitomi S, et al: A new method of intrathoracal biopsy using thoracoscope and tissue adhesive. Bronchopneumologie 26:161–173, 1976.

26. Kai T, Ikeda S, Hitomi S, et al: Lung biopsy using thoracoscopy application of a tissue adhesive. Jpn J Thorac Dis 10:450–455, 1972.

27. Takano Y: New treatment of spontaneous pneumothorax by liquid glue nebulization under thoracoscopic control. Bronchopneumologie 28:19–28, 1978.

28. Oakes D, Sherck J, Brodsky J, Mark J: Therapeutic thoracoscopy. J Thorac Cardiovasc Surg 87:269–273, 1984.

18

Thoracoscopy: Its Use for Diagnosis and Therapy

David D. Oakes, M.D.
John P. Sherck, M.D.
James B. D. Mark, M.D.

During the 19th century, attempts at endoscopy were initially frustrated by the inability to project light into deep recesses through hollow tubes. Modern endoscopy was born in 1883 when Newman incorporated the Edison electric light bulb into a contemporary cystoscope.[1] The discipline has matured with the development of fiberoptic systems for the transmission of "cold" light into almost any space.

H. C. Jacobaeus, Professor of Medicine at the University of Stockholm, is credited with the first use of the distally lighted cystoscope for examination of the pleural cavity in humans.[1] His studies began in 1911 when he used the device to investigate "idiopathic pleurisy"; most cases were found to be tuberculous in origin. He also attempted to distinguish between benign and malignant pleural masses by direct visualization and biopsy. Two years later he began applying thoracoscopy therapeutically to lyse adhesions that were preventing satisfactory collapse therapy for pulmonary tuberculosis, a technique subsequently termed "pneumonolysis."[2]

Jacobaeus referred to his procedure as "thoracoscopy." "Pleuroscopy" is probably a more precise designation, because bronchoscopy, esophagoscopy, and mediastinoscopy are also techniques for endoscopic examination of intrathoracic structures. Most authors, however, continue to use "thoracoscopy" to refer to instrument-assisted visualization of the pleural cavity, and we have retained this usage for the purpose of this discussion.

INDICATIONS

Thoracoscopy has both diagnostic and therapeutic indications (Table 18–1). In either situation it is employed to obviate the need for major thoracotomy or for empirical therapy based upon a suboptimal data base.

Diagnostic thoracoscopy is most useful in patients with chronic pleural effusions or pleural-based lesions that remain unexplained after the application of less invasive diagnostic techniques. Thoracentesis and cytologic examination of the pleural fluid is often positive in patients in whom malignancy is suspected. Needle biopsy of the pleura may likewise provide a definitive diagnosis, but a normal biopsy may be obtained by chance in patients whose pleural disease is not uniform in distribution. Nevertheless, 10% to 20% of patients with chronic pleural effusions will remain undiagnosed after the application of these two techniques. It is only in such cases that diagnostic thoracoscopy is indicated; that is, thoracoscopy should not be used as a substitute for thoracentesis or needle biopsy in the routine initial evaluation of pleural masses or effusions.

Less commonly, thoracoscopy may help in planning therapy for patients with known malignant disease. It may be useful for tumor staging in patients with mesothelioma or in some cases of lung cancer; for example, it may

Table 18–1. Indications for Thoracoscopy

DIAGNOSTIC
Cryptogenic pleural effusions
Pleural-based lesions
Tumor staging
Hormonal receptor determination

THERAPEUTIC
Pneumonolysis
Foreign body extraction
Pleurodesis
    Effusion
    Pneumothorax
Débridement of empyema cavity
    Post-pneumonectomy
    ?Other
Trauma
    Control of hemorrhage
    Evacuation of clot

aid in the search for residual intrathoracic disease in patients with oat cell carcinoma treated with radiation and chemotherapy in whom the need for further therapy is in question. In appropriate cases, thoracoscopy may be the best way of obtaining tissue for estrogen receptor analysis in patients with known metastatic breast cancer.[1]

We have recently reviewed the therapeutic applications of thoracoscopy.[3] Intrapleural pneumonolysis, as popularized by Jacobaeus, was once used to facilitate total collapse of the pulmonary parenchyma during the induction of pneumothorax for the treatment of tuberculosis. Although this application of thoracoscopy is now obsolete, the technique of pneumonolysis remains useful in certain patients in whom pleuropulmonary adhesions prevent full expansion of the adjacent lung, as in the case of a chronic, loculated pneumothorax.

Intrapleural foreign bodies may occasionally require removal—either to treat infection or to prevent it. Thoracoscopy, with or without fluoroscopic guidance, may supplant the need for major thoracotomy in this setting.

Chemical pleurodesis using tetracycline, asbestos-free talc, or other irritants is frequently used to prevent the recurrence of chronic pleural effusions and has been reported effective in the management of patients with spontaneous pneumothorax. In either setting, thoracoscopy is preferable to blind chemical pleurodesis because it allows pleural symphysis to be applied selectively to patients who will not require future thoracotomy—that is, only to those with proved unresectable malignancies or with recurrent pneumothorax without major blebs or bullae. The surgeon will thus be spared the difficult task of re-entering a hemithorax in which the pleural space has been previously obliterated.

We have found thoracoscopy useful in the management of patients with inadequately drained post-pneumonectomy empyema cavities. By providing direct visualization of the infected space, thoracoscopy permits safer removal of necrotic debris and allows direct inspection of the mediastinum to rule out foreign bodies, bronchopleural fistulas, or recurrent tumor.

From time to time, thoracoscopy has been advocated for the initial management of patients with chest trauma.[1,4] Proponents of this application have cited more complete visualization of the extent of intrathoracic injuries, determination of the integrity of the diaphragm, coagulation of bleeding vessels, and

Table 18–2. Technique of Thoracoscopy

1. General anesthesia
2. Endobronchial intubation: one-lung ventilation
3. Prepare and drape for thoracotomy
4. Single puncture
5. Rigid scope
6. Electrocautery
7. Intercostal drainage

better evacuation of clot than would be possible with tube thoracostomy alone. However, we have had no experience using thoracoscopy in the evaluation and management of patients with chest trauma and believe that further trials are needed before its widespread application in this setting can be recommended.

TECHNIQUE

We perform thoracoscopy with the patient under general anesthesia and intubated with a double-lumen tube to permit the selective deflation of the ipsilateral lung (Table 18–2). We believe that these measures permit optimal conditions for inspection of the hemithorax while assuring maximal patient comfort and safety. The patient also receives 100% oxygen during the period of one-lung ventilation, and arterial blood gas tensions are carefully monitored to assure adequate oxygenation and ventilation. We have found this approach to provide safe perioperative management in a wide variety of intrathoracic surgical procedures.[5]

The patient is prepared and draped for formal thoracotomy in case thoracoscopy proves unrevealing or major complications arise. Most examinations are performed with the patient in the lateral decubitus position, although other positioning may be used if indicated. We utilize a rigid Stortz thoracoscope (see Fig. 16–1), which is introduced through a 2 to 3 cm incision in the midaxillary line using a sheathed trocar. With the outer cannula remaining in place, the thoracoscope can be easily removed and reinserted if the lens becomes fogged or stained with blood.

Pleural fluid is aspirated and submitted for cytologic examination and culture. The lung is then collapsed, and the pleural surfaces are carefully inspected. Suspicious plaques or nodules are biopsied under direct vision; all large masses are aspirated prior to biopsy to ensure that they do not represent vascular lesions or major vessels. Bleeding points are visualized and controlled with suction and electric cautery.

If the malignant nature of an effusion is established or strongly suspected, chemical pleurodesis is performed. Prior to reinflation of the lung, 1 gm of tetracycline is dissolved in 50 ml of sterile saline and introduced into the pleural cavity. The patient is them moved about to assure uniform dispersal of the sclerosing solution. At the end of the procedure, the thoracoscope cannula is replaced by a 24 French chest tube, which is placed to suction drainage at a negative pressure of 20 cm H_2O, and the lung is re-expanded. We believe that patient discomfort is minimized during chemical pleurodesis if the sclerosing solution is introduced while the patient is under general anesthesia.

Although we prefer the Stortz rigid scope, thoracoscopy can be carried out using a variety of optical instruments. Senno has advocated use of a fiberoptic bronchoscope introduced through an intercostal tube.[6] Lewis has reported satisfactory results using a rigid bronchoscope,[7] and Radigan has employed a sterile sigmoidoscope.[8] Needle arthroscopes, mediastinoscopes, and laparoscopes have also been used for thoracoscopy. Some of the advantages of the rigid instruments include better illumination, a larger apparent field size, easier manipulation, capacity for larger biopsy forceps (yielding more adequate specimens), easier sterilization, and sturdier construction with lower maintenance costs.[1] As mentioned previously, instruments with an outer cannula allow the optical system to be withdrawn and reinserted at will.

It is apparent that thoracoscopy can be performed satisfactorily using any one of a wide variety of instruments. The most important consideration is that the surgeon be familiar with the particular system chosen for use.

COMPLICATIONS

In our series of over 50 thoracoscopies, there have been no deaths or major complications related to the procedure. The only complication of note was in a 61-year-old male with a massive right pleural effusion, who developed infection evidenced by contralateral lower lobe collapse, fever, and a positive sputum culture following thoracoscopy and removal of 3½ liters of serous effusion. His infection responded to oral penicillin, but bronchoscopy was required 3 weeks later for removal of a mucous plug.

Table 18–3 lists some of the complications

Table 18–3. Complications of Thoracoscopy

Bleeding
Empyema
Pyogenic
Tuberculous
Subcutaneous emphysema
Tumor "seeding"
Cardiac ischemia/arrhythmias
Pulmonary complications
Atelectasis
Pneumonia
Bronchopleural fistula

of thoracoscopy that have been reported by various authors. The report by Boutin and colleagues is indicative of the relative rarity of these complications:[9] Between 1970 and 1980 they performed 215 thoracoscopies with no deaths and only 12 complications. Six patients (four with mesothelioma and two with metastatic carcinoma) developed tumor implantation at the thoracoscopy site; these workers now refer such patients for local radiation therapy (1700 rad) to the scar, beginning 10 days postoperatively. Two patients developed extensive subcutaneous emphysema, which required no specific therapy. One patient had a moderate intrapleural hemorrhage requiring a single-unit blood transfusion. Another patient developed an empyema "responding well to three intrapleural antibiotic instillations." An 87-year-old man had transient asymptomatic ischemic changes on his electrocardiogram. The last of the 12 patients experienced postanesthetic hypotension and tremors lasting 30 minutes. We agree with Boutin and colleagues that thoracoscopy is an extremely safe procedure in which "complications are rare, minor, and not life-threatening"; this assessment is also supported by Bloomberg's extensive review.[1]

RESULTS

We have used thoracoscopy both in its diagnostic and in its therapeutic capacities. The following studies and case reports are representative of our experience and that of others with this technique.

Diagnostic Thoracoscopy

We have studied in detail 17 patients who underwent thoracoscopy for the diagnosis of cryptogenic pleural effusions or for the biopsy of pleural-based masses.[10] There were ten males and seven females, ranging in age from 21 to 76 years. Thoracoscopy was employed only after less invasive procedures, such as thoracentesis with culture and cytologic examination of the effusion or blind pleural biopsies with an Abrams' needle, had failed to yield a definitive diagnosis.

In 11 of the 17 patients, a firm diagnosis of malignancy was established by thoracoscopy: Four patients had metastatic carcinoma; three, carcinoma of the lung; three, lymphoma; and one, thymoma. In the remaining six patients, specimens gathered at thoracoscopy revealed only inflammation. In five of these six patients, the duration of follow-up has been more than 3 years; none has developed evidence of malignant disease. The sixth patient had a pleural-based mass that proved to be recurrent Hodgkin's disease at the time of thoracotomy 6 months later. This case represents the only false-negative result in our series; there were no false-positives. Overall, thoracoscopy was diagnostic in 16 of the 17 patients, yielding a diagnostic accuracy rate of 94%. This accuracy is especially significant in light of the difficulties in diagnosis typically presented by patients with cryptogenic effusions.

How many patients with recurrent pleural effusions will remain undiagnosed after needle biopsy of the pleura, pleural fluid cytology, or both? We cannot calculate this from our series because we do not have complete data for the group of patients with effusions from which our referral patients were drawn. Bloomberg, however, reviewed four large series reporting the use of pleural needle biopsies for the evaluation of chronic effusions;[1] needle biopsy was reported diagnostic in 75% to 80% of patients with tuberculosis and in 60% to 62.5% of patients with malignant disease. Rao collected 1294 cases from several studies and found that 41% of biopsies led to a diagnosis of either tuberculosis or carcinoma.[11] In his own series of 154 needle biopsies in 124 patients, a definitive diagnosis was established in 65%. In 95 patients with malignant effusions, Salyer found that one or two needle biopsies were diagnostic in 53 patients (56%).[12] He also noted that pleural fluid cytopathology (two specimens) was diagnostic in 61 patients (64%). By combining the two modalities, he achieved an overall diagnostic accuracy rate of 90%. This result is similar to the finding by Boutin and coworkers that 79.5% of 1000 consecutive patients with chronic pleural effusions could be diagnosed by one or two thoracenteses, combined with one (75%), two (16%), or three (11%) Abrams' needle biopsies.[9]

What should be done with patients whose effusions remain unexplained after initial thoracentesis for cytologic examination or a single Abrams' needle biopsy? Salyer found some yield from repeating the studies: among his 95 patients, six neoplasms were diagnosed on a second needle biopsy, but only 11 of 48 patients were so studied. Likewise, 19 cancers were diagnosed on repeat cytologies (two, three, four, or more specimens), but only 32 of 45 undiagnosed patients had these additional studies.[12] Boutin's group sought to answer this question—at least for patients later proved to have malignant effusions—by repeat pleural cytology and needle biopsies the day prior to thoracoscopy in 150 patients whose lesions remained undiagnosed after at least two prior thoracenteses.[9] All had had at least one negative needle biopsy. Repeat pleural cytology was positive in 22% of patients, and repeat needle biopsy in 36%. By contrast, thoracoscopy was diagnostic of malignancy by gross appearance in 134 patients (89%) and by biopsy in 131 (87%). Since 1978, using improved instrumentation, the accuracy of thoracoscopic biopsy in their hands has increased to 97%. This is essentially identical with the findings of Brandt and Mai that 97.5% of effusions could be diagnosed by a combination of cytology, bacteriology, and thoracoscopy.[13] Provided that the surgeon is facile in the use of thoracoscopy, only the very rare patient should require formal thoracotomy for the diagnosis of a chronic pleural effusion.

Therapeutic Thoracoscopy

We recently reviewed the clinical course in 13 patients in whom thoracoscopy played a therapeutic as well as a diagnostic role.[3] The aim of thoracoscopy in these patients was foreign body extraction (in three patients), chemical pleurodesis for effusion or recurrent pneumothorax (in eight patients), or débridement of inadequately drained post-pneumonectomy empyema cavities (in two patients).

Foreign Body Extraction

Three patients were referred to the thoracic surgical service because of the presence of intrapleural foreign bodies; in each case, a small segment of polyethylene catheter had sheared off during thoracentesis and remained within the pleural cavity.

Patient 1. The first patient was a 16-year-old girl with severe systemic lupus erythematosus, which produced encephalitis, polyarthritis, nephrotic syndrome, and polyserositis; consequently she was receiving prednisone, 60 mg orally per day, and azathioprine, 100 mg orally per day. Thoracentesis for relief of a right pleural effusion was complicated by loss of the distal six inches of the polyethylene catheter used for fluid withdrawal. Because of the patient's immunosuppressed state, removal of the catheter segment was deemed advisable. The catheter was easily visualized using a 30° lens and was removed with a pleural biopsy forceps.

Patient 2. The second patient had a much smaller piece of catheter (approximately 1.5 cm in length) in the pleural space (Fig. 18–1). Because the catheter piece represented a possible nidus for infection, and because the patient was scheduled to undergo insertion of orthopedic hardware (Harrington rods) to stabilize a recent T5 vertebral fracture, removal was indicated. Thoracoscopic retrieval was aided by the intraoperative use of fluoroscopy.

Patient 3. The third patient was a 47-year-old man with a pathologic fracture of the right tibia (later proved secondary to metastatic renal cell carcinoma) and a chronic undiagnosed pleural effusion. He presented in acute respiratory failure, which was not significantly relieved by thoracentesis. He was found to have pulmonary emboli requiring anticoagulation; removal of the intrapleural catheter was therefore indicated. It was retrieved without difficulty using thoracoscopy.

If thoracoscopy had been unsuccessful, each of these patients would have required formal thoracotomy for removal of the foreign body or faced increased risks of medical management with the object left in place. There were no perioperative complications.

Chemical Pleurodesis

Eight patients, aged 33 to 71 years, underwent thoracoscopically guided chemical pleurodesis for either pleural effusion of varying etiology (in seven patients) or recurrent pneumothorax (in one patient). Four of the patients were males, and four were females. In all cases we wished to determine that there were no

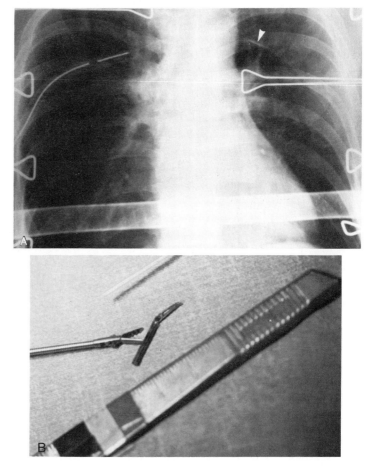

Figure 18–1. *A,* The chest roentgenogram of a 28-year-old man who fractured his fifth thoracic vertebra and became paraplegic secondary to a motorcycle accident. Thoracentesis to treat a left pleural effusion was complicated by loss of the distal 1.5 cm of the polyethylene catheter used for fluid withdrawal (see arrow). The fragment's intrapleural location was confirmed by its subsequent migration to the ipsilateral costophrenic sulcus. The foreign body represented a possible nidus for infection. Removal was therefore desirable prior to the placement of orthopedic hardware (Harrington rods) for spinal stabilization. *B,* Photograph showing the catheter fragment, the grasping forceps, and an undamaged catheter for comparison. Intraoperative fluoroscopy aided in the localization and removal of this small foreign body.

resectable lesions in the hemithorax prior to effecting pleural symphysis. We emphasize that blind obliteration of the pleural space will complicate thoracotomy if such later proves necessary; and in fact, although our results illustrate the value of thoracoscopy in ruling out the need for formal thoracotomy, two of our patients eventually did require thoracotomy.

Undiagnosed Effusion

In four of the seven patients with effusions, the underlying lesion remained undiagnosed in spite of multiple prior thoracenteses, pleural biopsies using the Abrams' needle, and other minimally invasive procedures, including bronchoscopy in two patients, needle aspirate of a lung nodule in the third patient, and needle aspiration of a pleural-based lesion in the fourth. In three of the four patients, a suspected diagnosis of malignancy was confirmed: metastatic breast carcinoma in two and metastatic renal cell carcinoma in the third. Satisfactory pleurodesis was achieved in all three patients, and they proceeded to chemotherapy without subsequent problems with pleural effusion (Fig. 18–2). Results in the fourth patient were less satisfactory:

Biopsy specimens from a 61-year-old man troubled by massive right pleural effusions of several months' duration revealed only nonspecific inflammation of the parietal pleura. A volume of 3½ liters of serous effusion was removed at thoracoscopy, which was complicated by infection as indicated by contralateral lower lobe collapse, fever,

and a positive sputum culture. The infection responded to oral penicillin, but the patient required bronchoscopy 3 weeks later for removal of a mucous plug. His effusion recurred in spite of two additional instillations of tetracycline. Four months after thoracoscopy he underwent open pleurectomy; histopathologic examination revealed only "chronic nonspecific pleuritis." One year later the patient died of a cerebral vascular accident. No malignancy was found at autopsy. Retrospective analysis suggested that his signs and symptoms were manifestations of the "yellow nail syndrome."[14]

Staging of Malignant Disease

Two patients with lung lesions had previously been found by cytologic examination to have malignant effusions:

A 57-year-old patient had undergone a 7-month course of multiple-drug chemotherapy for undifferentiated carcinoma, had no apparent distant metastases, and wished to be assured of the absolute unresectability of his disease. Thoracoscopy revealed widespread tumor implants involving both the visceral and parietal pleurae. Although chemical pleurodesis was performed, the patient continued to complain of severe fatigue, shortness of breath, and dyspnea on exertion. Roentgenograms showed near-total opacification of the right hemithorax. Loculated pleural fluid was suspected, and 6 weeks later the patient underwent exploratory thoracotomy to decorticate the right lung in hopes of lessening his symptoms. At operation, no free pleural cavity was found, indicating the success of the chemical pleurodesis; however, attempts to decorticate the lung were met with massive bleeding, and a pleuropneumonectomy was required for control. The patient survived operation only to succumb to

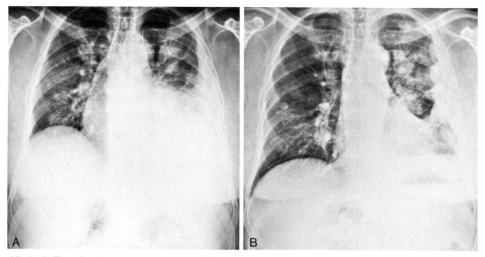

Figure 18–2. *A*, The chest roentgenogram of a 54-year-old man with a large pleural effusion that was undiagnosed in spite of two thoracenteses, an Abrams' needle biopsy of the pleura, and a needle biopsy of a left upper lobe nodule. Thoracoscopy revealed several pinkish-white nodules, which were then biopsied. Pathology was consistent with metastatic renal cell carcinoma, and a right renal mass was subsequently discovered. *B*, Chemical pleurodesis controlled the patient's effusion, even in the presence of considerable pleural disease.

his disease 9 months later in spite of continued multiple-drug chemotherapy.

A 68-year-old man with adenocarcinoma of the lung also insisted upon an "aggressive approach," not wishing to be declared categorically inoperable based upon cytologic studies alone. He too was found to have widespread intrapleural disease. Chemical pleurodesis was successful, and he was referred for palliative radiation and chemotherapy.

Removal of Postoperative Adhesions

A 63-year-old woman developed a left pleural effusion 5 years after mastectomy for breast carcinoma. Results of cytologic studies were positive, but the amount of effusion increased in spite of chemotherapy with cyclophosphamide, methotrexate, 5-fluorouracil, and doxorubicin. Because the effusion was loculated, pneumonolysis to allow full re-expansion of the involved lung was attempted thoracoscopically, but was only partially successful. The incision was therefore enlarged to about 10 cm in length to permit manual disruption of the remaining adhesions. The patient's disease progressed in spite of chemotherapy, hormonal therapy, and recombinant DNA interferon, but she remained asymptomatic with regard to her pleural effusion.

Pneumothorax

The eighth patient to undergo thoracoscopically directed chemical pleurodesis was a 33-year-old woman who presented with a recurrent left pneumothorax 3 years after thoracotomy and excision of apical blebs for a similar problem on the contralateral side. The patient, who liked to hike in remote areas, was willing to undergo pleurodesis in the hope of permanent cure, but she preferred to avoid thoracotomy if possible. Thoracoscopy was performed to rule out the presence of blebs or bullae prior to tetracycline instillation; at operation there were no adhesions or gross abnormalities of the pulmonary parenchyma. The parietal pleura overlying the second, third, and fourth ribs was scarified using the electrocautery, and 1 g of tetracycline was instilled. The chest tube was removed on the second postoperative day. Over a follow-up period of 5½ years, there has been no recurrence of pneumothorax.

Swierenga and colleagues, Vanderschueren, and Weissberg and Kaufman have all reported excellent results using thoracoscopy and insufflation of abestos-free talc (powdered anhydrous magnesium silicate) in the management of patients with *spontaneous* pneumothorax who do not have significant blebs or bullae.[15–17]

Therapeutic Failures

The two failures arose from incomplete pneumonolysis in one patient and from a recurrent massive effusion in the second. The procedure in the latter patient probably failed because of the large volume of his effusion and the apparent involvement of the entire pleural surface. The third patient to come to thoracotomy did so because he was incorrectly thought to have a persistent loculated effusion. In fact, his hemithorax was filled with malignant tumor; hence this case does not represent a failure or thoracoscopic pleurodesis.

DÉBRIDEMENT OF POST-PNEUMONECTOMY EMPYEMA CAVITIES

Two patients presented with signs and symptoms of continuing infection following open drainage of post-pneumonectomy empyema cavities. Using thoracoscopy, safe evaluation and drainage of the cavities was possible without resorting to extensive surgical procedures.

Patient 1. A 57-year-old man had his left lung removed in 1970 for oat cell carcinoma. He received postoperative radiation therapy and did well until October 1977, when he underwent creation of an Eloesser flap for drainage of an empyma. The flap was revised in August 1978, but the patient continued to be troubled by moderate to large amounts of foul-smelling drainage fluid. Cultures of the fluid grew multiple aerobic and anaerobic organisms. In July 1979, thoracoscopy was performed to débride the cavity, to evaluate the integrity of the bronchial closure, and to search for recurrent tumor. Under direct vision, approximately 50 ml of grumous material was removed; the bronchus was well healed, and there was no evidence of recurrent carcinoma. The pataient's symptoms abated, and he refused thoracoplasty.

Patient 2. A 56-year-old man underwent a right pneumonectomy in March 1978 for bronchogenic carcinoma. He received postoperative radiation therapy because of positive mediastinal nodes. In July 1980 he developed anorexia, fever, malaise, and anemia; a right-sided empyema was diagnosed and drained via chest tube. In September 1981 he underwent a seven-rib Schede thoracoplasty to obliterate the pleural space. Postoperatively he developed gram-negative sepsis and 5 weeks later was examined thoracoscopically to rule out a bronchopleural fistula, to search for recurrent tumor, and to débride the cavity (Fig. 18–3). Neither fistula nor tumor was encountered, and after débridement, thoracoscopic examination suggested the need for wider drainage of the posterolateral aspect of the cavity. This was accomplished, and the patient recovered uneventfully.

Weissberg has advocated thoracoscopy for all patients with loculated empyema not responding to drainage and antibiotics.[18] Among 19 such patients, he discovered one retained surgical sponge, one perforated esophageal tumor, and one bronchopleural fistula (all previously unsuspected). He believes that thora-

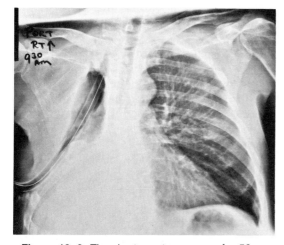

Figure 18–3. The chest roentgenogram of a 56-year-old man who developed an empyema 15 months after right pneumonectomy for bronchogenic carcinoma. Purulent discharge and systemic sepsis persisted in spite of tube drainage and subsequent seven-rib thoracoplasty. Thoracoscopy performed through the tube tract allowed the cavity to be inspected, safely débrided, and selectively enlarged. The patient did well without further surgical procedures.

coscopy allows better cleansing of empyema cavities and optimal positioning of drainage tubes. We have no experience using thoracoscopy in this clinical setting.

CONCLUSIONS

Obviously, any condition that can be diagnosed or treated by thoracoscopy can also be managed by thoracotomy. The purpose of thoracoscopy, however, is to spare selected patients the added morbidity and mortality of formal thoracotomy. Reported complications have been rare and well tolerated. Failures have been few when the technique has been employed for the indications discussed previously. Even if a few patients require thoracotomy because of a failure or complication of thoracoscopy, they are no worse off than if thoracotomy had been performed as the initial diagnostic or therapeutic procedure. We therefore believe that it is logical to attempt thoracoscopy in patients with appropriate indications for whom the only alternative is formal thoracotomy or empirical therapy based upon a suboptimal data base. We expect that the list of indications for thoracoscopy will increase as more surgeons gain familiarity and facility with this technique.

References

1. Bloomberg AE: Thoracoscopy in perspective. Surg. Gynecol Obstet 147:433–443, 1978.
2. Jacobaeus HC: The practical importance of thoracoscopy in surgery of the chest. Surg Gynecol Obstet 34:289–296, 1922.
3. Oakes DD, Sherck JP, Mark JBD: Therapeutic thoracoscopy. J Thorac Cardiovasc Surg 87:269–273, 1984.
4. Jones JW, Kitahama A, Webb WR, McSwain N: Emergency thoracoscopy: A logical approach to chest trauma management. J Trauma 21:280–284, 1981.
5. Burton NA, Watson DC, Brodsky JB, Mark JBD: Advantages of a new polyvinyl chloride double-lumen tube in thoracic surgery. Ann Thorac Surg 36:78–84, 1983.
6. Senno A, Moallem S, Quijano MD, et al: Thoracoscopy with the fiberoptic bronchoscope: A simple method in diagnosing pleuropulmonary diseases. J Thorac Cardiovasc Surg 67:606–611, 1974.
7. Lewis RJ, Kunderman PJ, Sisler GE, Mackenzie JW: Direct diagnostic thoracoscopy. Ann Thorac Surg 21:536–539, 1976.
8. Radigan LR, Glover JL: Thoracoscopy. Surgery 82:425–428, 1977.
9. Boutin C, Viallat JR, Cargnino P, Farisse P: Thoracoscopy in malignant pleural effusions. Am Rev Respir Dis 124:588–592, 1981.
10. Baumgartner WA, Mark JBD: The use of thoracoscopy in the diagnosis of pleural disease. Arch Surg 115:420–421, 1980.
11. Rao NV, Jones PO, Greenberg SD, et al: Needle biopsy of parietal pleura in 124 cases. Arch Intern Med 115:34–41, 1965.
12. Salyer WR, Eggleston JC, Erozan YS: Efficacy of pleural needle biopsy and pleural fluid cytopathology in the diagnosis of malignant neoplasm involving the pleura. Chest 67:536–539, 1975.
13. Brandt HJ, Mai J: Differential Diagnose des Pleuraergusses durch Thorakoskopie. Pneumonologie 145:192–203, 1971.
14. Hiller E, Rosenow EC, Olsen AM: Pulmonary manifestations of the yellow nail syndrome. Chest 61:452–458, 1972.
15. Swierenga J, Wagenaar JPM, Bergstein PGM: The value of thoracoscopy in the diagnosis and treatment of disease affecting the pleura and lung. Pneumonologie 151:11–18, 1974.
16. Vanderschueren RG: Le talcage pleural dans le pneumothorax spontané. Poumon Coeur 37:273–276, 1981.
17. Weissberg D, Kaufman M: Diagnostic and therapeutic pleuroscopy: Experience with 127 patients. Chest 78:732–735, 1980.
18. Weissberg D: Pleuroscopy in empyema: is it ever necessary? Poumon Coeur 37:269–272, 1981.

VI

The Use of Radionuclide Scans in Lung Cancer

Many pieces came together from many directions; some fit, and gradually a new discipline emerged—that of nuclear medicine. The new science grew by leaps and bounds with the explosion of knowledge and interest in atomic physics occasioned by World War II. Nuclear medicine has played an indispensable and vital role in medical progress during the past 40 years, with its involvement in countless areas of diagnosis and research.

The story began (1896) from one direction when Baumann observed that iodine was concentrated in the thyroid gland, a finding further substantiated by Oswald in his studies with thyroglobulin (1899). At almost the same time (1895) in another area Roentgen discovered invisible radiations that ionized the air and sensitized photographic emulsions. Because of their unknown character, he called them x-rays. The terms *radioactive* and *radioactivity* were introduced later (1898) by Pierre and Marie Curie.

Devices were developed, including the photographic plate, to register the emissions of these radioactive particles. And then in 1923, Hevesy investigated plant metabolism using a natural radioactive isotope of lead, the first recorded instance of a radioindicator in biology. Most importantly, Hevesy, sometimes termed the founder of nuclear medicine, recognized and demonstrated that the radioactivity of an element does not affect its biochemical characteristics. He understood that a radioactive atom could be used as a representative "tracer" along with its stable form in a biological system.

In 1924 Blumgart wanted to determine the speed of blood flow. "My attention was then brought to the possibility of the use of radioactive substances . . ." as material that could be injected and readily measured. He described (1927) an intravenous injection of saline and radon—the first "tracer" experiment in humans. In 1936, radiosodium was administered to three patients with leukemia. This was unsuccessful as regards benefit, but it was an introduction to therapeutic radioisotopes. The radiosodium had been produced in the cyclotron at Berkeley by the physicist, Ernest Lawrence. His physician brother John, realizing the preferential absorption of phosphorus in the hematopoietic tissues, introduced ^{32}P for the treatment of leukemia (1936).

Recalling the unique selectivity of the thyroid for iodine, Hertz, Roberts, and Evans (1938) did tracer studies with ^{128}I. Subsequently, ^{131}I was suggested and used for localized radiation to the thyroid, either as an alternative or an adjunct to surgery. Later it was given to thyroid cancer patients with functioning metastases (Seidlin, Marinelli, and Oshry).

The advent of the nuclear reactor ended the difficulty of producing and the scarcity of radioactive materials. With an announcement in *Science* (1946) of the public availability of radioactive isotopes, the modern era of nuclear medicine began. Radiochemicals emerged, new methods of scanning and recording (scintillation detectors) were designed, mechanical focusing by collimation was introduced, and imaging techniques for many different organs and disease states were developed. Clinical nuclear medicine was greatly assisted by the scintillation camera, invented by Anger (1958), in which a sodium iodide crystal is optically coupled with photomultiplier tubes. The data can be further enhanced by the addition of a computer.

Every thoracic surgeon would like to have a reliable method to diagnose and define bronchogenic carcinoma preoperatively both within and outside the chest. This is a continuing search, not yet ended. Meanwhile the controversies about scans still rage: *Which scans should be used? Which patients should be scanned?*

19

The Use of Radionuclide Scans in Lung Cancer: Gallium-67 Scanning for Preoperative Staging

Alex G. Little, M.D.
Tom R. DeMeester, M.D.
James W. Ryan, M.D.

It is important to emphasize accurate clinical staging in patients with lung cancer.[1] Use of a common staging system by all members of the medical community encourages precise, unambiguous communication and ensures the comparability of various modes of treatment.

The most important aspect of staging, however, is the direct relationship between stage of disease and the patient's prognosis: the more advanced the stage (i.e., the greater the extent of disease), the worse the prognosis. Knowledge of the extent or stage of disease therefore provides the most rational basis for selection of appropriate therapy. Precise and dependable clinical staging is particularly important in the selection of patients for surgical intervention, for two reasons: First, surgical resection, either alone or as part of a multimodality therapeutic approach, is essential for the possibility of cure. No patient should be denied operation because of inaccurate or incomplete clinical staging. Second, accurate clinical staging that reliably identifies absolute contraindications to surgical intervention, such as widespread metastatic disease, or relative contraindications, such as mediastinal nodal metastases or invasion of extrapulmonary structures by the primary tumor, is important so that the patient is spared an unnecessary or fruitless operation.

Recognizing the importance of accurate clinical staging, we have routinely employed gallium-67 scanning for 8 years in the staging of lung cancer patients in the Chest Oncology Group at the University of Chicago Hospitals and Clinics. Our extensive experience with the use of gallium scanning has convinced us that it is an invaluable component of the staging process.

INDICATIONS AND TECHNIQUE

We do not recommend that gallium-67 scanning be used as a screening examination for the detection of lung carcinoma. In addition to having a high affinity for lung cancer cells, gallium-67 also concentrates in some inflammatory cells and certain other tumor cells.[2] Abnormal foci of gallium accumulation may therefore be present in patients with acute bacterial infections, sarcoidosis, Hodgkin's disease, lymphoma, and melanoma; such patients, though usually identifiable clinically, will often have positive gallium-67 scans. The best use of gallium-67 scanning in lung cancer patients is for staging the extent of disease prior to initiation of therapy.

Our technique is described here in detail because our results and conclusions are dependent upon our methods. Inappropriate criticisms have come from others who have used different techniques and, not surprisingly, have failed to duplicate our results.[3]

A frequent complaint regarding gallium-67 scanning is poor image quality. We have achieved considerable improvement by several steps:[4]

1. Using an injected dose of 10 mCi to increase the number of photons that generate the image.
2. Using three separate pulse height analyzers for simultaneous detection of the 93-, 184-, and 300-kev photon emissions of gallium-67.
3. Increasing the scanning time.
4. Increasing the time interval from tracer injection to scanning from 48 to 72 hours to allow a decrease in "background" activity to

occur, while further gallium concentration in the abnormal site takes place, so that contrast is enhanced.

5. Employing tomographic imaging routinely in our institution for gallium scanning. Currently we use a Pho/Con scanner with 12 longitudinal projections per study. This delineates the abnormal sites in the chest and allows their differentiation from the sternum, spine, and ribs. This technique also aids interpretation of tracer uptake in the abdomen caused by residual gallium in the colon, which can occur despite routine bowel cleansing with laxatives prior to scanning.

In general, the minimal abnormality size required for detection with gallium-67 scanning is about 2 cm. Smaller abnormalities cannot be consistently separated from the background. If other radionuclide scans are planned in addition to gallium scanning, they should be obtained prior to the gallium study because gallium-67 is retained by the tissues for several days and, once in place, may necessitate a delay before other scans can be performed.

RESULTS

It is useful to analyze our results with gallium-67 scanning from three aspects: First, what can be learned from a gallium scan about the primary tumor? Second, what is the reliability regarding evaluation of the mediastinum for nodal metastases? Finally, can metastatic tumor—especially when clinically occult—be identified?

Primary Tumor. Although we do not advocate gallium scanning as a routine screening test for detection of lung carcinoma, it is useful to know the accuracy regarding lung cancer primary tumors because important information regarding the nature of a lung mass can be obtained. Prospective evaluation of 123 patients with abnormal chest roentgenograms suggestive of primary carcinoma of the lung was carried out at the University of Chicago by our Chest Oncology Group between July 1, 1976 and August 1, 1977.[4] Of these 123 patients, 23 were ultimately proved to have a lesion metastatic to the lung from another primary tumor or benign pulmonary disease. There was discrete gallium uptake in the primary tumor (i.e., the scan was positive in the primary) in 96 of the 100 patients with histologically proved carcinoma of the lung. A representative example is shown in Figure 19–1. In other words, the sensitivity (the probability that gallium-67 scanning will identify lung cancer when it is present) is 96%. Of the 23 patients without lung cancer, 13 had a single pulmonary metastasis from a primary tumor elsewhere and in 7 the lesion was gallium-positive. Of 10 of these patients with benign abnormality, 3 had positive gallium scans. In sum, of 106 patients with positive scans, 96 had a primary carcinoma of the lung. This means that a positive gallium-67 scan has a predictive value of 91%.

What about so-called "negative scans," i.e., those with no abnormal focal gallium accumulations? Of the 17 patients with a negative gallium scan, only 4 had a primary lung carcinoma. This means that the predictive value of a negative scan for the absence of primary carcinoma of the lung is 76%, and that the specificity (the probability a scan will be negative when lung cancer is not present) is 59%.

Mediastinal and Hilar Evaluation. Of the prospectively evaluated 100 lung cancer patients, 66 had invasive mediastinal staging by mediastinoscopy or thoracotomy in addition to gallium-67 scanning. The presence of contralateral hilar node uptake of gallium-67 is considered synonymous with mediastinal lymph node uptake. The results are shown in Tables 19–1 and 19–2. Although overall results are given, it is important to separate results for paramediastinal tumors from those for more peripherally located tumors because of the difficulty in distinguishing gallium-67 uptake by mediastinal lymph nodes when the primary tumor is adjacent to the mediastinum (Fig. 19–2).

Table 19–1. Results of Gallium-67 Scanning for Mediastinal Staging Compared with Biopsy Results

| | Gallium Scan Results | | | | | | | | |
| | Peripheral Primaries | | | Paramediastinal Primaries | | | All Tumors | | |
Biopsy Results	Positive	Negative	Total	Positive	Negative	Total	Positive	Negative	Total
Mediastinum positive	7	5	12	12	10	22	19	15	34
Mediastinum negative	1	25	26	1	5	6	2	30	32
All tumors	8	30	38	13	15	28	21	45	66

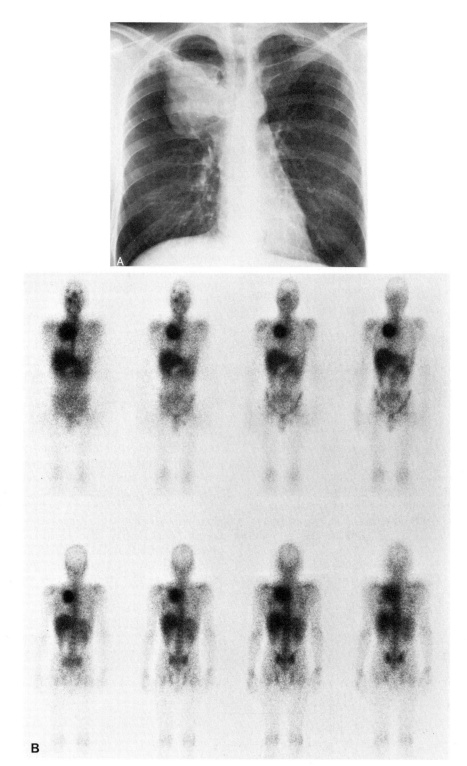

Figure 19–1. The patient was a 47-year-old man with a long smoking history who presented with a cough. *A,* Chest roentgenogram showing a right upper lobe mass. Bronchoscopy was performed; examination of the tissue obtained revealed squamous cell carcinoma. *B,* Gallium-67 scan showing the series of tomographic images routinely obtained. The only abnormal activity is in the primary tumor. The patient subsequently underwent right upper lobectomy. The final pathologic classification was Stage I, $T_2N_0M_{0x}$.

Table 19–2. Accuracy and Predictive Value of Gallium-67 Scanning in Mediastinal Staging[a]

Location of Primary Tumor	Sensitivity (%)	Specificity (%)	Accuracy (%)	Predictive Value	
				Positive Scan (%)	Negative Scan (%)
Peripheral primaries	58	96	84	86	83
Paramediastinal primaries	55	83	61	92	33
All tumors	56	94	74	90	67

[a]Data derived from Table 1.

Fifteen of the 66 patients had false-negative gallium-67 scans of the mediastinum. In seven of these patients the involved nodes were adjacent to a paramediastinal primary tumor. In four patients, small, intranodal mediastinal metastases were present; these lesions measured less than the 2-cm threshold size for detection by gallium scanning. Four of the false-negative scans were in patients who had supraclavicular lymph node metastases, which could not be differentiated from normal gallium uptake by the sternoclavicular joint.

Distant Organ Evaluation. Forty of the 100 lung cancer patients were found to have one or more distant organ metastases during the initial staging evaluation. In 28 of these 40

Figure 19–2. The patient was a 52-year-old female who presented with a change in her chronic cough. *A,* Chest roentgenogram showing a left suprahilar mass. *B,* Gallium-67 scan reveals uptake in the primary lesion and definite, separate mediastinal activity. Subsequent mediastinoscopy proved the presence of mediastinal nodal metastases.

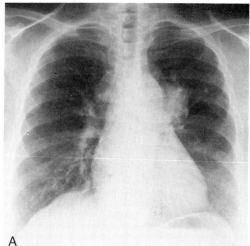

A

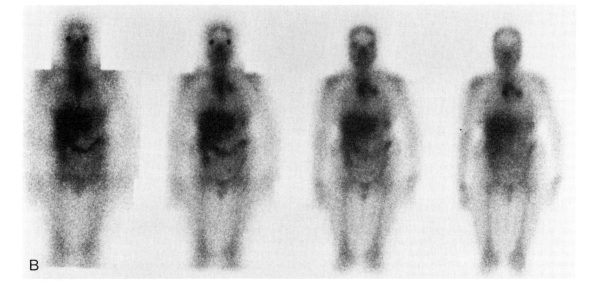

B

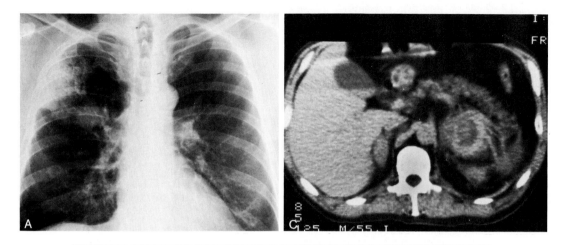

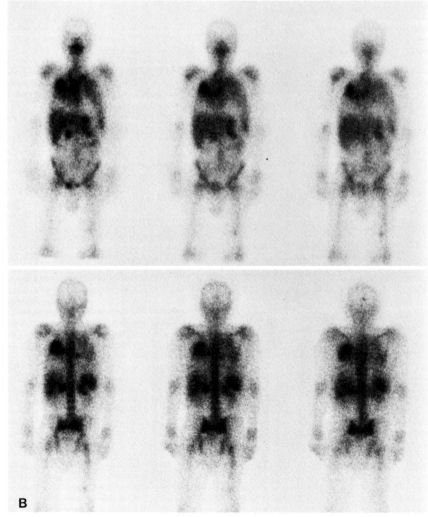

Figure 19–3. The patient was a 61-year-old male smoker who presented to the hospital with pneumonia. *A*, The chest roentgenogram shows a right upper lobe mass with a distal, obstructive pneumonia. Bronchoscopy proved this to be an adenocarcinoma. There were no signs or symptoms of metastatic disease. *B*, The gallium-67 scan reveals typical activity in the primary tumor site (and the pneumonitic region as well) and definite abnormal activity in the region of the right adrenal gland (*arrow*). *C*, Subsequent CT scan demonstrated a necrotic metastasis within the left adrenal gland (*open arrow*) as well as the solid metastasis, causing the gallium-67 uptake, in the right adrenal gland (*solid arrow*).

patients (70%), the distant metastases were symptomatic. In 12 (30%), however, the distant metastases were occult and were detected solely by radionuclide imaging studies. Of these 12 patients with clinically occult metastatic disease, 11 (92%) were detected by gallium-67 scanning alone, and the addition of other scans offered no clinical benefit (Fig. 19–3). In the larger group of 40 patients, gallium-67 scanning had a sensitivity for detecting distant organ metastasis of 88%, a specificity of 100%, and an accuracy of 92%. That is, there were no false-positive scans in these 40 patients.

CONCLUSIONS

We have derived three general principles from our experience with gallium scanning that are applicable to staging of patients with bronchogenic carcinoma.

1. If a mass seen on chest roentgenogram is clinically suspicious for carcinoma of the lung and the gallium scan is discretely positive, the probability that this lesion represents a bronchogenic carcinoma is 91%. Conversely, if the gallium scan is normal, there is a 76% probability that this mass does not represent a primary bronchogenic carcinoma.

2. When the primary tumor has discrete gallium positivity and the mediastinum or contralateral hilum or both also demonstrate gallium uptake, the probability that a mediastinal or contralateral hilar node metastasis is present is 90%. On the other hand, if the primary tumor is gallium-positive and neither the mediastinum nor the contralateral hilum has discrete uptake, there is a 67% probability that mediastinal or contralateral hilar lymph node metastases are not present.

3. When the primary tumor is gallium-positive, the probability that discrete areas of extrapulmonary gallium uptake represent metastatic disease is greater than 90%.

The results that we have obtained by incorporating gallium-67 scanning as a standard part of our clinical staging approach to patients with lung cancer are shown in Figures 19–4 and 19–5. It is clear from Figure 19–4 that addition of gallium-67 scanning to initial clinical staging provides valuable information. Figure 19–5 shows that clinical staging incorporating gallium-67 scanning is very accurate when compared with surgical/pathologic staging.

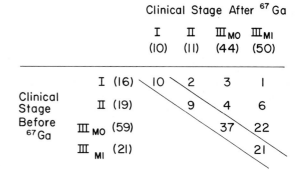

| | | Clinical Stage After ^{67}Ga | | | |
		I (10)	II (11)	III$_{MO}$ (44)	III$_{MI}$ (50)
Clinical Stage Before ^{67}Ga	I (16)	10	2	3	1
	II (19)		9	4	6
	III$_{MO}$ (59)			37	22
	III$_{MI}$ (21)				21

Figure 19–4. The impact of gallium-67 scanning on clinical staging of 115 patients with proved lung cancer in a University of Chicago series. (Numbers refer to numbers of patients.) The clinical information used to classify patients before use of gallium-67 scanning came from history-taking, physical examination, and standard clinical laboratory tests such as liver function tests, peripheral blood counts, and urinalysis. (From Little AG et al: The staging of lung cancer. Semin Oncol 10:56–70, 1983.)

Figure 19–5. The accuracy of clinical staging incorporating gallium-67 scanning compared with final staging utilizing biopsy results and findings at surgical exploration and/or resection. (The series of patients is the same as that in Fig. 19–4; numbers refer to numbers of patients.) (From Little AG et al: The staging of lung cancer. Semin Oncol 10:56–70, 1983.)

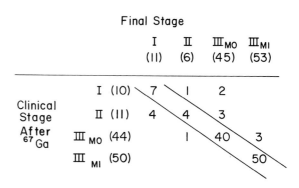

| | | Final Stage | | | |
		I (11)	II (6)	III$_{MO}$ (45)	III$_{MI}$ (53)
Clinical Stage After ^{67}Ga	I (10)	7	1	2	
	II (11)	4	4	3	
	III$_{MO}$ (44)		1	40	3
	III$_{MI}$ (50)				50

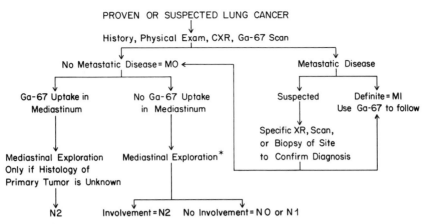

Figure 19–6. Flow diagram representing the approach to clinical staging of patients with lung cancer at the University of Chicago. In patients without mediastinal uptake of gallium-67, mediastinal exploration is not performed prior to thoracotomy in those with T₁ primary tumors because of the low yield.

We have established a sequential approach to clinical staging in patients with proved or suspected lung cancer, using gallium-67 scanning as an integral component, which is based on the experience presented here. This approach is outlined in Figure 19–6.

COMPUTED TOMOGRAPHY VERSUS GALLIUM-67 SCANNING

Several groups have evaluated computed tomographic (CT) scanning of the chest in lung cancer patients, primarily for mediastinal staging. Results have varied, primarily depending upon the criteria utilized for definition of abnormal lymph nodes. For example, where the identification of any mediastinal lymph node by CT scanning was considered evidence of abnormality, a sensitivity of 80% and a specificity of 76% were achieved based on final histologic staging.[5] According to this evaluation, a CT scan showing no mediastinal abnormality is sufficient evidence that mediastinal lymph node metastases are not present and that mediastinoscopy prior to thoracotomy is not required. However, when a lymph node size of 15 mm or greater is chosen as the definition of abnormal, different results and conclusions are reported.[6] Selecting this larger node size to represent an abnormal finding decreases sensitivity, but specificity rises to greater than 90%. This still does not solve the dilemma of identified nodes that are smaller than 15 mm.

Apparently, a completely normal CT scan of the mediastinum is a reliable clinical indicator that mediastinal lymph nodes do not contain metastatic deposits. Positive CT scans are a diagnostic problem, however, because enlarged, reactive processes secondary to pulmonary infection or inflammation may be responsible for the identified adenopathy. It would be unfortunate if potentially curative resection were withheld in such cases.

It is possible that the two procedures of CT scanning and gallium scanning for mediastinal staging may be complementary, because gallium scanning is most predictive when it is positive, with a specificity of greater than 90%, whereas CT scans are most accurate when they demonstrate a normal mediastinum (i.e., when they are negative). We are presently evaluating this possibility at our institution. It is a consideration that CT scanning is slightly more expensive than gallium scanning and does not provide as extensive a screen for distant organ metastatic disease.

References

1. Little AG, DeMeester TR, MacMahon H: The staging of lung cancer. Semin Oncol 10:56–70, 1983.
2. Alazraki N: Usefulness of gallium imaging in the evaluation of lung cancer. CRC Crit Rev Diagn Imaging, 13:249–267, 1980.
3. Nieweg OE, Beekhuis H, Piers DA, et al: ⁵⁷Co-bleomycin and ⁶⁷Ga-citrate in detecting and staging lung cancer. Thorax 38:16–21, 1983.
4. DeMeester TR, Golomb HM, Kirchner P, et al: The role of gallium-67 scanning in the clinical staging and preoperative evaluation of patients with carcinoma of the lung. Ann Thorac Surg 28:451–464, 1979.
5. Rea HH, Shevland JE, House AJS: Accuracy of computed tomographic scanning in assessment of the mediastinum in bronchial carcinoma. J Thorac Cardiovasc Surg 81:826–829, 1981.
6. Modini C, Passariello R, Iascone C, et al: TNM staging in lung cancer: role of computed tomography. J Thorac Cardiovasc Surg 84:569–574, 1982.

20

The Use of Radionuclide Scans in Lung Cancer: The Case Against Routine Multiorgan Scans

James B. D. Mark, M.D.

It is generally agreed that surgical resection provides the best chance of cure in patients with non–oat cell, T_1 or T_2, N_0 or N_1 (Stage I or II), M_0 carcinoma of the lung. There are some patients with T_3 lesions (those with attachment to the chest wall, for example) or even N_2 lesions who might be considered for resection, but such cases are more controversial. Some patients with oat cell carcinoma are also candidates for resection, particularly those rare patients with peripheral, localized oat cell carcinoma and those with limited disease who have responded well to chemotherapy. As a rule, however, operation is contraindicated in patients with distant metastases from lung cancer. There are rare exceptions to this rule; for example, a patient with a peripheral lung cancer, a single metastasis in the liver, and major hemoptysis from the cancer would probably be best served by palliative lobectomy. Nonetheless, the rule is a good one. The problem is, then, how to confirm the presence or absence of distant metastases in patients with otherwise operable lung cancer.

PRINCIPLES OF EVALUATION

Each patient with a lung mass referred for diagnosis and treatment presents a different combination of problems, each has a different attitude or set of mind, and each requires judgment in management, but evaluation must always be directed at answering the following questions:

1. What is the mass?
2. What is the local extent of disease?
3. Will the patient's general condition, especially cardiorespiratory reserve, allow the proposed operation to be carried out safely?
4. Are there distant metastases that would preclude resection?

The full array of possible investigative procedures is not indicated in every patient. For example, in a patient with a hard supraclavicular node and a lung lesion, biopsy of the node rather than bronchoscopy is the diagnostic procedure of choice, and pulmonary function tests are unnecessary.

Definitive Diagnosis

Obtaining a definitive diagnosis is the most frequently overlooked part of the evaluation; at least, its importance is undervalued. Many physicians are apt to do various laboratory tests and scanning procedures before determining what the lesion is. Although many suspicious peripheral lesions are resected for both diagnosis and treatment, certain others, particularly proximal lesions, deserve more local and less peripheral evaluation, at least initially.

For lesions within the reach of the flexible bronchoscope, bronchoscopy is the diagnostic procedure of choice. With proper technique, biopsy of a lesion under direct vision is essentially 100% accurate in determining the cell type of the tumor. Lesions beyond the reach of the bronchoscope may be biopsied transbronchoscopically under fluoroscopic guidance with a diagnostic accuracy of 50% or 60%. For such peripheral lesions, percutaneous needle aspiration of the lesion under fluoroscopic control provides a specific diagnosis in over 80% of lung cancer patients.

Histologic or cytologic diagnosis of carcinoma is not necessary prior to thoracotomy in every patient with a peripheral lesion. We recommend thoracotomy with resection for diagnosis and treatment in any new, noncalcified peripheral lesion over 1 cm in diameter in any adult smoker, male or female, judged able to tolerate the appropriate resection. We do not, however, perform routine multiorgan scanning prior to thoracotomy in such patients if they are asymptomatic and have normal results on neurologic examination and liver function tests.

Local Extent of Disease

Computed tomography of the chest is the best examination for determination of the local extent of disease.[8] Bronchoscopy for this purpose by the thoracic surgeon is mandatory if the result is critical in the decision for or against operation. Computed tomography (CT) in our institution has been highly sensitive and almost as highly specific in the detection of mediastinal adenopathy due to metastatic cancer and of other reasons for local unresectability. We do not do chest CT scanning in all patients prior to thoracotomy. A normal-appearing mediastinum on posteroanterior and lateral chest films in a patient with a peripheral lesion serves to rule out the need for further radiographic investigation. In those patients found to have enlarged mediastinal nodes on the CT scan, we recommend mediastinoscopy or anterior mediastinotomy for proof of diagnosis in most instances.

General Condition of the Patient

The most critical aspect of the general condition of the patient is cardiorespiratory reserve. Since most patients with lung cancer are cigarette smokers, they are apt to have cardiac and pulmonary disease in addition to the cancer. History and physical examination are of critical importance. If a patient has good respiratory reserve clinically and the planned resection is almost certainly lobectomy, then we do not do routine pulmonary function tests. If there is a question of adequate pulmonary reserve or if pneumonectomy is contemplated, then pulmonary function tests are carried out. On occasion, quantitative perfusion lung scans for determining differential pulmonary function will be indicated.

Investigation for Distant Metastases

Symptoms suggestive of distant metastases, such as bone pain or dizziness, deserve closer investigation. However, our position on patients with no suggestion of metastases on careful history and physical examination is that routine radionuclide and/or CT scanning is not justified.

The most frequent sites of occult metastases in patients with carcinoma of the lung are liver, adrenal, brain, and bone. These are therefore areas to which most attention should be directed in the history and physical examination. Has there been anorexia, weight loss, or fatigue to suggest systemic disease? Has there been recent dizziness or localized weakness, loss of memory or sensation, or headache? Is there evidence of deficit on neurologic examination? Has there been bone pain? Is there jaundice or is the liver enlarged? Are liver function tests and serum electrolytes normal? Clearly if there is any clinical suspicion of metastatic disease, appropriate investigations should be pursued. If not, the strong preponderance of evidence shows that performance of routine multiorgan scans is neither clinically rewarding nor economically justified.[1–7, 9–14]

Experience with over 1000 patients with lung cancer at Stanford Medical Center over the past 10 years, several hundred of whom have been patients with Stage I or II disease, has led us to adopt the following plan. If the tumor is a peripheral lung carcinoma amenable to "clean" lobectomy (clinical Stage I or II) as indicated on chest films or CT scans or both and if there is no suggestion by history, physical examination, or routine laboratory examination that metastases are present, we do not obtain brain, bone, or liver scans in order to search for occult metastatic disease, although any abnormality is investigated further. This approach has yielded satisfactory results. No patient with pathologic Stage I disease showed clinical evidence of distant metastases during the first postoperative year. A small number of patients with pathologic Stage II disease developed brain metastases during the first postoperative year, but none within the first 6 months, making it unlikely that preoperative scanning would have detected the problem.

Preoperative multiorgan scanning is more appropriate in patients with proximal lesions, that is, those who will require pneumonectomy. Even in these patients, the incidence of occult metastases is low, but the risks and benefits of the operation that they face are such that even low-yield procedures of little or no risk and moderate cost may be justified.

SELECTION OF APPROPRIATE SCANS

Our selection of scanning procedure is based on its sensitivity and specificity for the specific organ. In the brain, CT scan is more sensitive and more specific than radionuclide scan and is therefore our choice. Radionuclide bone scan is far more sensitive than an x-ray bone survey for bone metastases. Any abnormality on bone scan should be pursued by radiographs of the area in question to help detect or rule out metastatic disease; old fractures and osteoarthritis are the most common reasons for false-positive results. Old rib fractures may be especially confusing: if the "hot spots" are all in a row or grouped, they are more likely to be the result of old fractures than if they are scattered in a random fashion; x-ray confirmation is frequently helpful. On occasion, needle biopsy or even open biopsy may be necessary.

When liver scanning is indicated, we use radionuclide scanning for initial screening. This is a relatively inexpensive procedure of moderate sensitivity but relatively low specificity. If obvious metastases are present, they may be confirmed by needle biopsy of the liver. If the radionuclide scan is equivocal, CT liver scan with contrast may help to clarify the problem.

Other investigators recommend gallium scans for detection of both primary and metastatic disease. Our experience with these scans is limited and relatively unfavorable, so we do not use them.

CONCLUSIONS

The literature is replete with articles for and against the use of routine multiorgan scanning in patients with lung cancer. Very few of the studies reported in these articles relate the clinical stage of the disease to the incidence of positive scans in asymptomatic patients. Even more important, few of the studies include the incidence of positive scans in those patients whose other screening tests were negative for metastatic disease. We agree with Rossi, who states, "Scanning (liver, brain, bone) has been abandoned for surgical patients because the yield has been too low to justify routine use."[11]

He goes on to say that ". . .the incidence of positive scan in asymptomatic Stage I and Stage II patients [is] less than 1%."[11]

Because of satisfaction with our plan for the past 10 years and because of widespread support from the available literature, we do not perform routine multiorgan scanning in asymptomatic patients with operable lung cancer.

References

1. Benfield JR: III. Staging, operations and adjuvant therapy. Curr Probl Cancer 1:22–34, 1977.
2. Bone RC, Balk R: Staging of bronchogenic carcinoma. Chest 82:473–480, 1982.
3. Butler AR, Leo JS, Lin JP, et al: The value of routine cranial computed tomography in neurologically intact patients with primary carcinoma of the lung. Radiology 131:339–401, 1979.
4. Gravenstein S, Peltz MA, Pories W: How ominous is an abnormal scan in bronchogenic carcinoma? JAMA 241:2523–2524, 1979.
5. Hooper RG, Beechler C, Johnson MC: Radioisotope scanning in the initial staging of bronchogenic carcinoma. Am Rev Resp Dis 118:279–286, 1978.
6. Johnson DH, Windham WW, Allen JH, Greco FA: Limited value of CT brain scans in the staging of small cell lung cancer. AJR 140:37–40, 1983.
7. Kies MS, Baker AW, Kennedy PS: Radionuclide scans in staging of carcinoma of the lung. Surg Gynecol Obstet 147:175–176, 1978.
8. Modini C, Passariello R, Iascone C, et al: TNM staging in lung cancer: Role of computed tomography. J Thorac Cardiovasc Surg 84:569–574, 1982.
9. Poon PY, Feld R, Evans WK, et al: Computed tomography of the brain, liver, and upper abdomen in the staging of small cell carcinoma of the lung. J Comput Assist Tomogr 6:963–965, 1982.
10. Ramsdell JV, Peters RM, Taylor AT Jr, et al: Multiorgan scans for staging lung cancer. J Thorac Cardiovasc Surg 73:653–659, 1977.
11. Rossi NP: Radionuclide scans. Postgraduate Course in Thoracic Surgery, American College of Surgeons, 69th Annual Clinical Congress, 1983.
12. Smalley RV, Malmud LS, Ritchie WGM: Pre-operative scanning: Evaluation for metastatic disease in carcinoma of the breast, lung, colon, bladder, and prostate. Semin Oncol 7:358–369, 1980.
13. Turner P, Haggith JW: Pre-operative radionuclide scanning in bronchogenic carcinoma. Br J Dis Chest 75:291–294, 1981.
14. White DM, McMahon LJ, Denny WF: Usefulness outcome in evaluating the utility of nuclear scans of the bone, brain, and liver in bronchogenic carcinoma patients. Am J Med Sci 283:114–118, 1982.

21

The Use of Radionuclide Scans in Lung Cancer: The Case for Routine Multiorgan Scans

Ernest W. Fordham, M.D.
Amjad Ali, M.D.

With lung cancer the leading cause of cancer deaths in males and rapidly becoming the same in females, and with the majority of lung cancer patients failing because of multiorgan metastases, there has been considerable interest in developing a reliable test to detect metastases at the initial evaluation of these patients. Radionuclide imaging has been used for this purpose with varying success.

GENERALLY ACCEPTED CRITERIA FOR SCANS

There is general agreement that the appropriate evaluation of the patient with lung cancer includes multiorgan imaging when (1) the cell type is oat cell (small cell), (2) the patient has symptoms, signs, or biochemical evidence of metastases, or (3) the patient is asymptomatic but the primary lesion is extensive, with radiographic or other clinical evidence of regionally advanced disease.[1–6]

Some authors suggest that scanning should be limited to those organs suspected to be involved, as indicated by abnormal symptoms, signs, or biochemical abnormalities. However, one group of investigators has suggested that the presence of any one of a brief but comprehensive list of clinical findings should precipitate the spectrum of imaging studies, since in their study correlation with organ-specific findings was not reliable, whereas correlation with the spectrum of clinical findings was excellent.[3] For example, weight loss was noted in 47.6%, hepatomegaly in 43%, and elevated serum alkaline phosphatase level in 66.6% of patients with positive liver scans. One or more of these findings were present in 76% of patients, but 24% patients with "true-positive" liver scans did not exhibit any clinical evidence of liver disease. Similarly, central nervous system (CNS) symptoms were present in 50% and

neurologic abnormalities in 56% of patients with positive brain scans. One or both of these findings were noted in 62% of the patients, but both were absent in 38%. However, all patients with positive brain and liver scans had other non-organ-specific clinical evidence of metastases. Of patients with positive bone scans, a history of bone pain was noted in 47.6%, bone tenderness was elicited by physical examination in 14.3%, and increased serum alkaline phosphatase concentrations were found in 47.6%. Again, one or more of these findings were noted in 75% of patients with a positive bone scan, while 25% showed no clinical evidence of osseous metastases. In contrast with brain and liver imaging, 8% of the positive bone scans were from patients with *none* of the clinical indicators of metastatic disease, but half of these were considered false-positives. Thus, only 4% of the bone scans from the completely asymptomatic patients were true-positives.

SCANNING IN THE ASYMPTOMATIC PATIENT

There is great variance of opinion regarding the value of multiorgan imaging in asymptomatic lung cancer patients, particularly those with stage I or II bronchogenic carcinoma. Most authors believe that the yield from routine multiple-organ imaging in this group is too low to warrant the additional hospitalization time and expense involved.[3, 7, 8] However Kelly and colleagues reported that 18.4% of their patients with no clinical evidence of metastatic disease to bone, liver, or brain had at least one kind of abnormal radionuclide study.[1]

A typical example of this view is found in a prospective study of 100 patients with clinical findings suggesting resectable bronchogenic carcinoma who had multiorgan imaging (brain, liver, and bone scans).[7] In the 52 patients of this group who had resectable disease, there was discordance between scans and clinical evaluation in 25 of 153 scans (16%). Two of 22 negative studies were false-negative. Sixteen of 17 positive studies unsupported by clinical findings proved to be false-positive. Only one scan in the face of absent clinical findings proved to be true-positive. In the face of such evidence it is readily apparent why routine multiorgan imaging in the asymptomatic patient with early disease has been abandoned at many institutions. Identification of early metastases in these patients has been limited to no more than a few percent, often at the cost of false-positive rates equaling or even exceeding true-positive rates. For example, Hooper and coworkers did not find any patients with brain or liver metastases on scanning without one or more clinical findings of metastatic disease (not necessarily pointing to the involved organ). Only 4% of the bone scans identified disease in the absence of clinical findings, and then only at the cost of a 4% false-positive rate.

Yet the majority of the patients with lung cancer (including those with resectable bronchogenic carcinoma) fail, and they fail primarily because of distant metastases that must have been present at the time of surgery (Fig. 21–1). Obviously, more sensitive indicators of the metastatic distribution of disease than those heretofore available are needed.

EXPERIENCES AND RESULTS

Our experience, gained through routine multiorgan imaging in all of our lung cancer patients in the late 1970s and early 1980s, is somewhat at variance with most clinical studies reported in the literature but closely parallels that reported by Kelly and colleagues.[1] The pickup rate for silent metastases in the patient with resectable bronchogenic carcinoma is low even in our experience, but it is high enough to warrant the routine use of liver, brain, and bone imaging. Exact figures are, as yet, not available, but it is quite clear that a pickup rate of about 10% can be expected in these patients when all three organs are imaged without incurring comparable false-positive rates (as with bone scanning). The pickup of the silent, clinically unsuspected disease is distributed evenly among the three organs, with perhaps a slightly greater pickup on skeletal scintigraphy; only rarely have we found more

than one organ to be involved in any given patient with asymptomatic disease.

We have wondered at the disparity between our experience and that reported in the literature and believe that it can be related to the methodology. Most of the articles recommending omission of routine multiorgan imaging in the asymptomatic patient were generated in the mid- to late 1970s, from studies performed in the mid- and earlier 1970s. Marked changes in nuclear medicine technology occurred rapidly during this period. Indeed, when procedures employed in these studies are examined it is apparent that the radiopharmaceuticals and, particularly, the equipment were strikingly inferior to those that became available shortly thereafter. The old dual-probe scanners, so necessary for the high-energy emission of strontium-85 of the 1960s and fluorine-18 of the early 1970s in skeletal imaging, are totally inadequate when compared with the superior characteristics of the technetium-99m (^{99m}Tc) labeled bone-seeking radiopharmaceuticals of today. The scintillation cameras of that era, requiring three passes—producing two seams—to cover the average patient, were even worse, not so much because of the seams themselves but because of poor uniformity, which routinely produced gross artifacts at the seams and undoubtedly contributed to both high false-positive and false-negative rates. Poor resolution prevented precise assessment of the *location* of lesions and robbed the observer of the most important tool in differentiating various osseous disorders: pattern recognition.

Modern instrumentation permits single-pass scanning with "jumbo" cameras and two-pass imaging with large-field cameras and provides a more accurate assessment of patterns of abnormality. This improved uniformity has eliminated much of the troublesome artifacts, especially at seams, and has improved resolution to allow more precise localization and better definition of lesions. The focal lesion on a bone scan is a nonspecific finding representing osseous reaction to a focus of tumor, infection, trauma, and so on. However, when lesions become more diffuse in extent, number, or both, the *pattern* generated is usually a very reliable indicator of the underlying insult (Fig. 21–2).

Similarly, the radiopharmaceuticals employed in that era left much to be desired. The ^{99m}Tc-labeled polyphosphates, which brought routine bone scanning to the community hospital, were extremely variable in quality. These

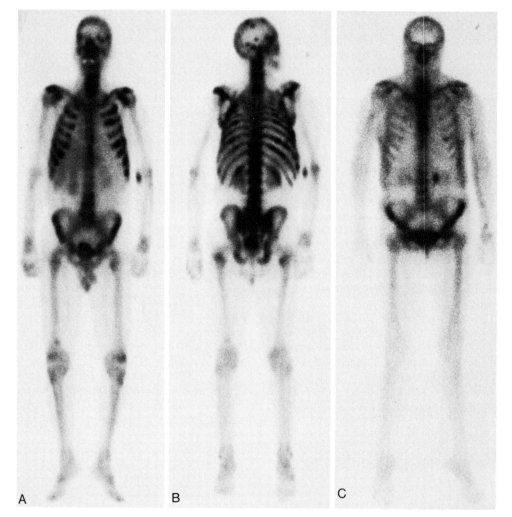

Figure 21–1. Bone scans may reveal diagnostic lesion configurations as well as more subtle evidence of tumors.

A, In a patient with skeletal metastases from a lung primary, the scan demonstrated the typical pattern of metastatic tumor: multiple lesions, randomly scattered, involving primarily the axial skeleton. This pattern is mimicked only by that seen with metastatic infection. Note the radiation defect involving the thoracic spine from a prior attempt to control an extensive primary lesion.

B, In another patient, the scan demonstrated a much less common and diagnostically more difficult pattern of skeletal metastases: diffuse confluent involvement of the entire skeleton, producing an axioperipheral disproportion. This configuration is also seen occasionally in the anemic patient, in whom the scan may show marked stimulation of central bone marrow without the usual pattern of peripheral bone marrow expansion. A simple marrow biopsy will differentiate between the two diseases. In this case the asymmetry of proximal femoral uptake and the irregularity of uptake in scattered ribs speak strongly for tumor.

C, The patient was totally asymptomatic, and indeed, the bone scan failed to demonstrate osseous metastases. However, the subtly increased soft-tissue retention of radionuclide in the arms, neck, and shoulders correctly pointed to slight fluid accumulation (clinically inapparent), secondary to early compromise of the superior vena cava by regionally advanced tumor.

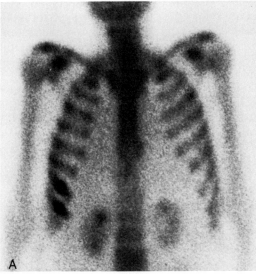

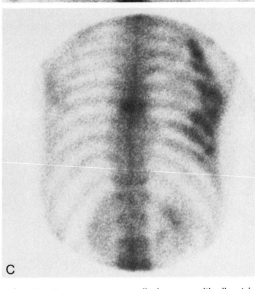

Figure 21–2. Although any given focal lesion in radionuclide skeletal imaging is highly nonspecific, the finding of a second lesion or extension of the focal lesion provides a pattern of involvement that commonly allows accurate diagnosis of the responsible disease, as demonstrated by these scans.

A and *B,* Both patients were middle-aged men with bronchogenic carcinoma who underwent bone scanning in the search for metastatic disease. In both patients, the scan demonstrated only two lesions limited to the right lower anterior rib cage. *A,* The two lesions in adjacent ribs were confidently and correctly ascribed to trauma. Rib lesions configured in rows are always due to trauma. *B,* The two (coalescing) lesions in a single rib were correctly ascribed with even greater confidence to tumor. By contrast, traumatic lesions are widely separated and usually are accompanied by other lesions in adjacent ribs to give the telltale row configuration. Trauma, however, rarely produces two lesions in a single rib.

C, A third patient had multiple lesions concentrated in the posterolateral aspect of one hemithorax. This pattern of regional metastases usually is seen with direct invasion of chest wall, as in this case, but occasionally may be seen without demonstrable pleural disease.

yielded an image quality decidedly inferior to that obtainable with the diphosphonates, which became available in the mid-1970s and are still the front-line radiopharmaceutical employed for high-quality skeletal imaging.

For similar reasons there has been significant (if not as great) improvement in the quality of brain and liver imaging. Improvement has been related primarily to the development of better uniformity, finer resolution, and larger fields for scintillation cameras, which with appropriate collimation offer higher efficiency and higher-count density images. Radiopharmaceutical quality in these areas is unchanged; better logistics in brain scanning have been achieved since the reduction of the injection-

scan interval to one hour with the advent of (^{99m}Tc)technetium-tagged DTPA.

The improvement in imaging quality has been marked, particularly in the case of liver scans. In our experience, the smallest lesions in right and left lobes of the liver detected by scanning and documented at laparotomy measured 12 mm and 5 mm across, respectively; these were perceived only on motion-corrected (for respiration) scans. Note that the correction technique was not yet available in the mid-1970s, when the scanning reported in many series was performed. A study done at our institution showed very significant improvement in liver lesion detectability with the use of motion correction, by all of five observers with experience in the interpretation of scans ranging from a few months to more than a decade. The most experienced observer picked up 94% of the lesions, with a false-positive rate of only 4%.[9] We have repeatedly identified an early, silent liver lesion in the patient with a resectable bronchogenic carcinoma.

The detectability of silent brain lesions has not improved as much. It is true that the resolution of standard-field-of-view cameras has improved markedly since the mid-1970s, with an even greater increase in resolution and efficiency for converging collimator–equipped, large-field cameras. These advances have improved the quality of brain scans, if at the cost of some distortion. None of the methods previously described include radionuclide angiography performed at the time of administration of the radiopharmaceutical used for brain scanning—a procedure that has always been *routine*

in our laboratory. Note that use of this procedure does little or nothing to increase *lesion detectability* in cerebral metastases, but it does give valuable information regarding the nature of lesions, particularly nonmetastatic lesions, and reduces the risk of false-positives for metastatic disease. The radionuclide angiogram occasionally also provides valuable adjunctive information. Our clinical experience suggests that of lung cancer patients with a positive brain scan, only half will exhibit any clinical evidence of brain metastases; this is similar to the experience reported by Hooper and colleagues.[3]

Systematic multiorgan imaging at the time of initial work-up of patients suspected of having lung cancer has been successfully employed at our institution—even in asymptomatic patients with resectable disease. The yield in this latter group is relatively low but nevertheless enough to justify the time and

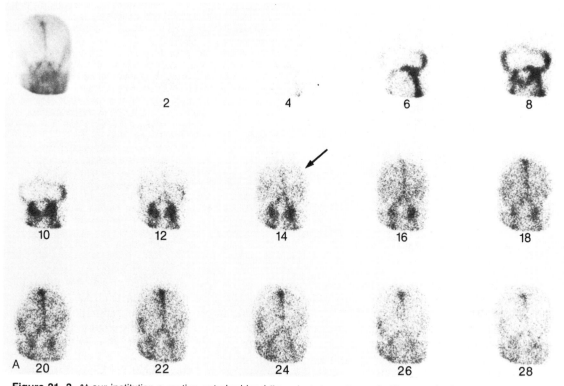

Figure 21–3. At our institution a routine anterior blood flow study is performed with every brain scan.

A, This study of a patient with bronchogenic carcinoma demonstrates the striking appearance of early collateral flow in a pattern seen only with blockage of the left innominate vein, most commonly occurring in patients with mediastinal involvement by lung cancer. Numbers represent seconds after injection of contrast. Following injection of radionuclide in the left antecubital fossa, activity is faintly seen in the left jugular vein as early as 4 seconds; clear demonstration of the left jugular vein and sigmoid sinus occurs on the 6-second frame; and flow across the lateral vein into the right sigmoid sinus and jugular vein is seen by 8 seconds, with most of the bolus having passed through by 10 seconds. Note the normal pattern of flow through anterior (*midline*) and middle (*lateral, arrow*) cerebral arteries on the 14-second frame, and appearance of radionuclide in the superior sagittal sinus by 18 seconds. For reference, a static image of the brain (anterior view) collected in exactly the same position is shown in the upper left corner.

Illustration continued on opposite page

expense incurred. We believe that the use of multiorgan imaging in all patients with lung cancer offers several advantages. First, it permits more comprehensive understanding of the magnitude of the patient's problem and occasionally modifies the approach taken with the asymptomatic patient with presumed resectable disease. Second, the primary surgical therapy in most patients with lung cancer—even those with resectable lesions—commonly fails, and other therapeutic modalities must thereafter be used in many of these patients. In this regard, a baseline imaging series obtained early in the course of the disease can be of great advantage. Third, imaging studies provide useful adjunctive information. For example, the radionuclide angiogram obtained as part of brain imaging procedure can demonstrate abnormalities in cerebral blood flow and identify the patient at greater risk for a cerebrovascular accident during the operative procedure. It will also identify mediastinal involvement by tumor as demonstrated by obstruction of the innominate system (Fig. 21–3). Indeed, we have seen many patients with CNS complaints referred for brain scanning, which subsequently revealed an innominate block caused by a previously unsuspected lung primary. Similarly, a pattern of soft-tissue retention of the bone-scanning radiopharmaceutical in the upper torso and arms has correctly identified an early unsuspected and clinically inapparent superior vena cava syndrome (Fig. 21–1C). In any patient with lung cancer undergoing bone scintigraphy who has distended veins in the neck or arms, radionuclide angiography of the chest can be performed with little additional effort utilizing the

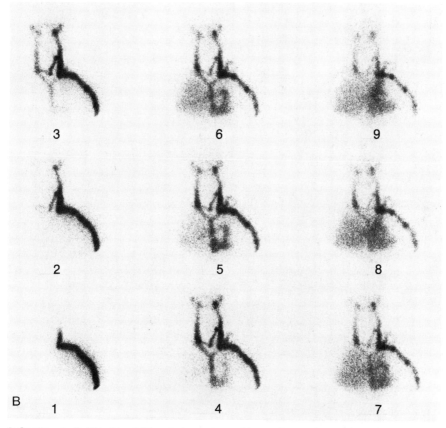

Figure 21–3 *Continued. B,* This blood flow study, performed in another patient under a large camera on a field-of-view that includes both the head and the upper thorax demonstrates a similar abnormality. On the first frame flow can be seen passing through the left axillary and subclavian veins to the junction with the left jugular and innominate veins; flow then starts to proceed up the jugular, rather than through the innominate across the mediastinum and down the superior vena cava. On the second frame, flow can be seen moving into thyroid veins and up the jugular into the sigmoid veins, with flow reaching the right side through these collaterals on the third frame. On the fourth frame, sharply diminished flow can be recognized reaching the right side of the heart through a markedly compromised superior vena cava. This study implies a complete left innominate block and at least a severely compromised superior vena cava. Note also the perfusion defect in the left upper lung laterally on late images, when most of the bolus has passed.

dose of bone-seeking radiopharmaceutical. The bone scan will also frequently identify other problems producing skeletal pain (degenerative arthropathy or hypertrophic osteoarthropathy) or serum alkaline phosphatase elevation (Paget's disease or healing fracture), thus ruling out metastatic disease. Hypertrophic osteoarthropathy (HO) is a case in point. The majority of patients with HO have pulmonary disease, usually lung cancer. In our experience, when HO is caused by lung cancer, the symptoms bringing the patient to the physician are related to the HO in approximately 10%; the discovery of lung cancer is incidentally made in half of these (5%) on the admitting chest film, and in the other half (5%) it is suggested by the finding of HO on the bone scan. The *return* of HO on the follow-up bone

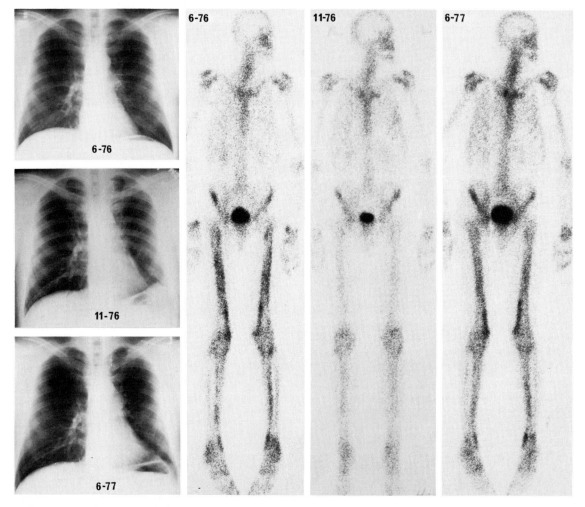

Figure 21–4. Serial radiographic and scintigraphic studies in a 52-year-old man with lung cancer, including plain films of the chest and whole-body bone scans.

The patient initially presented with a 4-month history of cough producing blood-flecked sputum. Initial work-up, including chest roentgenography, bronchography, and bronchoscopy, failed to demonstrate evidence of tumor, and the patient was discharged on therapy for bronchitis. Two months later (*6-76*) he was readmitted with progression of cough and the onset of discomfort in joints of lower extremities. The plain chest roentgenogram was considered normal, but the bone scan revealed the typical periosteal changes of hypertrophic osteoarthropathy, limited in this case to the symptomatic lower extremities, adding additional impetus to the search for pulmonary tumor. A left apical lesion was suspected on an apical lordotic chest x-ray film and was thereafter confirmed by tomography (*not shown*).

Five months following resection of the left upper lobe, when the patient was asymptomatic (*11-76*), the chest film and bone scan were normal except for expected postoperative changes. Note resolution of the hypertrophic osteoarthropathy.

The final studies (*6-77*) were obtained shortly after recurrence of cough. Note the new left hilar mass on the chest film and the reappearance of hypertrophic osteoarthropathy on the bone scan. At no time through the series were skeletal lesions apparent in a metastatic pattern.

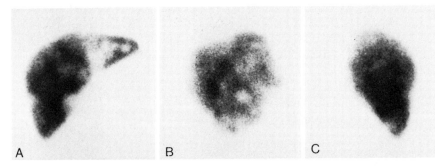

Figure 21–5. Normal biochemical determinations are not a reliable indicator of freedom from metastases. These liver scans of a patient with normal serum alkaline phosphatase and other liver function studies clearly demonstrate multiple metastases from bronchogenic carcinoma. A, anterior view; B, right lateral view; C, posterior view.

In a survey of our patients with liver metastases demonstrated by radionuclide imaging, over 10% had serum alkaline phosphatase levels well within normal limits.

scan suggests with high probability the recurrence of lung cancer, even when it is not clinically apparent (Fig. 21–4).

Most authors suggest that liver scanning is unrewarding and unnecessary in patients with normal liver function studies (particularly the serum alkaline phosphatase). Our experience sharply differs: in more than 10% of *all* patients with unequivocal space-occupying disease (99% due to metastasizing tumor) in the liver, results of liver function studies are entirely normal (Fig. 21–5). This experience is sharply skewed by the preponderance of patients with extensive disease under evaluation and treatment by the medical oncology services. The smaller size and number of lesions in the earliest stages of the metastasizing tumor can be expected to result in a far higher rate of clinically and biochemically silent tumors. Indeed, Hooper and coworkers reported that serum alkaline phosphatase concentrations were normal in one third of patients with liver involvement; this included all patients undergoing initial staging of bronchogenic carcinoma.[3] Liver function studies are quite sensitive in the detection of hepatocellular disease, are somewhat less reliable in establishing biliary obstruction, but are by no means reliable indicators of the presence of space-occupying disease.[10]

Clinical evaluation of liver size is also a rather unreliable method of detection. In most cases, the clinical "hepatomegaly" seen in our laboratory is found to be merely an inferiorly displaced liver.

Even the "gold standard" of laparotomy and open biopsy for determining the presence of liver metastases is not completely reliable. Surgeons have as much difficulty identifying a 2-cm-diameter lesion deep in the right lobe of the liver at operation as we do in radionuclide imaging. Since many space-occupying lesions have the same consistency as that of normal liver, they can become quite large and still escape detection at laparotomy. We have seen apple-sized lesions in the left lobe, and on one occasion, we identified a football-sized lesion bisecting the right lobe—the presence of which correlated well with findings on computed tomography (CT), angiography, and ultrasonography—subsequently missed at laparotomy specifically undertaken to define those lesions.

Gallium-67 (^{67}Ga) has been utilized for routine staging of the primary lung lesion as well as in the search for distant metastases.[8, 11] It offers several distinct advantages over other tracers, related particularly to its ability to demonstrate soft-tissue abnormality in organs and sites not amenable to the use of other tracers (Fig. 21–6). Thus, the local and regional extent of tumor in the lung and mediastinum can be appreciated. Whole-body imaging with ^{67}Ga allows evaluation of all organs with one tracer, in a single procedure. It offers the only practical method utilizing radionuclides for evaluating disease in adrenals—a very common site of metastases from lung primaries (Fig. 21–7).

^{67}Ga also suffers from several disadvantages. Pickup rates are variable with different cell types, being better for epidermoid than for adenocarcinoma. Small lesions can escape detection despite their reasonable affinity for ^{67}Ga. The radiation burden is the highest and the injection-scan interval is the longest (2 to 4 days) of any routine radionuclide imaging procedure. The physical characteristics of ^{67}Ga are such that it must be employed *last* in any multiorgan imaging approach employing radio-

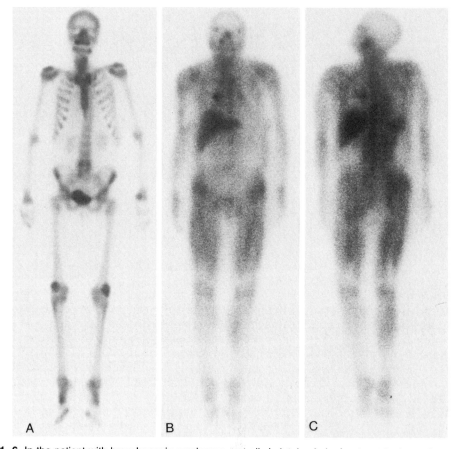

Figure 21–6. In the patient with bronchogenic carcinoma, not all skeletal pain is due to metastases (most is not), nor is all extremity pain due to hypertrophic osteoarthropathy—nor is all "skeletal" pain even osseous in origin.

A patient with a right hilar bronchogenic carcinoma underwent bone scanning for investigation of diffuse skeletal pain, thought to be of metastatic origin, rather than from hypertrophic osteoarthropathy in which skeletal pain typically is limited to the extremities. The bone scan (A, anterior view) is normal except for mild abnormality at L5–S1, wrists, hands, and feet in a typical degenerative arthropathy pattern; no lesions were seen to suggest either metastases or hypertrophic osteoarthropathy. However, ^{67}Ga imaging (B and C) reveal the probable explanation for diffuse skeletal pain. Note the pattern of diffuse ^{67}Ga uptake in major muscle groups, particularly those in the back, buttock, and thigh, suggesting "myositis"—a diagnosis not confirmed as it was not pursued. Note focal uptake in the right hilar tumor.

nuclides. Finally, although ^{67}Ga offers diagnostic information about all organs, lesion detection rates are greater when organ-specific agents are employed. For example, ^{67}Ga may demonstrate osseous metastases, but these are better perceived by bone scanning, which often will show additional osseous lesions.

Logistically, when a multiorgan radionuclide search for metastases is undertaken, we recommend scanning the liver first, as unperturbed resolution is most important in evaluating this organ, followed the same day by the brain scan. Skeletal scintigraphy can be done the following day with minimal interference. When ^{67}Ga is used, the administration of this radionuclide can proceed immediately on completion of the bone scan, with whole-body

scanning of ^{67}Ga distribution optimally undertaken 72 to 96 hours later.

Ventilation-perfusion imaging of lung to derive quantitative assessment of regional function can occasionally be helpful in planning resection limits in patients with compromised pulmonary function. When required, this study should either precede or follow the other (non-^{67}Ga) studies by one day, but it can be done on the same day as the bone scan if the latter is done early.

McNeil and colleagues[12] have presented a rationale for screening lung cancer patients for occult metastases. For their study, they analyzed the results of two diagnostic and therapeutic strategies, including (1) a test strategy, in which extensive staging tests (including mul-

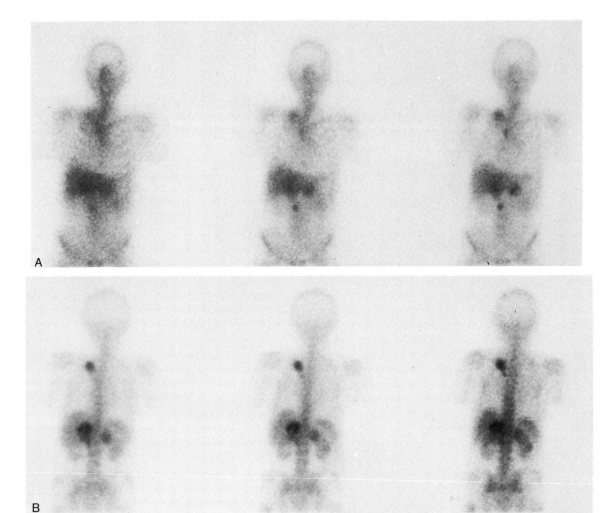

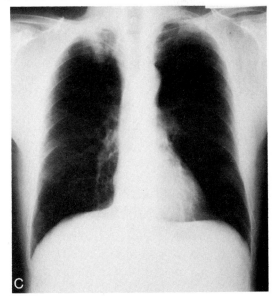

Figure 21–7. [67]Ga scanning in a patient with a posterior right upper lobe carcinoma demonstrates not only the primary lesion clearly but also a small, satellite (lymph node?) lesion lying inferomedial to the primary lesion, as well as anterior upper mediastinal adenopathy. Note also involvement of both adrenal glands (particularly the right) on posterior planes along with less striking left renal, epigastric, and liver (left lobe) lesions; these findings correlated with the chest roentgenogram (C). Finally, note a faint but probable lesion in pelvis just lateral to the left sacroiliac joint and a more prominent lesion in the greater trochanter of the right femur. It has been our experience that adrenal metastases are rather common, though seldom expected, and are demonstrable only by ^{67}Ga or upper abdominal CT imaging; among those patients in whom distant metastases can be demonstrated by ^{67}Ga, the adrenal glands are involved in approximately 50%.

tiorgan scanning) were performed preoperatively on patients with stage I or II lesions, and (2) a no-test strategy, in which such examinations were not performed. In comparing the two strategies, these investigators noted the following:

1. The average survival was little affected;
2. The greatest benefits of the test strategy were the avoidance of unnecessary operation, and thus of the risk of perioperative death, and a better possibility of long-term cure in selected patients;
3. The overall financial cost was similar.

SUMMARY

There appears to be agreement that the symptomatic patient with lung cancer should undergo multiorgan imaging, but that yields are low in multiorgan imaging of the asymptomatic patient with a resectable lesion. We have pointed out the benefits of such imaging—using carefully performed studies with modern, state-of-the-art equipment and radiopharmaceuticals—in all patients with lung cancer.

References

1. Kelly RJ, Cowan RJ, Ferree CB, et al: Efficacy of radionuclide scanning in patients with lung cancer. JAMA 242:2855–2857, 1979.
2. McNeil BJ: Value of bone scanning in neoplastic disease. Semin Nucl Med 14:277–286, 1984.
3. Hooper RG, Beechler CR, Johnson MC: Radioisotope scanning in the initial staging of bronchogenic carcinoma. Am Rev Resp Dis 118:279–286, 1978.
4. Donato AT, Ammerman EG, Sullesta O: Bone scanning in evaluation of patients with lung cancer. Ann Thorac Surg 27:300–304, 1979.
5. McNeil BJ: Rationale for the use of bone scans in selected metastatic and primary bone tumors. Semin Nucl Med 8:336–345, 1978.
6. Levenson RM Jr, Sauerbrunn BJ, Ihde DC: Small cell lung cancer: radionuclide bone scan for assessment of tumor extent and response. Am J Radiol 137:31–35, 1981.
7. Ramsdell JW, Peters RM, Taylor AT, et al: Multiorgan scans for staging lung cancer—correlation with clinical evaluation. J Thorac Cardiovasc Surg 73:653–659, 1977.
8. Smalley RV, Malmud LS, Ritchie WGM: Preoperative scanning: evaluation for metastatic disease in carcinoma of the breast, lung, colon, bladder and prostate. Semin Oncol 7:358–369, 1980.
9. Turner DA, Fordham EW, Ali A: Motion corrected hepatic scintigraphy: an objective clinical evaluation. J Nucl Med 19:142–148, 1978.
10. Gutman AB: Serum alkaline phosphatase activity in diseases of skeletal and hepatobiliary system. A consideration of the current status. Am J Med 27:875–901, 1959.
11. Deland FH, Sauerbrunn BJL, Boyd C, et al: Gallium-67 citrate imaging in untreated primary lung cancer: preliminary report of cooperative group. J Nucl Med 15:408–411, 1974.
12. McNeil BJ, Collins JJ, Adelstein SJ: Rationale for seeking occult metastases in patients with bronchial carcinoma. Surg Gynecol Obstet 14:389–393, 1977.

VII

The Use of Mediastinoscopy in Lung Cancer

Despite the many aggressive surgical exploits of German and French surgeons during the 1800's, procedures involving the mediastinum were not developed until the turn of this century. With the increasing frequency of occurrence of intrathoracic tumors and infections, invasive and noninvasive techniques for the investigation of mediastinal disease have become numerous and varied.

A surgical approach to the anterior mediastinum was first performed by Heidenhain (1899) and Rasumowski (1899). In both of their patients a collar incision was made to surgically treat mediastinitis secondary to esophageal perforation by a bone in one patient and to a gunshot wound of the esophagus and trachea in the other. Both patients recovered successfully.

The success and application of this type of mediastinotomy continued (Eiselsberg, 1909) and reached its peak during World War I. Marschik (1916, 1919, and 1940) introduced the concept of prophylactic mediastinotomy for war wounds of the neck and mediastinum. These experiences provided the foundation for further surgical efforts when interest in the mediastinum shifted from therapy to diagnosis.

Milton, an English surgeon practicing in Cairo, had thought about the problems of mediastinal and thoracic surgery (1897). Taking a cue from the pathologist, he suggested median thoracic section, or midline sternotomy, to see whether or not ". . . the general cavity of the thorax must remain a *terra incognita* to the operating surgeon." After numerous anatomic and animal studies, he successfully used this incision in a patient with a large tuberculous tumor of the sternum. He emphasized the convenience of this incision and predicted its utility: "I have no doubt that it will constitute the most generally useful route to the thoracic organs." Although Milton's article appeared in the *Lancet,* it obviously was either poorly received or went unnoticed.

The technique of mediastinoscopy was preceded by the classic study of Daniels, who reported on scalene fat pad biopsy to diagnose ". . . deep, nonpalpable lymph nodes of the lower neck and upper mediastinum." At present the surgeon has his choice of several types of mediastinoscopy: the Harken cervicomediastinal mediastinoscopy (1954), the Carlens collar mediastinoscopy (1959), the Specht expanded mediastinoscopy (1965), the Mihaljevic lateral mediastinoscopy (1968), and the Weber hiloscopy (1968). Of all these and other modifications (Storey and Reynolds, 1953; Steele and Marable, 1959), the procedure devised by Carlens is most commonly used.

Harken initiated use of the Jackson *laryngoscope* through a cervical incision to better visualize the mediastinum and to biopsy tissue under direct vision. His series of 300 such operations established the efficacy and safety of this procedure (1954). The lymph nodes were not palpably enlarged in any of his patients. Harken promoted another important concept when he argued that extirpative therapy for carcinoma of the lung might not be indicated if there is mediastinal node involvement. "If a resection has a small chance of curing the patient and increases his likelihood of dying or of suffering from operative complications, such an operation should be avoided. . . . This policy of excluding from radical surgery patients with cervicomediastinal lymphatic metastases has been called defeatist. However, since the surgeon is bound to be defeated at times, it behooves one to seek critical methods of predestined defeat. If this simple and painless technic can spare some incurable patients the risk and discomfort of thoracotomy it is distinctly useful."

This followed similar reasoning by Bricker and Modlin (1951) in their philosophy about pelvic malignancy and pelvic exenteration and was parallel to the opinion of Haagensen (1956) regarding carcinoma of the breast: ". . . *when carcinoma has involved the lymph nodes at the apex of the axilla, the supraclavicular nodes, or the internal mammary nodes in the first interspace, no conceivable form of surgical attack will succeed.*" The success of the surgeon by mastering the problems of operative techniques enabled him to refocus his attention on consideration of the factors determining length and quality of survival.

Bronchogenic carcinoma is the most common fatal carcinoma in the United States. Mediastinoscopy has been repeatedly demonstrated to be a safe and convenient method for determining mediastinal node involvement. However, the questions continue:

Should mediastinoscopy be routinely done preoperatively in every patient with bronchogenic carcinoma?

Does mediastinal node involvement contraindicate pulmonary resection in bronchogenic carcinoma?

22

The Use of Mediastinoscopy in Lung Cancer: The Dilemma of Mediastinal Lymph Nodes

Thomas W. Shields, M.D.

The prognosis of the patient with carcinoma of the lung is markedly worsened when metastatic disease is present in the mediastinal lymph nodes. Numerous series have reported 5-year survival rates ranging between 8% and 28%[1, 17, 25, 38, 46, 59, 60] (Table 22–1) when surgical resection alone has been carried out. The status of the nodal involvement—that is, grossly normal but microscopically positive nodes, grossly enlarged nodes but with the nodal capsule intact, or the presence of extracapsular growth, as well as the number of nodes and nodal stations involved—has been unreported in most of these long-term survivors. Therefore, it would appear to be important to determine which patients with metastatic mediastinal nodal involvement (N_2) should undergo resection for potential cure and which patients should be considered to have nonresectable disease.

Several aspects of management of the patient with carcinoma of the lung remain controversial: whether mediastinal nodal involvement should be sought for routinely or selectively preoperatively; the choice of diagnostic modalities in determining such involvement; and the therapeutic implications of a preoperative, intraoperative, or postoperative positive finding of metastatic disease. To gain insight into these problems and to approach a rational solution, the first essential steps are to define anatomically the mediastinal nodal groups and to define their possible involvement with carcinoma arising in each of the five lobes of the lungs.

ANATOMY OF THE MEDIASTINAL LYMPH NODES

The mediastinal lymph nodes may be divided into four major groups: the anterior mediastinal nodes, the posterior mediastinal nodes, the tracheobronchial nodes, and the paratracheal nodes.[43]

The *anterior mediastinal nodes* overlie the upper portions of the pericardium; on the right these are parallel and anterior to the phrenic nerve and on the left are in close proximity to the origin of the pulmonary artery and the ligamentum arteriosum. They extend upward along the phrenic nerve to the inferior border of the left innominate vein. These nodes on either side, right or left, lie anterior to the great vessels in the superior mediastinum.

The *posterior mediastinal nodes* are largely paraesophageal and are more common in the lower half of the mediastinum than in the superior portion, although a paraesophageal node is ocasionally found to lie retrotracheally in the area of the vena azygos arch. In the lower half of the mediastinum these nodes are adjacent to the esophagus and are most often present in the pulmonary ligament just caudad to the inferior pulmonary vein.

The *tracheobronchial nodes* lie in three

Table 22–1. Long-Term Survival in Lung Cancer Patients with Mediastinal Lymph Node Involvement

Author(s) of Published Study	5-Year Survival (% of Patients)
Shields et al[59]	8.9
Paulson and Reisch[46]	8.0
Smith[1]	28.5
Friese et al[17]	13.2
Kemeny et al[25]	11.0
Mountain et al[38]	16.0
Shimizu et al[60]	19.3

groups about the bifurcation of the trachea: The *inferior tracheobronchial nodes,* or the *subcarinal nodes,* lie in the angle of the bifurcation of the trachea and are within the pretracheal fascial envelope. The *superior tracheobronchial nodes,* right and left, are located in the obtuse angle between the trachea and corresponding main bronchus. These nodes lie outside the pretracheal fascial envelope, in contrast to the subcarinal nodes. On the right the superior tracheobronchial nodes are medial to the arch of the vena azygos and above the right pulmonary artery. The left group lies within the concavity of the aortic arch; these are the *aortic window nodes,* or *Botallo's nodes.* Some are related to the left recurrent nerve and others are situated more anteriorly and join the anterior mediastinal nodes in the region of the ligamentum arteriosum. A connection between the right and left nodal groups is reported[9] via an anterior tracheal group that lies in front of the lowest part of the trachea.

The *paratracheal nodes* are located higher in the superior mediastinum. On the right these nodes lie anterolateral to the trachea, inferior and to the right of the innominate artery, and are overlapped by the superior vena cava. On the left these nodes lie similarly anterolateral to the trachea.

Unfortunately, the aforementioned designations, proposed by Nohl-Oser,[43] have not been routinely used in the literature; as a result, some confusion exists. Naruke and colleagues[40] for example, have designated these groups somewhat differently, as shown in Table 22–2. The schematic map of the location of these nodal groups is seen in Figure 22–1.

PATTERNS OF METASTASIS TO MEDIASTINAL NODES

The metastatic involvement of the mediastinal lymph nodes by the tumors of the lung varies with the lobar location of the lesion. Tumors of the right upper lobe metastasize initially to the right superior tracheobronchial nodal group (azygos nodes). From these nodes, the more superior nodes in the paratracheal group become involved. Involvement of lymph nodes in the contralateral mediastinum from tumors in the right upper lobe is infrequent, being seen in only 3% of patients; likewise, subcarinal node involvement is relatively rare, with an incidence of 2%.[43] However, it is to be noted that some investigators[19, 56] have recorded a higher incidence of

Table 22–2. Comparison of Terminologies for Mediastinal Lymph Node Designation

Anatomic Location[a]	Nodal Station[b] Name	Number
Paratracheal	Superior	1
	Paratracheal	2
	Retrotracheal	3p
	Pretracheal	3p
Anterior mediastinal	Anterior mediastinal	3a
	Para-aortic (phrenic)	6
Superior tracheobronchial	Tracheobronchial	4
	Subaortic	5
Inferior tracheobronchial (subcarinal)	Subcarinal	7
Posterior mediastinal	Paraesophageal	8
	Pulmonary ligament	9

[a]Data from Nohl-Oser HC: Lymphatics of the lung. In Shields TW (ed): General Thoracic Surgery, 2nd ed. Philadelphia, Lea & Febiger, 1983.
[b]Data from Naruke T et al: Lymph node mapping and curability at various levels of metastasis in resection lung cancer. J Thorac Cardiovasc Surg 76:832, 1978.

subcarinal node involvement with tumors in the right upper lobe. Lesions arising in the right lower lobe, as well as those in the middle lobe, drain to both the right superior and the inferior tracheobronchial (subcarinal) nodal groups. Lower lobe tumors also drain to the posterior mediastinal node group adjacent to the esophagus and in the pulmonary ligament. Crossover lymphatic metastasis to the contralateral (left) side is infrequent with tumors arising in the right lower lobe, the incidence being approximately 4%.[43]

Tumors of the left upper lobe spread to the left superior tracheobronchial (aortic window) nodes, the anterior mediastinal nodes, and the inferior tracheobronchial node groups. Lesions in the left lower lobe spread to the superior and inferior tracheobronchial nodes and to the posterior mediastinal node groups. In contrast to the case with lesions arising in the right lung, crossover of metastatic disease from tumors of the left lung to the contralateral (right) side of the mediastinum is not unusual. Nohl-Oser[43] has reported an 11% incidence with left upper lobe lesions and a 25% incidence with left lower lobe tumors.

The incidence of metastatic involvement of the aforementioned nodal groups and the magnitude of this involvement, of course, vary with the aggressiveness of the tumor and the resistance of the host. The cell type of the tumor, as well as the clinical stage of the disease at the time of examination of the

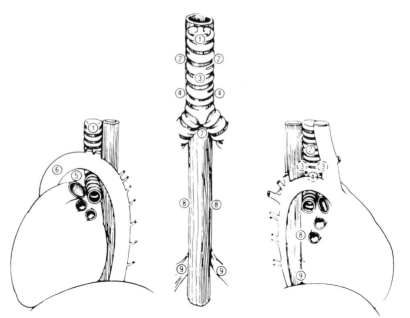

N2 NODES

Figure 22–1. Location of mediastinal lymph nodes. Numbers correspond to those listed in Table 22–2. (From Nohl-Oser HC: Lymphatics of the lung. In Shicedo TW (ed): General Thoracic Surgery. 2nd ed. Philadelphia, Lea & Febiger, 1983.)

CELL TYPE AND MEDIASTINAL NODE INVOLVEMENT

The incidence of mediastinal node involvement by metastatic disease in patients with carcinoma of the lung varies with the series reported. Autopsy series represent late disease, and surgical series represent selected series of patients in earlier stages of the disease. In the autopsy study reported by Ochsner and DeBakey,[44] regional—that is, hilar and mediastinal—nodal metastases were reported in 72.2% of the patients studied, and the tumor cell types included undifferentiated small cell carcinoma, undifferentiated large cell carcinoma, adenocarcinoma, and squamous cell carcinoma, listed in the order of decreasing frequency. Larsson,[29] in a series of mediastinoscopies, found mediastinal lymph node metastases to be present in 33.1% of the centrally located tumors and in 28.4% of the peripheral lesions. The incidence related to cell type was essentially as noted in the aforementioned autopsy study; the data reported by Jolly[23] and Whitcomb[67] and their coworkers were also similar in this regard. In contrast, in a series of 2341 men who had undergone a resection

mediastinum for such involvement, influences the incidence of positive findings.

of a carcinoma of the lung reported by the Veterans Administration Oncology Group (VASOG),[59] the incidence of mediastinal lymph node involvement was found to be the same in each cell type category, being just slightly greater than 11%. The data in this latter series reflect only a highly selected population relative to the incidence of nodal involvement. However, review of the data relative to prognoses of the 268 patients with metastatic involvement of the mediastinal lymph nodes revealed that cell type was an important factor. Patients with squamous cell tumors had the best 5- and 10-year survival experience (11.5% and 5.4%, respectively) among the three cell types reported (Table 22–3). In a series of 132 patients with undifferentiated small cell cancer, also reported by the VASOG,[58] only one patient with mediastinal node metastases of the 28 patients with either T_3 or N_2 disease, or both, survived for 5 years. Similar experiences relative to mediastinal node involvement and cell type have been reported by others.[1, 37, 46, 54] When postoperative adjuvant irradiation has been given, the survival experiences as reported by Kirsh and Sloan[28] and Martini and coworkers[33] are dissimilar, being much more favorable than in patients undergoing resection alone (Table 22–4).

Notwithstanding these latter reports, the

Table 22–3. Cell Type and Survival in 268 Lung Cancer Patients Following Resection of N$_2$ Lesions

Cell Type	5-Year Survival (% of Patients)	10-Year Survival (% of Patients)
Squamous cell carcinoma	11.5	5.4
Adenocarcinoma	2.7	0
Undifferentiated carcinoma	6.1	4.1

Data from Shields TW et al: Relationship of cell type and lymph node metastasis to survival after resection of bronchial carcinoma. Ann Thorac Surg 20:501, 1975.

survival after resection in the presence of involved mediastinal nodes is poor, and it is therefore appropriate to exclude those patients in whom a resection provides little hope for salvage. The identification of mediastinal nodal involvement prior to definitive exploration for resection is probably advisable. As noted, however, the questions of which diagnostic procedures are indicated to accomplish this most efficiently and of which groups of patients with carcinoma of the lung should be subjected to such studies remain to be completely resolved.

EVALUATION OF THE MEDIASTINUM

Noninvasive Diagnostic Procedures

The major noninvasive diagnostic tools available for evaluation of mediastinal lymph node involvement are roentgenographic examinations, computed tomography (CT), and radionuclide studies. Roentgenographic examinations include standard roentgenograms of the chest, the esophagogram, and tomography of the mediastinum.

Standard roentgenograms of the chest are considered by most investigators to have the

Table 22–4. Survival Following Postoperative Radiation Therapy in Two Groups of Patients with Resected N$_2$ Lesions

Cell Type	5-Year Survival (% of Patients) Group 1	Group 2
Squamous cell	36	44
Adenocarcinoma	13	56
All cell types	26	49

[a]Series of Kirsch and Sloan.[28]
[b]Series of Martini et al.[33]

Table 22–5. Comparison of Noninvasive Methods for Preoperative Lung Cancer Staging

	Chest Roentgenogram	Tomogram	CT Scan
Sensitivity (%)	50	75	87
Specificity (%)	85	85	77
Accuracy (%)	70	80	82
Predictive value (%)			
Positive results	80	80	68
Negative results	60	80	94
False-positive rate (%)	20	20	32
False-negative rate (%)	40	20	6

Adapted with permission from Swett HA: Personal communication.

least sensitivity and accuracy when compared to standard or computed tomographic examination of the mediastinum (Table 22–5). Nonetheless, the posteroanterior and lateral roentgenograms of the chest are excellent guides not only to whether or not additional studies are indicated but to the selection of such studies to resolve further the issue of possible involvement of the mediastinal nodes. On the standard films, five categories may be readily established: (1) an abnormal mediastinal shadow or silhouette, (2) a suspiciously abnormal mediastinal silhouette, (3) a normal mediastinal shadow but an abnormal (enlarged) hilus, (4) both a normal mediastinal shadow and hilus, and (5) either the mediastinal shadow or hilus, or both, obscured by adjacent or overlying parenchymal disease.

In the patient with an abnormal mediastinal shadow (Fig. 22–2), even in the absence of clinical findings of metastatic involvement (e.g., superior vena caval obstruction, recurrent nerve involvement, or hemidiaphragmatic paralysis), metastatic involvement of the mediastinal nodes (N$_2$ disease) should be considered present. The patient should be considered to have nonresectable disease until proved otherwise by appropriate diagnostic invasive mediastinal exploration. Parenthetically, the high incidence of involvement of mediastinal nodes in some series of up to or even exceeding 30%[3, 23, 29, 50] in patients considered to be operable may be the result of the inclusion of a number of such patients in the population under review.

A suspiciously abnormal mediastinal shadow (Fig. 22–3) as the result of subtle changes on the roentgenogram, such as widening of the

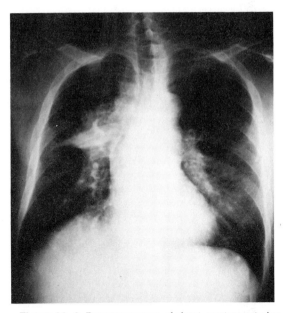

Figure 22–2. Roentgenogram of chest, posteroanterior projection, demonstrating a large central infiltrate on the right with an enlarged abnormal mediastinum to the right of the trachea. Mediastinal exploration revealed metastatic squamous cell carcinoma.

tracheal carina, a silhouette change of the normal aortic arch, tracheal air column narrowing, or widening of the superior mediastinal shadow just lateral to the trachea, suggests the possibility of mediastinal node involvement. In this situation additional studies should be done to rule out metastatic disease. Computed tomography (CT) may be done, or the clinician may proceed directly to surgical exploration of the mediastinum; the implications of this former study will be discussed subsequently.

In the patient with a normal mediastinal shadow but with an abnormal hilus (Fig. 22–4), additional roentgenographic studies such as hilar tomography with 30° and 55° oblique views may be done (Figs. 22–5, 22–6, and 22–7). These studies are reported[34, 36, 42] to permit the visualization of anterotracheal, subcarinal, subaortic, and para-aortic nodes as well as nodal enlargement in the hilus (Fig. 22–8). When any of these nodal groups or the hilar nodes are found to be enlarged, surgical exploration of the mediastinum is indicated. As in patients with suspiciously abnormal mediastinal shadow, CT of the mediastinum may be done as the initial step prior to an invasive procedure.

In patients with both a normal-appearing mediastinal shadow and a normal hilus (Fig. 22–9), marked differences of opinion exist about the need for and choice of additional diagnostic studies prior to thoracotomy for resection. Many surgeons[18, 23, 26, 29, 47, 50, 55, 63, 67] believe all patients considered to have a resectable lesion should undergo routine surgical examination of the mediastinum regardless of the roentgenographic features. However, in such patients with "normal" mediastinal shadows, Baker and colleagues[5] and others[4, 22] have reported the incidence of mediastinal nodal

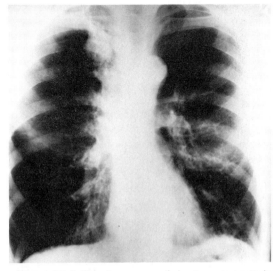

Figure 22–3. Roentgenogram of chest, posteroanterior projection, revealing a solitary peripheral mass in apex of right lung with a suspiciously abnormal mediastinal shadow. Results of mediastinal exploration were negative, and patient underwent lobectomy for an undifferentiated large cell carcinoma.

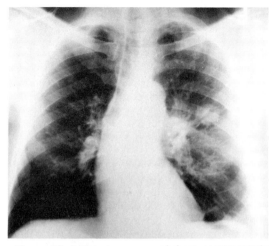

Figure 22–4. Roentgenogram of chest, posteroanterior projection, demonstrating enlarged left hilar shadow and a peripheral solitary lesion in the left mid-lung field. Surgical exploration revealed metastatic adenocarcinoma in anterior mediastinal lymph nodes.

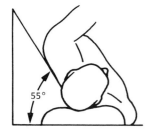
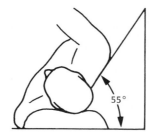
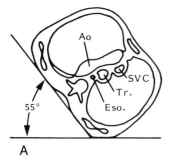
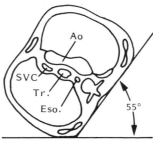

A   B

Figure 22–5. Patient positions for right posterior (*A*) and left posterior (*B*) 55° oblique tomography of the hilar areas.

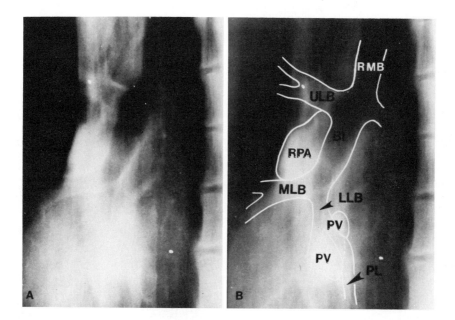

Figure 22–6. A 55° oblique tomogram of the right hilus (*A*) with anatomic structures identified (*B*). The bronchial angles are presented in this normal study. (From Hughes RA et al: Management of the hilar mass. Chest 79:85, 1981.)

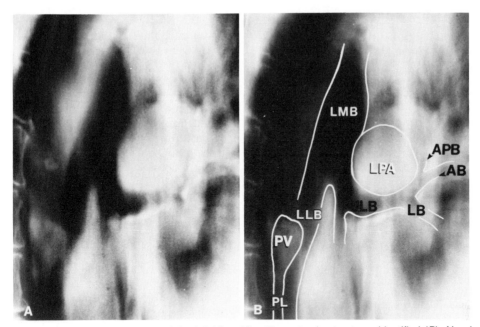

Figure 22–7. A 55° oblique tomogram of the left hilus (*A*) with anatomic structures identified (*B*). No abnormalities were present in the patient with prominence of the left hilus on a routine chest radiograph. (From Hughes RA et al: Management of the hilar mass. Chest 79:85, 1981.)

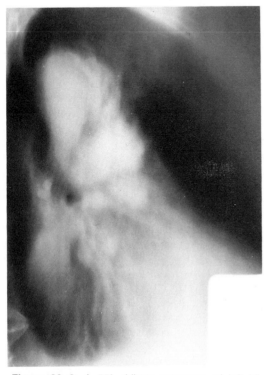

Figure 22–8. A 55° oblique tomogram of left hilus revealing abnormal enlargement of the lymph nodes surrounding the left upper lobe bronchus.

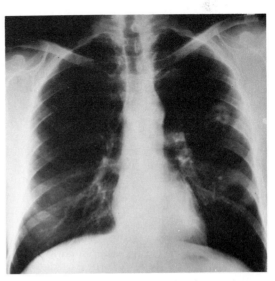

Figure 22–9. Roentgenogram of the chest, posteroanterior projection, with peripheral mass in left lung field with normal hilar and mediastinal shadows. There were no involved lymph nodes at the time of resection.

Table 22–6. Resection of N_2 Lesions by
Pretreatment Clinical Stage

| Clinical Stage | No. of Patients | | |
	Total	*Explored*	*Complete Resection*
N_0 or N_1 Lesions			
$T_1N_0M_0$	22	22	21
$T_2N_0M_0$	44	44	27
$T_1N_1M_0$	2	2	2
$T_2N_1M_0$	11	11	7
$T_3N_0M_0$	35	35	9
$T_3N_1M_0$	2	2	0
Total	116	116	66
N_2 Lesions			
$T_1N_2M_0$	16	13	1
$T_2N_2M_0$	45	30	9
$T_3N_2M_0$	135	58	4
Total	196	101	14
All Lesions	312	217	80

Adapted from Martini et al: Prospective study of 445
lung carcinomas with mediastinal lymph node metastases.
J Thorac Cardiovasc Surg 80:390, 1980.

involvement to be approximately only 5% in
patients with peripheral T_1 lesions (3-cm size
or less). Recently, Murray and coworkers[39]
have reported an incidence of only 4% of
superior mediastinal node involvement discovered by routine mediastinoscopy in patients
with right lower lobe lesions that were considered to be clinically resectable. These reports
have supported my own observation that in
clinically operable patients with a normal mediastinal shadow and hilus on standard roentgenographic study, the incidence of mediastinal metastases is well under 10%. Martini
and colleagues[33] believe that mediastinal exploration is not indicated in patients with clinical
Stage I disease. Of 22 patients in their series
with clinical signs suggesting T_1N_0 disease who
on exploration had N_2 disease, complete resection was possible in all but one patient. Of the
44 patients with T_2N_0 disease, however, complete resection was possible in only 27 (Table
22–6); it is probable in this T_2N_0 group that
some patients did not in fact have normal
mediastinal and hilar shadows prior to surgery.
The aforementioned data suggest that in patients with T_1 disease and normal hilar and
mediastinal shadows, no further evaluation of
the mediastinum is indicated. However, in
patients with T_2 disease, further examination
of the mediastinum by CT appears to be appropriate before decision for or against surgical
exploration of the mediastinum is made.

In the last group of patients, those with
either the mediastinal or hilar shadow, or both
(Fig. 22–10), obscured by adjacent or overlying parenchymal changes, initial investigation
by CT may be beneficial. However, whether
the observed findings on the scan are due to
enlarged nodes or to adjacent parenchymal
changes may be difficult to ascertain. Therefore, many, if not all, patients in this group
should undergo surgical exploration of the
mediastinum prior to the final therapeutic decision.

The *esophagogram* (Fig. 22–11) is a useful
supplement for evaluating the posterior–
inferior tracheobronchial (posterior subcarinal) and retrotracheal nodes. Enlargement of
these nodes will displace the barium-filled
esophagus posteriorly. This examination
should be done in any patient with a widened
tracheal carina visualized on standard roentgenograms of the chest. Possibly it might routinely be employed effectively in patients with
lower lobe tumors, especially on the left.

Standard tomography of the mediastinum,
although of more value than the standard
roentgenograms of the chest, has a significantly
high false-negative rate so that it is better
replaced by CT of the mediastinum. The use
of oblique tomograms has been discussed previously. Unfortunately, I have found these to
be difficult to interpret at times and find their
use limited. *Xerotomography* yields clear silhouettes of much of the bronchial wall, the
pulmonary vessels, and the aorta;[11, 61] therefore, it has been suggested as a very satisfactory method of evaluating the mediastinum.
However, experience with its use has been
limited, and its role is yet to be defined.

Computed tomography (CT) of the chest
permits distinct imaging of the upper mediastinum, aortic arch, superior vena cava, right
brachiocephalic artery, left carotid artery, trachea, and esophagus. When a contrast medium
is added, the mediastinal lymph nodes may be
clearly delineated (Fig. 22–12). The paratracheal nodes, aortic window nodes (Botallo's
nodes), and superior and inferior tracheobronchial nodes may be recognized. Studies of
numerous investigators[13, 14, 31, 36, 45, 51, 53, 62] have
evaluated the use of CT in identifying nodal
enlargement. In most reports a node 1 cm or
greater in size has been considered to be
enlarged and thus possibly involved in metastatic disease,[13, 14, 31, 53] although Osborne and
coworkers[45] have considered nodes as small as
5 to 6 mm to be positive. In most of the
studies, the sensitivity and accuracy of CT are

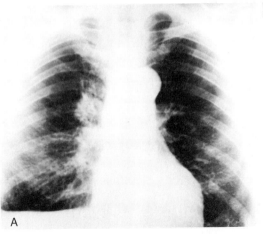

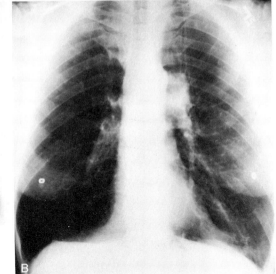

Figure 22–10. Parenchymal changes may obscure roentgenographic detail. *A,* Inferior portion of the right superior mediastinum just above the right hilus obscured by parenchymal mass. There was no evidence of metastasis on mediastinotomy, and right upper lobectomy was performed to resect an undifferentiated large cell carcinoma. *B,* Aortic window area obscured by parenchymal infiltrate in left upper lobe. Mediastinotomy with histopathologic examination revealed metastatic squamous cell carcinoma.

acceptable (Table 22–7). The predictive value of a negative CT is generally over 90%. However, the predictive value of a positive CT is less, being frequently below 80%. Therefore, it may be concluded that when the CT is negative, surgical exploration of the mediastinum is not necessary, but that when it is positive, surgical exploration of the mediastinum is indicated to rule out the significant incidence of false-positive results.

Radionuclide studies utilizing gallium-67 (^{67}Ga) to identify metastatic nodal involvement in the mediastinum are controversial, and their ultimate role remains undetermined. Hoffer[21] has reported that approximately 90% of the carcinomas of the lung of all cell types will take up the [67]Ga. Unfortunately, there is a considerable variation in the percentages reported for the detection of mediastinal metastases with this isotope.[2, 8, 12, 30] Tumors near the mediastinum appear to be the most difficult to evaluate and have a higher false-positive rate than is seen with peripheral lesions. The sensitivity of detecting involved nodes ranges from 55% to 100%, with a range of specificity of 63% to 94%. In contrast to CT, a positive scan appears to be more accurate than a negative one. Nonetheless, it is suggested that when the primary tumor is positive and the mediastinum is negative, surgical evaluation is not indicated, and that when the mediastinum is positive, such evaluation is necessary. Despite the enthusiasm voiced in some reports such as those of DeMeester[12] and Fosburg[15] and their colleagues, my experience has been less than satisfactory with this examination, and I rarely use it in the preoperative evaluation of the mediastinum in patients with carcinoma of the lung.

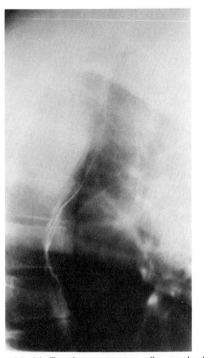

Figure 22–11. Esophagogram revealing marked deviation of the barium column caused by enlarged subcarinal nodes.

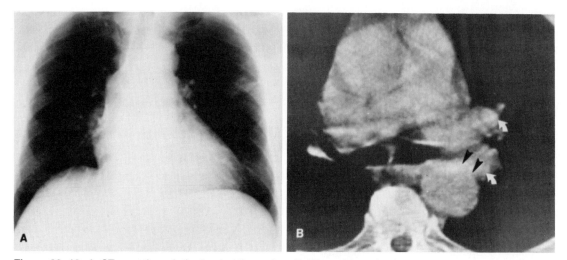

Figure 22–12. *A,* CT scan through the level of the carina. *B,* Hilar adenopathy (*curved arrows*) and invasion of the aorta (*arrowheads*). (From Mintzer RA et al: Computed vs conventional tomography in evaluation of primary and secondary neoplasms. Radiology 132:653, 1979.)

Invasive Diagnostic Procedures

The standard invasive procedures to evaluate the mediastinum have been either cervical mediastinoscopy or anterior mediastinotomy. However, the value of bronchoscopy with or without transbronchial needle aspiration and percutaneous needle biopsy of suspicious mediastinal masses should not be forgotten.

Bronchoscopy may yield indirect evidence of mediastinal lymph node enlargement, such as widening and fixation of the tracheal carina or rigidity and fixation of either main-stem bronchus. In the former situation, transcarinal needle aspiration may be helpful in demonstrating metastatic disease in the subcarinal nodes.[16] This now may be accomplished with safety by use of the appropriate aspiration needles for use with the fiberoptic bronchoscope.[24, 64, 65]

Percutaneous aspiration needle biopsy of suspected mediastinal metastatic lesions is not popular. When the area of involvement may be readily located, the use of a fine, thin-walled needle may be used to obtain material for cytologic examination. The danger of bleeding from puncture of a major vessel is minimal; in fact, I have used this technique without incident in patients with superior vena caval syndrome (Fig. 22–13).

Direct surgical exploration of the mediastinum, however, continues to be the most often employed invasive diagnostic method. *Cervical mediastinoscopy,* introduced by Carlens,[10] or *anterior mediastinotomy,* suggested by McNeill and Chamberlain,[35] or a combination of the two, is the approach used. The operative techniques, precautions, and complications have been reviewed recently by Hashim and coworkers.[20] Cervical mediastinoscopy permits biopsy of the paratracheal groups on both the right and the left, the superior tracheobronchial nodes on the right and the anterior subcarinal nodes; however, the anterior medias-

Table 22–7. Results of Computed Tomography in Identification of Involved Mediastinal Nodes

Authors of Published Study	Criteria for Positive Node	Sensitivity/ Specificity (%)	Accuracy (%)	Predictive Value (%) Positive Scan	Negative Scan
Underwood et al[62]	?	44/88	66	80	61
Mintzer et al[36]	?	75/100	93	100	91
Ekholm et al[13]	1 cm	26/46	42	11	72
Rea et al[53]	All visible nodes	80/76	77	50	93
Faling et al[14]	1.5 cm	88/94	92	88	94
Osborne et al[45]	5–6 mm	94/62	76	65	94
Lewis et al[31]	1 cm	91/94		88	95

Adapted with permission from Swett HA: Personal communication.

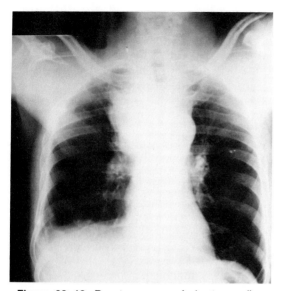

Figure 22–13. Roentgenogram of chest revealing a large superior mediastinal mass in a patient with superior vena caval syndrome. Percutaneous needle biopsy revealed undifferentiated small cell carcinoma.

tinal nodes on the left and most of the superior tracheobronchial (aortic window) nodes on the left are inaccessible. Anterior mediastinotomy permits only unilateral exploration, and it is difficult to biopsy the subcarinal nodes by this procedure. However, it does permit better visualization of the ipsilateral mediastinum, as well as palpation of the pulmonary artery in the superior hilar area. Neither procedure permits examination of the posterior inferior tracheobronchial (posterior subcarinal) or posterior mediastinal (lower paraesophageal or pulmonary ligament) lymph nodes.

Despite the limitations of cervical mediastinoscopy, many surgeons routinely use this procedure regardless of the location of the primary tumor. However, as pointed out by Jolly and colleagues,[23] anterior mediastinotomy should be the procedure of choice in patients with left upper lobe lesions. Actually, I prefer an anterior mediastinotomy when I believe mediastinal exploration is indicated regardless of whether the lesion is in the right or left lung. A more thorough examination is possible, and it affords palpation of the superior aspect of the hilus. This yields additional information in respect to resectability of the tumor under consideration. This in my opinion offsets the disadvantage of a unilateral exploration. When there is suspicion of contralateral spread, primarily when the left lower lobe is the site of the carcinoma, the tracheal carina should be evaluated; if it is seen to be widened, a trans-

carinal needle aspiration may be carried out. A combination of a cervical mediastinotomy and a left anterior mediastinotomy may also be done in such situations.

The results of the use of either one of these invasive diagnostic procedures varies with the selection of the patient population under study and the cell type of the primary tumor. The yield in patients with undifferentiated small cell tumors far exceeds the incidence of positive biopsies in patients with non–small cell tumors. Because of this fact, almost all surgeons, including myself, believe that surgical mediastinal exploration is mandatory in any patient with a small cell tumor considered clinically to be a resectable lesion $(T_1N_0M_0)$.[58]

In patients with non–small cell tumors, selection as outlined in the previous section on noninvasive procedures is appropriate, and surgical mediastinal exploration should not be done routinely. However, a question that has not yet been resolved is whether an exception to this rule should be made, as suggested by Kirsh and Sloan,[28] as well as by Hashim and colleagues,[20] in patients with an adenocarcinoma or undifferentiated large cell tumor of any size that is centrally located or that is over 3 cm and is located peripherally (T_2 lesion). The use of CT in such patients prior to a final decision would appear to be indicated.

The routine use of mediastinal exploration in poor-risk patients because of age, debility, or poor pulmonary function in the hopes of finding a reason *not* to operate is to be condemned. A decision as to whether or not to explore the chest in such a patient for possible resection should be based on more appropriate reasons.

As noted, depending upon the operative indications chosen, the cell type of the tumor, and the procedure employed, the incidence of positive biopsies revealing metastatic involvement of one or more mediastinal nodes varies, ranging from 5% to over 30%. The therapeutic significance of such involvement discovered by mediastinal exploration has been interpreted differently by the various surgeons who have reported on the problem.

THE SIGNIFICANCE OF POSITIVE MEDIASTINAL NODES

Positive Nodes Discovered on Mediastinal Exploration

All authors agree that the finding of a mediastinal node involved by an undifferentiated small cell carcinoma at mediastinoscopy or mediastinotomy is an absolute contraindication to exploration for possible resection. Similarly, the finding of either adenocarcinoma or undifferentiated carcinoma also is considered by most to be a contraindication to further surgical intervention. However, when the node or nodes are involved by a squamous cell carcinoma, marked differences in opinion exist about whether further surgical consideration is appropriate and, if so, in which patients.

The status of the metastatic growth is important. Extension of the disease outside the capsule (perinodal growth) significantly worsens the prognosis of the patient. This observation initially was recorded by a surgical group from Sweden.[6, 7, 29] In 62 patients with perinodal metastatic growth discovered on mediastinoscopy, there were no long-term survivors in the 49 patients who subsequently had undergone a resection. The mortality rate was high (25%) in this group of patients. In contrast, in nine patients with intranodal growth only (the capsule intact), there was one postoperative death, and five patients were alive without disease at 3 years postoperatively. The significance of intranodal versus extracapsular growth also is apparent in the report of Abbey Smith,[1] although in a somewhat differently selected group. Following resection only one of 16 patients with N_2 disease surviving 5 years or longer had perinodal involvement, whereas the other 15 had intranodal growth only. Thus, I believe patients in whom there is perinodal growth or fixation to surrounding mediastinal structures, regardless of cell type, should be excluded from further surgical intervention. In the early studies, by Pearson and coworkers,[50] this contraindication to resection was present in 39.5% of the patients with non–small cell tumors who were deemed inoperable by mediastinoscopy regardless of the position of the node within the mediastinum.

Location of the involved nodes in the mediastinum, even without perinodal growth, also influences the therapeutic decision. The presence of involved contralateral nodes or high ipsilateral paratracheal nodes (those just inferior to the innominate artery) on the right side is considered a contraindication to resection. Nodal involvement in the anterior mediastinum on the left likewise is considered a contraindication. However, patients with squamous cell carcinoma and involved nodes without extensive extracapsular spread in the low paratracheal area, the ipsilateral superior tracheobronchial area, or anterior subcarinal area are considered by Pearson[48] to have potentially resectable lesions. Bergh and Larsson[6] concur with this opinion when the growth is intranodal. However, with the exception of these latter patients (intranodal growth only), the results of resection of involved subcarinal or paratracheal nodes discovered initially by mediastinal exploration have not been overly encouraging. Pearson and colleagues,[49] proponents of such an approach, have recently reported a series of patients in which a resection could be accomplished in 85% of a highly selected positive mediastinoscopy group. Of these resections, 75% (64% of all patients) were thought to be curative. Most patients also received adjuvant irradiation. In the 35 patients with squamous cell carcinoma who underwent a curative resection, the actuarial 5-year survival was 18%. In the 12 patients with either adenocarcinoma or undifferentiated large cell carcinoma the survival was 7%. There was only one 5-year survival in 17 patients with subcarinal node involvement, and only one 5-year survival was observed in 17 patients with low paratracheal node involvement. In 48 patients with superior tracheobronchial node involvement, 4 patients (one of whom was the aforementioned patient who also had subcarinal node involvement) survived for over 5 years. In the series reported by Gibbons[18] and Fosburg and coworkers,[15] none of the patients with mediastinoscopically positive nodes and subsequent resection (no adjuvant therapy) survived for 5 years.

After consideration of the aforementioned data, I believe that any prethoracotomy positive mediastinal exploration, regardless of cell type or location of the involved lymph node or nodes, is a contraindication to resection. An exception may be the infrequently encountered patient with squamous cell carcinoma with only intranodal growth, especially in a node or nodes in the ipsilateral superior tracheobronchial area. This recommendation, however, does not apply to those patients in whom a positive mediastinal node (N_2) is initially discovered at the time of thoracotomy and in whom either a surgical mediastinal exploration has been negative or was not performed preoperatively.

Positive Nodes Discovered at Thoracotomy

Mediastinal nodal metastasis is sometimes discovered initially at thoracotomy performed with the aim of curative resection. This unfortunate finding is seen not only in patients in

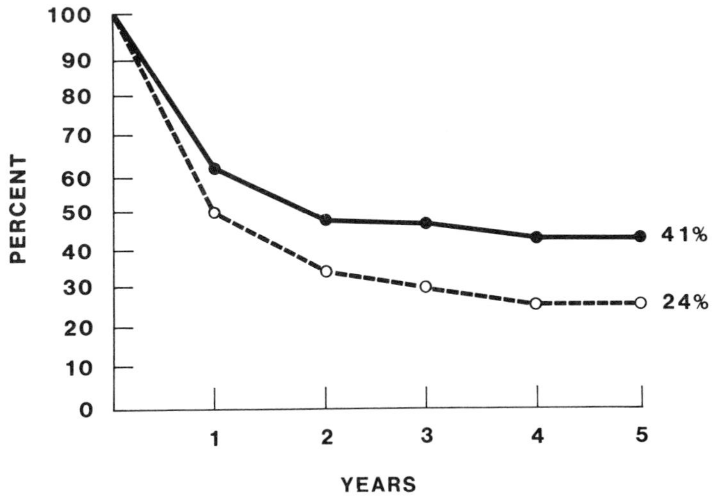

Figure 22–14. Actuarial survival curves for all patients (-------) undergoing resection with N$_2$ disease and for all those undergoing a "curative" resection in the presence of N$_2$ disease (———). (From Pearson FG et al: Significance of positive superior mediastinal nodes identified at mediastinoscopy in patients with resectable cancer of the lung. J Thorac Cardiovasc Surg 83:1, 1982.)

whom clinical signs suggested merely localized disease but also in patients in whom diagnostic mediastinal exploration was in fact negative.

As does any diagnostic procedure, mediastinal exploration yields occasional false-negative results. Such results may be due to failure to recognize an involved node, either because it is small or the capsule is intact, or because the nodal involvement is in an area not visualized during the procedure. The latter is true of the aortic window nodes and anterior mediastinal nodes in patients with left upper lobe lesions who are evaluated by mediastinoscopy. The use of mediastinotomy in patients with left upper lobe lesions should obviate some of false-negative findings noted in the past. Posterior subcarinal and posterior (paraesophageal) mediastinal nodes, important in patients with middle lobe or lower lesions, are inaccessible using either procedure.

The reported incidence of false-negative results ranges from 8% to 20% in studies of patients undergoing routine mediastinoscopy prior to thoracotomy.[29, 50] Three quarters or more of the false-negative results were due to inaccessibility of the involved nodes with the procedure employed. Yet the results of resection in the false-negative group are much more encouraging than in those patients who had an initially positive mediastinal exploration. Pearson and coworkers[49] reported a higher resectability rate in the mediastinoscopy false-negative group than in the initially positive group (92% and 85%, respectively), although the number of curative resections was less (40% versus 65%). The actuarial survival of all patients undergoing resection in the false-negative group was 24% at 5 years. The unfavorable influence of a subcarinal location of the

involved node or nodes was noted. Only 1 of 32 patients with such involvement survived 5 years. In the patients in whom the resection was considered to be curative, the actuarial survival was 41% (Fig. 22–14). Of interest is that 18 of the 25 patients who were thought to have had a curative resection did not receive adjuvant radiation therapy; yet the actuarial survival in this group was 48%. A similar survival experience (55% at 3 years postoperatively) was noted by Bergh and Larsson[6] in patients with false-negative N$_2$ disease when the growth was intranodal.

Thoracotomy also occasionally reveals involved mediastinal nodes in patients whose clinical signs suggested only limited disease, so that prethoracotomy mediastinal exploration was judged unnecessary. Of course, the incidence of N$_2$ disease in patients who have not undergone mediastinal exploration varies with the selectivity exercised in choosing the patients submitted to thoracotomy. In patients in whom surgical mediastinal exploration is used selectively, the incidence of positive mediastinal (N$_2$) disease should be no more than 5% to 10%. In patients in whom exploration is not performed, the incidence of N$_2$ disease in those patients who subsequently are considered to have had complete removal of all tumor (a curative resection) ranges from as low as 10% to as high as 30%.[1, 17, 33, 40] Most patients who fall into the curative resection group are those in whom the N$_2$ disease was not suspected clinically. In a large series reported by Martini and colleagues,[33] 66 of the 80 patients who underwent curative resections of N$_2$ disease were not considered to have such disease preoperatively (Table 22–6). In this series, the lesions most promising for resection were those classified preoperatively as T_1N_0 disease, and the least were those classified as N_2 disease with any T (Table 22–6). The rates of curative resection were equal in patients with lesions classified cytopathologically (postoperatively) as either T_1N_2 or T_2N_2 (50%), but complete resection was possible in only 10% of those with T_3N_2 disease. In this series a greater number of patients had adenocarcinoma than squamous cell carcinoma. A similar observation was reported by Naruke and coworkers;[40] in fact, in their series there were 35 patients with either adenocarcinoma or alveolar cell tumors, compared to only 17 with squamous cell carcinoma. In contrast, Kirsch and Sloan[28] had an essentially equal distribution of these two cell types in their patients with N_2 disease who underwent resection.

In these three reported series, adjuvant therapy (in most instances irradiation) was used postoperatively. In the series of Naruke and colleagues,[40] a 5-year survival of 18.8% was recorded for the 64 patients with N_2 disease who underwent resection; a salutary effect of adjuvant therapy was not noted. In a series of 80 patients with N_2 disease reported by Martini and coworkers,[33] the 3-year survival following complete resection was 49%, and the use of postoperative irradiation was thought to be beneficial. In patients with squamous cell carcinoma the 3-year survival was 44%; in those with adenocarcinoma it was 56%. In their 136 patients with N_2 disease in whom postoperative irradiation was used, Kirsh and Sloan[28] reported a 21.3% 5-year survival, but in contrast to the experience of Martini's group, those patients with squamous cell tumors did better than those with adenocarcinoma: 36% and 12.7% 5-year survival rates, respectively.

In the series reported by Abbey Smith[1] and Paulson and Reisch,[46] postoperative irradiation was not used. In the former series a 28.5% 5-year survival was recorded, but in the latter it was only 8%.

In these five series there is general, although not absolute, agreement that some of the unfavorable preoperative features of resected N_2 lesions are a subcarinal location of the metastatic disease, extracapsular spread of the disease, involvement of more than two nodal stations, and a large primary tumor (T_2) or one that has invaded beyond the visceral pleural envelope (T_3). Unfortunately, there is little agreement about the influence of cell type or the use of postoperative adjuvant therapy.

The discrepancies among these reports are difficult to explain. Undoubtedly, patient selection and the relative distribution of the various final cytopathologic stages of the resected disease play predominant roles. However, combining the experience in these reports with those of patients found to have N_2 disease after a false-negative mediastinal exploration permits several conclusions regarding the prognoses of patients with N_2 disease who have undergone a resection for potential cure.

PROGNOSTIC IMPLICATIONS OF MEDIASTINAL NODE METASTASES INITIALLY IDENTIFIED AT OPERATION

As noted, it is suggested or inferred by most authors that the prognostic outlook is far better for patients with intranodal metastatic disease (gross or microscopic) than for those with extracapsular extension.[1, 27, 29, 46, 66] The location of the nodal station or stations involved also affects the prognosis. Positive nodes in the subcarinal area are less favorable than in the other nodal stations.[33, 40, 49] Location of the primary tumor on the left side is even less favorable.[40] The more nodal stations involved, the fewer long-term survivals are recorded.[33, 66] The size of the primary tumor (T_1 or T_2), as well as the extent of the disease within the hemithorax (T_3), plays a role. Patients with T_1N_2 lesions do better than those with T_2N_2 lesions, and those with T_3N_2 disease rarely survive for 5 years.[6, 33, 40, 66]

The influence of cell type on prognosis of patients with N_2 disease is generally agreed upon. Patients with squamous cell tumors do better than those with either adenocarcinoma or undifferentiated large cell carcinoma, and those with undifferentiated small cell tumors do worst of all.[41, 46, 59]

The use of postoperative adjuvant radiation therapy has been reported to improve the prognosis of patients with N_2 disease. Many investigators[28, 40, 41] believe this beneficial effect is confined to those patients with squamous cell tumors, although Martini and coworkers[33] report its use to alter even the poor prognostic outlook of patients with adenocarcinoma. Actually, in some series[40, 49] the patients who received no adjuvant therapy did better than those who did. The reason for these differences undoubtedly is dependent upon the selection of the patient population.

It is obvious that better definition of nodal involvement is necessary before any dogmatic statements may be made about the proper surgical management of patients with metastatic involvement of the mediastinal lymph nodes discovered at thoracotomy. Likewise, prospective studies to evaluate potentially beneficial adjuvant therapy (e.g., postoperative irradiation) are also indicated to define its true role. Nonetheless, a rational approach applicable in most patients may be suggested after consideration of the aforementioned data.

SELECTION OF PATIENTS WITH N$_2$ DISEASE

In patients in whom metastatic mediastinal lymph node involvement is discovered at the time of exploration for resection, the status of the nodal disease and the location of the nodal stations and the number of stations involved rather than the cell type, with the exception of undifferentiated small cell carcinoma, should determine whether or not a resection is carried out. When there is evidence of extracapsular growth, resection in most if not all instances should be abandoned. The occasional long-term survival in such cases is anecdotal at best. An incomplete (palliative) resection is generally of little or no benefit. The patient is exposed to the morbidity and mortality of the procedure with little chance of meaningful survival.[6, 28, 33, 49, 56] When the metastatic disease is confined within the capsule of the node, even when the node is enlarged, the surgeon should proceed with the appropriate resection and mediastinal dissection that will encompass the disease process. In instances of right upper lobe disease, a radical right upper lobectomy is as satisfactory as a pneumonectomy.[52] The only contraindication to resection is involvement of more than two nodal stations, particularly when the inferior tracheobronchial (subcarinal) station is one of the nodal groups involved.

In a small number of patients, the N$_2$ disease is not suspected, the nodes being normal grossly, and is not discovered until histopathologic examination of the resected specimen. Such patients indeed may have the most favorable prognosis among all patients with N$_2$ disease. Thus, it is necessary in all resections to inspect and sample each lymph node station that may be primarily involved by a tumor arising within a specific lobe.[32] When this is done, the patient may be placed into the appropriate TNM category prognostically, and a more meaningful decision may be made about the possible use of postoperative adjuvant therapy.

The question of postoperative adjuvant therapy remains unsettled. Neither chemotherapy nor immunotherapy has been shown to be beneficial. However, as noted, postoperative irradiation has been reported to improve the prognosis of patients with N$_2$ disease. Despite the lack of a prospective controlled study that might reveal its purported value either as a true adjunctive modality or only as an aberration of selection, the use of postoperative irradiation at this time appears to be indicated. Perhaps the strongest support of this approach is not the increased long-term survivals reported but rather the observation that mediastinal recurrence is rare after irradiation but is almost routinely observed in patients with resected N$_2$ disease who have not received such therapy.[28, 33]

References

1. A. Smith R: The importance of mediastinal lymph node invasion by pulmonary carcinoma in selection of patients for resection. Ann Thorac Surg 25:5, 1978.
2. Alazraki NP, Ramsdell JW, Taylor A, et al: Reliability of gallium scan chest radiography compared to mediastinoscopy for evaluating mediastinal spread in lung cancer. Am Rev Respir Dis 117:415, 1978.
3. Ashraf MH, Milson PL, Walesby RK: Selection of mediastinoscopy and long-term survival in bronchial carcinoma. Ann Thorac Surg 30:208, 1980.
4. Baggs, KJ, Raun RA: An evaluation of mediastinoscopy as a guide to diagnosis and therapy. Arch Surg 111:703, 1976.
5. Baker RR, Lillemoe KD, Tockman MS: The indications for transcervical mediastinoscopy in patients with small peripheral bronchial carcinoma. Surg Gynecol Obstet 148:860, 1979.
6. Bergh NP, Larsson S: The significance of various types of mediastinal lymph-node metastases in lung cancer. In Jepsen O, Sorenson HR (eds): Mediastinoscopy. Proceedings of an International Symposium, Odense University, Odense University Press, 1971.
7. Bergh NP, Schersten T: Bronchogenic carcinoma: A follow-up study of a surgically treated series with special references to prognostic significance of lymph node metastases. Acta Chir Scand (Suppl) 129:347, 1965.
8. Brereton HD, Line BR, Londer HN, et al: Gallium scans for staging small cell lung cancer. JAMA 240:666, 1978.
9. Brock RC, Whytehead LL: Radical pneumonectomy for bronchial carcinoma. Br J Surg 43:8, 1955.
10. Carlens E: Mediastinoscopy: A method for inspection and tissue biopsy in the superior mediastinum. Dis Chest 36:343, 1959.
11. Chuang VP, Doust BD, Ting YM: Xerotomography of the mediastinum and tracheobronchial tree. Radiology 111:475, 1974.

12. DeMeester TR, Golomb HM, Kirschner P, et al: The role of gallium-67 scanning in the clinical staging and preoperative evaluation of patients with carcinoma of the lung. Ann Thorac Surg 28:451, 1979.

13. Ekholm S, Albrechtsson U, Kugelberg J, et al.: Computed tomography in preoperative staging of bronchogenic carcinoma. J Comput Assist Tomogr 7:763, 1980.

14. Faling LJ, Pugatch RD, Jung-Legg Y, et al: Computed tomographic scanning of the mediastinum in the staging of bronchogenic carcinoma. Am Rev Resp Dis 124:690, 1981.

15. Fosburg RG, Hopkins GB, Kan MK: Evaluation of mediastinum by gallium-67 scintography in lung cancer. J Thorac Cardiovasc Surg 77:76, 1979.

16. Fox RT, Lees WM, Shields TW: Transcarinal bronchoscopic needle biopsy. Ann Thorac Surg 1:92, 1965.

17. Friese G, Gabler A, Liebig S: Bronchial carcinoma and long-term survival: Retrospective study of 433 patients who underwent resection. Thorax 33:228, 1978.

18. Gibbons JPR: The value of mediastinoscopy in assessing operability of carcinoma of the lung. Br J Dis Chest 66:162, 1972.

19. Greschuchna R, Maasen W: Die lymphogenen absiedlungswege des Bronchialkarzinomas. Stuttgart, Georg Thieme Verlag, 1973.

20. Hashim SW, Baue AE, Geha AS: The role of mediastinoscopy and mediastinotomy in lung cancer. Clin Chest Med 3:353, 1982.

21. Hoffer PB: Status of gallium-67 in tumor detection. J Nucl Med 21:394, 1980.

22. Hutchinson CM, Mills NL: The selection of patients with bronchogenic carcinoma for mediastinoscopy. J Thorac Cardiovasc Surg 71:768, 1971.

23. Jolly PC, Li W, Anderson RP: Anterior and cervical mediastinoscopy for determining operability and predicting resectability in lung cancer. J Thorac Cardiovasc Surg 79:366, 1980.

24. Kato H, Ono J: Transbronchial aspiration cytology (TBAC). In Hayata Y (ed): Lung Cancer Diagnosis. Tokyo–New York, Igaku-Shoi, 1982, p 127.

25. Kemeny MM, Block LR, Braun DW Jr, et al: Results of surgical treatment of carcinoma of the lung by stage and cell type. Surg Gynecol Obstet 147:865, 1978.

26. Kirschner PA: Mediastinoscopy; guide to management of lung cancer. NY State J Med 71:2041, 1971.

27. Kirsh MM, Kahn DR, Gago O, et al: Treatment of bronchogenic carcinoma with mediastinal masses. Ann Thorac Surg 12:11, 1971.

28. Kirsh MM, Sloan H: Mediastinal metastases in bronchogenic carcinoma: Influence of postoperative irradiation, cell type, and location. Ann Thorac Surg 33:459, 1982.

29. Larsson S: Pretreatment classification and staging of bronchogenic carcinoma. Scand J Thorac Cardiovasc Surg 7:1, 1973.

30. Lesk DM, Wood TE, Carroll SE, et al: The application of ^{67}Ga scanning in determining the operability of bronchogenic carcinoma. Radiology 128:707, 1978.

31. Lewis JR Jr, Madrazo BL, Gross SC, et al: The value of radiographic and computed tomography in the staging of lung carcinoma. Ann Thorac Surg 34:553, 1982.

32. Martini N: Improved methods of recording data in lung cancer. Clinical Bulletin of Memorial Sloan-Kettering Cancer Center 6:93, 1976.

33. Martini N, Flehinger BJ, Zaman MB, et al: Prospective study of 445 lung carcinomas with mediastinal lymph node metastases. J Thorac Cardiovasc Surg 80:390, 1980.

34. McLeod RA, Brown LR, Miller WE, et al: Evaluation of the pulmonary hila by tomography. Radiol Clin North Am 14:51, 1976.

35. McNeill TM, Chamberlain JM: Diagnostic anterior mediastinoscopy. Ann Thorac Surg 2:532, 1966.

36. Mintzer RA, Malave SR, Neiman HL, et al: Computed vs conventional tomography in evaluation of primary and secondary pulmonary neoplasms. Radiology 132:653, 1979.

37. Mountain CF: Surgery of lung cancer including adjunctive therapy. In Hansen HH, Rorth M (eds): Proceedings of the Second World Conference on Lung Cancer. Copenhagen, 1980.

38. Mountain CF, Hermes KE: Management implications of surgical staging studies. In Muggia F, Rozencweig M (eds): Lung Cancer; Progress in Therapeutic Research. New York, Raven Press, 1979.

39. Murray GF, Mendes OC, Wilcox BR: Bronchial carcinoma and the lymphatic sump: The importance of bronchoscopic findings. Ann Thorac Surg 34:634, 1982.

40. Naruke T, Suemasu K, Ishikawa S: Lymph node mapping and curability at various levels of metastasis in resection lung cancer. J Thorac Cardiovasc Surg 76:832, 1978.

41. Naruke T, Suemasu K, Ishikawa S: Surgical therapy for N_2 disease. Presented at The III World Conference on Lung Cancer, The Secretariat of the III World Conference on Cancer, National Cancer Center, Tsukiji, Tokyo, Japan, 1982 (abstract).

42. Nishiwaki Y, Nishiyama H: Oblique tomography and xerotomography. In Hayata Y (ed): Lung Cancer Diagnosis. Tokyo–New York, Igaku-Shoin, 1982, p 204.

43. Nohl-Oser HC: Lymphatics of the lung. In Shields TW (ed): General Thoracic Surgery, 2nd ed. Philadelphia, Lea & Febiger, 1983.

44. Ochsner A, Debakey M: Significance of metastasis in primary carcinoma of the lung. J Thorac Surg 11:357, 1942.

45. Osborne DR, Korobkin M, Putman CE, et al: Comparison of plain radiography, conventional tomography and computed tomography in detecting intrathoracic lymph node metastasis from lung carcinoma. Radiology 142:157, 1982.

46. Paulson DL, Reisch JS: Long-term survival after resection for bronchogenic carcinoma. Ann Surg 184:324, 1976.

47. Paulson DL, Urschel HC: Selectivity in the surgical treatment of bronchogenic carcinoma. J Thorac Cardiovasc Surg 62:554, 1971.

48. Pearson FG: Use of mediastinoscopy in the selection of patients for lung cancer operation. Ann Thorac Surg 39:205, 1980.

49. Pearson FG, DeLarue NC, Ilves R, et al: Significance of positive superior mediastinal nodes identified at mediastinoscopy in patients with resectable cancer of the lung. J Thorac Cardiovasc Surg 83:1, 1982.

50. Pearson FG, Nelems JM, Henderson RD, et al: The role of mediastinoscopy in the selection of treatment

for bronchial carcinoma with involvement of superior mediastinal lymph nodes. J Thorac Cardiovasc Surg 64:382, 1972.

51. Pugatch RD, Faling LJ, Jung-Legg Y, et al: CT scanning of the mediastinum in the staging of bronchogenic carcinoma. Am Rev Respir Dis 121:179, 1980.

52. Ramsey HE, Cahan WG, Beattie EJ, et al: The importance of radical lobectomy in lung cancer. J Thorac Cardiovasc Surg 58:225, 1969.

53. Rea HH, Shevland JE, House AJS: Accuracy of computed tomographic scanning in assessment of the mediastinum in bronchial carcinoma. J Thorac Cardiovasc Surg 81:825, 1981.

54. Rubenstein I, Baum GL, Kalter Y, et al: Resectional surgery in the treatment of primary carcinoma of the lung with mediastinal lymph node metastases. Thorax 34:33, 1979.

55. Sarin CL, Nohl-Oser HC: Mediastinoscopy: A clinical evaluation of 400 consecutive cases. Thorax 24:585, 1969.

56. Sarrazin R, Voog R, Dyon JF: Contribution a l'étude des lymphatiques du poumon. Poumon Coeur 30:289, 1974.

57. Shields TW: The fate of patients after incomplete resection of bronchial carcinoma. Surg Gynecol Obstet 139:569, 1974.

58. Shields TW, Higgins GA Jr, Matthew MJ, et al: Surgical resection in the management of small cell carcinoma of the lung. J Thorac Cardiovasc Surg 84:481, 1982.

59. Shields TW, Yee J, Conn JH, et al: Relationship of cell type and lymph node metastasis to survival after resection of bronchial carcinoma. Ann Thorac Surg 20:501, 1975.

60. Shimizu N, Matsumoto S, Ogino K, et al: The surgical treatment of N_2 lung cancer. Presented at The III World Conference on Lung Cancer, The Secretariat of the III World Conference on Cancer, National Cancer Center, Tsukiji, Tokyo, Japan, 1982, p 114 (abstract).

61. Tsuchiya R, Suemasu K, Matsuyama T, et al: Evaluation of mediastinal abnormality by xerotomography. Jpn J Clin Oncol 9:49, 1979.

62. Underwood GH Jr, Hooper RG, Axelbaum SP, et al: Computed tomographic scanning of the thorax in the staging of bronchogenic carcinoma. N Engl J Med 300:777, 1979.

63. Viikari SJ, Inberg MN, Puhakka H: The role of mediastinoscopy in the treatment of lung carcinoma. Bull Soc Int Chir 2:119, 1974.

64. Wang KP, Marsh BR, Summer WR, et al: Transbronchial needle aspiration for diagnosis of lung cancer. Chest 80:48, 1981.

65. Wang KP, Terry P, Marsh B: Bronchoscopic needle aspiration biopsy of paratracheal tumors. Am Rev Respir Dis 118:17, 1978.

66. Watanabe Y, Iwa T, Kobayashi H, et al: Results of surgical treatment for lung cancer with N_2 disease. Presented at The III World Conference on Lung Cancer, The Secretariat of the III World Conference on Cancer, National Cancer Center, Tsukiji, Tokyo, Japan, 1982 (abstract).

67. Whitcomb ME, Barham E, Goldman AL, et al: Indications for mediastinoscopy in bronchogenic carcinoma. Am Rev Respir Dis 113:189, 1976.

23

The Use of Mediastinoscopy in Lung Cancer: Preoperative Evaluation

Joel D. Cooper, M.D.
Robert J. Ginsberg, M.D.

Resectional surgery as a method of curing lung cancer has been in use for more than 50 years. It was recognized early that when lymph node involvement occurs in the disease, the prognosis following resection is worse. Initially, attempts were made to identity those patients with lymphatic spread to the supraclavicular area. For this purpose, scalene node biopsy was advocated since any patient with involvement of scalene nodes was believed to be beyond hope of surgical cure. For disease involving intrathoracic mediastinal lymph nodes, many early authors, including Allison in 1946,[2] Brock in 1948,[5] and Caham and colleagues in 1951,[6] recommended radical pneumonectomy, although this did not appear to improve currability. Indeed, Bergh and Schersten[3] later demonstrated that once mediastinal lymph nodes are involved, few patients survive 5 years.

Carlens in 1959[7] first proposed the use of cervical mediastinal exploration in an attempt to identify preoperatively those patients who would not benefit from surgical resection. This became popularized in Europe. Pearson[15] reported his experience in North America in 1965.

Since the introduction of mediastinoscopy, controversies have appeared over its proper place in the preoperative assessment prior to thoracotomy. Many surgeons believe that mediastinal nodal involvement identified at mediastinoscopy indicates inoperability. Others believe that only those patients with "intranodal" disease low in the mediastinum benefit from surgical resection. Finally, there remains a group of surgeons who believe in radical surgical resection of involved mediastinal nodes, even if only to offer palliation.

Many investigators have attempted to replace mediastinoscopy with less invasive techniques. Initially, mediastinal tomography[8] and hilar oblique tomography[11] were proposed as possible alternatives. Most recently, computed tomography[4] (CT), radioisotope studies, and magnetic resonance imagine have been advocated. With each of these modalities, it was hoped that sensitivity and specificity would be good enough to identify patients with involved superior mediastinal nodes without requiring an invasive technique such as mediastinoscopy.

Wang and associates[18] have developed a technique of transbronchoscopic needle aspiration of mediastinal lymph nodes. This technique is used to sample enlarged mediastinal lymph nodes previously identified on CT scan.

It is our belief that mediastinoscopy plays a vital role in the preoperative staging of disease in patients with lung cancer. The following discussion includes our technique and our results with this procedure.

THE IMPORTANCE OF NODAL STAGING

The prognosis in patients with lung cancer depends on the stage of the disease at the time of treatment as well as the cell type. It is now well recognized that for patients with N_0 disease, the prognosis is excellent if a curative resection is performed. It can be expected that a T_1N_0 tumor will be cured in about 80% of patients. Although absolute survival rates approach only 70% at 5 years, many of these patients die from other diseases without evidence of recurrent tumor. For patients with T_2N_0 tumors, the prognosis is less favorable.

Once tumor spreads to lymph nodes, the ultimate prognosis is significantly worse. As long as the involved lymph nodes are within the confines of the lung (N_1) and tumor has not spread to mediastinal lymph nodes, there is a reasonable chance of curability, approaching 30% to 40% at 5 years. In patients with adenocarcinoma, the prognosis is worse than with squamous cell carcinoma. Mediastinal lymph node involvement (N_2 disease) indicates an ominous prognosis, whatever the cell type. Although the 5-year survival figures culled from the literature range from 0% to 35%, it is difficult to assess the exact prognosis following resection for N_2 disease because of selectivity of the reports describing curative resection. Moreover, in most series accurate staging methods for N_2 disease have not been utilized.

Naruke and coworkers[13] in Japan and Martini and colleagues[12] in the United States were the first to perform intraoperative lymph node mapping for accurate staging of each tumor in order to identify the ultimate prognosis. The Lung Cancer Study Group similarly has adopted this procedure, as reported by Weisenberger and coauthors.[20] Only with the use of accurate staging can results be compared and prognoses be identified. Mediastinal lymph node mapping can be done quite accurately at the time of surgery. However, for left-sided tumors, superior mediastinal lymph node mapping is difficult without the use of mediastinoscopy.

As well as its value in identifying prognosis, accurate staging may be important in the future in considering adjuvant treatment before or after resection. Current studies[9, 12, 13, 20] seem to indicate that adjuvant radiotherapy and possibly adjuvant chemotherapy delay the time to recurrence in patients with N_1 and N_2 disease and may possibly improve survival. With our present state of knowledge, it is apparent that patients with N_0 disease do not require adjuvant therapy except perhaps for T_3 tumors. Until a large number of accurately staged tumors (especially the N_2 component) can be followed in well-constructed prospective clinical trials to evaluate adjuvant therapy, the value of such treatment will remain unclear.

MEDIASTINOSCOPY FOR ASSESSMENT OF N_2 DISEASE

The use of preoperative mediastinoscopy for assessing patients with lung carcinoma remains controversial. The choice of some centers not to employ preoperative mediastinoscopy in the assessment of patients with lung cancer is based upon one or more of the following considerations: (1) the belief that delineation of superior mediastinal lymph node status is not essential to the decision-making process; (2) the feeling that noninvasive diagnostic methods may give equivalent information; and (3) the concern regarding the morbidity and mortality of this invasive diagnostic procedure.

We have routinely employed mediastinoscopy for the preoperative assessment of patients with presumably operable cancer of the lung for more than 20 years. Our experience with this technique continues to persuade us that the information so obtained is critical to informed decision-making regarding operability, as well as to the selection of adjuvant therapies combined with surgical resection. In evaluating the significance of mediastinoscopy, it is important to address two issues: First, is the status of superior mediastinal lymph nodes important in selecting treatment and assessing prognosis? Second, can other nondiagnostic modalities replace mediastinoscopy in making this assessment?

To answer the first question it is necessary to review the experience with surgical resection in patients having positive mediastinal lymph nodes at the time of resection. Most such reports are based upon mediastinal lymph node involvement identified at the time of thoracotomy.[1, 3, 10, 12–14, 17] The 5-year survival rate in such patients averages between 20% and 30%, a very respectable figure under the circumstances. These reports, however, are largely based upon retrospective analysis of pathology reports rather than on prospective, careful lymph node mapping at the time of surgery. Two exceptions are the series reported by Naruke[13] and Martini[12] and their colleagues, which did involve such prospective mapping. In none of these series, however, was preoperative mediastinoscopy used for the assessment of mediastinal lymph nodes.

Our own experience with the results of surgical resection in patients having positive mediastinal lymph nodes identified at preoperative mediastinoscopy suggested a far worse prognosis and prompted a review of our experience several years ago.[16] We compared results of thoracotomy in patients with positive findings on preoperative mediastinoscopy with results in patients having mediastinal lymph node involvement not identified until thoracotomy. The patients having positive findings on preoperative mediastinoscopy and subsequent thoracotomy represented a highly selected subset of a much larger group of patients having positive mediastinoscopy, most of whom were not operated upon. Approximately one out of every five patients with a positive mediastinoscopy was selected for surgical therapy. Thus, in most patients in whom metastases in the superior mediastinal lymph nodes were identified at mediastinoscopy, disease was not considered operable. This group included patients with the finding of small cell anaplastic carcinoma, contralateral mediastinal involvement, extensive lymph node extracapsular spread, fixation to mediastinal structures, or gross nodal involvement in high paratracheal locations. Over a 16-year period, 79 patients were selected for thoracotomy in spite of mediastinal lymph node involvement as determined at preoperative mediastinoscopy. Most of these received adjuvant radiotherapy. The overall result in this highly selected group of patients showed a cumulative 5-year survival rate of 9%.

During the same time period, we evaluated another group of 62 patients in whom positive mediastinal lymph nodes were found at thoracotomy despite negative findings on preoperative mediastinoscopy. The results in this group of patients showed an actuarial 5-year survival of 24%. In both series, survival figures included postoperative deaths and unresectable cases.

It must be emphasized that our results with surgical resection in patients with positive findings on preoperative mediastinoscopy included only a highly selected group. Had all patients with positive mediastinoscopy been subjected to thoracotomy, it seems obvious that the overall results for this group of patients would indeed have been dismal. Furthermore, had we not used mediastinoscopy to determine the N_2 status prior to proceeding with surgical resections, approximately a fourth of the patients operated on during this period of time would have had N_2 disease in the superior mediastinum that was either nonresectable or amenable only to palliative resection. This would significantly lower both the overall resectability rate and the rate of curative resection for patients with lung carcinoma. A review of approximately 700 consecutive thoracotomies for primary lung cancer in our hospital demonstrated a resectability rate of 93%, with 84% of the total having complete or curative resections.

We have therefore concluded from our own experience that the presence of lymph node metastases in the superior mediastinum confers a much more ominous prognosis than the finding of involved mediastinal lymph nodes at the time of thoracotomy. Although each case must be assessed individually regarding the merits of resection, the status of superior mediastinal lymph nodes is of significance regarding both prognosis and decision-making. Perhaps this can best be illustrated by reviewing two well-documented series of thoracotomies for lung carcinoma performed without preoperative mediastinoscopy. Naruke and coworkers[13] reported on 464 resections for lung cancer. They

claimed a 19% cumulative 5-year survival in patients who had positive mediastinal lymph nodes (most of whom received adjuvant chemo- or radiotherapy). An analysis of this series is instructive: Of the 464 patients, there were 24 postoperative deaths, which are not included in the survival figures. Of the 440 patients remaining, 170 underwent resections that were deemed "noncurative"; these patients were also eliminated from analysis of the results. The remaining 270 patients underwent resections judged curative or "relatively curative." Of the 270 patients, 64 were found to have a positive mediastinal lymph node at thoracotomy; among these, there were 12 who were 5-year survivors (19%).

Several conclusions are inescapable: the elimination of operative deaths and of those patients who had unfavorable findings at thoracotomy greatly affected the authors' analysis of survival with positive mediastinal lymph nodes; the true figure, including all cases, would probably be well under 8%. Moreover, 37% of the patients underwent a fruitless thoracotomy; in many of these, disease could probably have been identified as unresectable with the use of preoperative mediastinoscopy.

The report by Martini and colleagues[12] is similarly instructive. They described their experience with surgical treatment of lung cancer in 241 patients found to have mediastinal lymph node metastases at operation. For the patients in whom resection of tumor was "complete," the actuarial survival rate was 49% at 3 years. However, 135 of the 241 patients had extensive tumor involvement precluding complete excision. Resection with mediastinal lymph node dissection was carried out in the remaining 106 patients (44%); resection was considered merely palliative in 26 of these patients because of persistent disease at the completion of the surgical treatment. Only 80 of the 241 patients (33%), therefore, had a complete resection. The 49% 5-year survival rate is based solely on these 80 patients. This type of retrospective, selective analysis of patients with mediastinal lymph node involvement clearly gives a far different picture from that obtained by assessing the entire group. Notwithstanding the fact that these workers employed intraoperative radioisotope implant therapy in some of their unresected or incompletely resected cases, it seems apparent that the routine preoperative use of mediastinoscopy would have provided useful information that almost certainly would have reduced the number of fruitless thoracotomies and correspondingly improved the overall resectability rate.

NONINVASIVE STAGING

It is well know that plain posteroanterior and lateral chest x-ray films are much too insensitive to be useful for N_2 assessment. *Mediastinal tomography* has been suggested as a more precise technique. We evaluated this method in a prospective, "blind" study[8] and found it to lack both specificity and sensitivity, with a false-positive rate of about 30% and a false-negative rate of 10%. These findings have been confirmed by others.[7a, 9a] If mediastinal tomography is used alone to assess N_2 disease, at least 20% of patients will have inappropriate therapy—either unnecessary thoracotomy or no surgery when indeed the tumor is resectable and the disease potentially curable. Oblique tomograms are reliable for early detection of nodal involvement (N_1) in the hilum but not in the subaortic region, where they reveal only more advanced metastases (N_2). They are not useful for detecting superior mediastinal involvement.

It had been hoped that *computed tomography* (CT) would provide improved specificity and sensitivity. However, enlarged lymph nodes detected by CT in the mediastinum are not necessarily tumor-laden lymph nodes; rather, such enlargement may reflect merely benign inflammatory change. Some authors, therefore, advocate mediastinoscopy only in those patients with positive findings on mediastinal CT scan, in order to avoid unnecessary operation. On the other hand, of the patients with no evidence of involvement on CT scan (i.e., without node enlargement), 10% will ultimately be proved to have nodal metastases despite the initial negative findings, because the scan cannot detect microscopic involvement by tumor.

Magnetic resonance imaging is currently being investigated as a staging tool.[4] It may have an advantage over CT examination in that it permits distinction among various tissue densities, perhaps allowing differentiation among nodal involvement with tumor, fibrosis, and inflammation.

Nuclear imaging using either gallium-67-labeled[19] or cobalt-57-bleomycin[13a] has even less sensitivity and similar problems with specificity. Compounding these inadequacies is the fact that only in those tumors that take up the isotope will there be any correlation with mediastinal nodal involvement. Unfortunately, inflammatory as well as neoplastic processes have an affinity for gallium-67, causing problems with sensitivity.

A newer semi-invasive method of determining mediastinal involvement is that of *transbronchoscopic needle aspiration* of subcarinal and paratracheal lymph nodes, as described by Wang.[18] Mediastinal lymphadenopathy in association with a "positive" transbronchoscopic needle aspirate is absolute proof of N_2 disease. However, if the decision for resection depends on unilaterality or limited intranodal rather than extranodal involvement, operability cannot always be assessed by this technique.

Although some centers depend solely upon noninvasive imaging to estimate N_2 status prior to surgery, it must be realized that there are significant inaccuracies with these techniques. Although false-negative results may be as low as 10%, the false-positive rate may be as high as 30%; if "positive" imaging implies inoperability, curative therapy may be denied to many patients with potentially curable disease. Thoracotomy without mediastinoscopy should be performed only if the surgeon intends to perform accurate superior mediastinal node staging at that time.

TECHNIQUE OF MEDIASTINOSCOPY

We generally combine bronchoscopy with mediastinoscopy, using general anesthesia, whether or not a preliminary bronchoscopy with a flexible instrument has been performed using local anesthesia. Both rigid and flexible bronchoscopes are utilized to assess the anatomy of the tracheobronchial tree as well as the direct or indirect effects of tumor.

The endotracheal tube is positioned at the left corner of the mouth, and the anesthetic tubing and apparatus are located to the left of the patient's head to permit unimpeded access and visualization of the sternal notch from the head of the table. The neck is extended and the shoulders are elevated. We use an inflatable balloon placed under the shoulders prior to induction of general anesthesia, though a sandbag can be used for the same purpose. The patient's occiput is stabilized with the use of a "donut" ring placed under the head. The neck and anterior chest are prepped and draped. The table may be either level or slightly tilted, foot downward, to lessen venous congestion.

A small (4-cm) transverse incision is made just above the suprasternal notch. The pretracheal muscles are separated vertically in the midline to expose the anterior surface of the trachea. The trachea is exposed to just below the thyroid isthmus, which is then retracted superiorly. The trachea is thus exposed to just below the cricoid cartilage. There is often a tendency to expose the anterior trachea more inferiorly, thus dissecting down into the mediastinum at the same time. Such a dissection, however, is not as safe or simple, particularly in an obese patient.

The pretracheal fascia is incised and separated from the anterior surface of the trachea using the tip of the surgeon's index finger. Blunt finger dissection is then extended down into the mediastinum, keeping the back of the finger tip in direct contact with the anterior surface of the trachea until the carina has been reached (usually palpable as the beginning of a cleft in the anterior trachea as felt with the dorsum of the extended index finger). Flexing the finger tip slightly to the left will identify the back of the aortic arch. Withdrawing the finger tip 2 to 3 cm and flexing it toward the right will identify the back of the innominate artery. Further blunt dissection should then be carried out with the finger tip to open a channel to the right and left of the trachea in the mid-tracheal plane.

The finger is then withdrawn, and the mediastinoscope is inserted into the pretracheal plane in the midline. This may be facilitated by retracting upward on the lower flap of the pretracheal fascia with a small right-angled retractor. Dissection through the channel of the mediastinoscope is best performed using the mediastinoscopy sucker. An insulated sucker is useful as it permits cautery to be applied to the tip of the sucker only. Lymph nodes in the right paratracheal and tracheobronchial area may not be immediately apparent, because they are often imbedded in fat and must be dissected free. Attention will be initially directed to any firm or enlarged nodes identified by the palpating finger; however, positive mediastinal nodes not grossly abnormal to palpation or on inspection are common. Accessible areas for dissection and biopsy of lymph nodes include the anterior subcarinal nodes and both right and left tracheobronchial angle lymph nodes and paratracheal lymph nodes. Potential hazards include vascular injury to the azygos vein (just lateral to the

trachea above the right tracheobronchial angle), the innominate artery (to the right and anterior to the trachea at the mid-tracheal level), the right pulmonary artery (just anterior to the subcarinal and right main bronchial area), or the aorta. Dissection of the subcarinal lymph nodes is frequently associated with bleeding from bronchial arteries, which on occasion can be significant. Long, narrow gauze packing should always be immediately available prior to starting a mediastinoscopy dissection. Most instances of hemorrhage can be dealt with by packing through the mediastinoscope until the bleeding has subsided.

The left recurrent nerve lies just lateral to the trachea on the left side and can be routinely visualized about 3 cm proximal to the carina, 1 cm lateral to the trachea in the mid-tracheal plane, heading obliquely toward the left at a slight angle. Just above the left tracheobronchial angle is commonly found a lymph node immediately medial to the left recurrent nerve. Biopsy of this lymph node should be done from the medial aspect of the node because approach from its lateral aspect may incur injury to the recurrent nerve.

Following exposure of lymph nodes to be biopsied, aspiration of the specimen through a long, thin aspirating needle is advised even for the experienced operator. The use of aspiration rather than more drastic retrieval methods avoids catastrophic injury to vascular structures when they are not readily distinguishable from lymph nodes, as when a flattened node covers the surface of a vein or an artery.

At our institution all biopsy specimens are sent for quick section analysis as soon as they are taken, and immediate, accurate reporting is available.

For right-sided tumors, subcarinal and right paratracheal and tracheobronchial lymph nodes are assessed, with more cursory assessment of the left paratracheal area. For left-sided tumors however, both right and left paratracheal areas are carefully examined, as well as the subcarinal area. Unfortunately, posterior subcarinal nodes cannot be assessed by mediastinoscopy.

For patients with left upper lobe tumors, left anterior mediastinotomy is performed along with cervical mediastinoscopy, if the cervical mediastinoscopy has yielded negative findings. In such cases the cervical incision is left open following the mediastinoscopy, and a small transverse incision is made in the second left interspace just lateral to the sternal border. Dissection is carried down to the intercostal membrane, which is carefully incised to expose pre-pleural fatty tissue. Care should be taken to avoid injury to the internal mammary vessels at this point. The anterior mediastinal area is then explored with the surgeon's right index finger, best accomplished with the surgeon standing on the right side of the table. The pleura is not entered at this point but is swept to the left. The superior anterior mediastinum is best explord by palpation. With the right index finger still in place, the surgeon's left index finger is inserted through the cervical mediastinoscopy incision, and the tip of the left index finger is positioned posterior to the aortic arch. With this finger tip as a guide, the surgeon's right index finger, inserted through the anterior mediastinal incision, can easily palpate the anterior surface of the aortic arch and the subaortic area. At this point, the right and left index fingers are virtually encircling the aorta for assessment of the subaortic nodes. Following palpation, the mediastinoscope can be inserted to visualize, aspirate, and biopsy any palpated abnormalities. If the left pleural space has not been inadvertently opened at this stage, it can be incised for more thorough examination of the left hilar area.

Upon completion of the procedure, the platysma is closed with a running suture, and the skin is closed with a subcuticular suture. We do not routinely reapproximate the pretracheal muscles.

Though it is common for surgeons to continue immediately with thoracotomy upon completion of the mediastinoscopy procedure, it is not our practice to routinely do so. The reason for this is a logistic one: Of patients undergoing mediastinoscopy, 30% are found to have positive mediastinal lymph nodes, and most of these are eliminated from consideration for thoracotomy. We therefore perform thoracotomy as a separate procedure several days following mediastinoscopy. Because we utilize mediastinoscopy as one of the initial steps in evaluating patients with lung carcinoma, this interval also permits further investigations prior to thoracotomy if required. In addition, our practice of separating mediastinoscopy from thoracotomy allows further evaluation of patients with positive findings at mediastinoscopy to select those for whom thoracotomy may still be deemed advisable. This separate scheduling also permits discussions with the patient and family members about the rationale, risks, and expectations specific to each procedure. Furthermore, this practice avoids the psychological stress experienced by the patient who awakens from anesthesia to discover that the anticipated thoracotomy has in fact been found to be contraindicated; it also eliminates possible pressure on the surgeon to proceed with thoracotomy merely to fulfil the patient's expectation of a definitive result.

The majority of mediastinoscopies at our institution are performed by the resident staff, indicating that with proper teaching and supervision, mediastinoscopy can be performed without the need for extensive experience on the part of the operating surgeon.

COMPLICATIONS

Anticipated complications from mediastinoscopy include hemorrhage from injury of major vessels; pneumothorax (usually on the right, from dissection through the mediastinal pleural surface); left recurrent nerve palsy (usually transient); and wound infection.

We have recently reviewed our 5-year experience with mediastinoscopy between 1979 and 1984. During this time 1559 patients were admitted to the thoracic surgical service at our hospital for lung carcinoma. Of these, 960 (62%) underwent mediastinoscopy, with 127 concomitant anterior mediastinotomies. Positive mediastinal lymph nodes were found in 30% of patients. Complication rate was 2% overall, with no mortality. Complications included significant hemorrhage in three patients, pneumothorax in four, and wound infection in five. In this series there were no recurrent nerve palsies, although in our previous series, transient recurrent nerve palsy from injury at mediastinoscopy was noted.

References

1. A. Smith R: The importance of mediastinal lymph patients for resection. Ann Thorac Surg 25:5–11, 1978.
2. Allison PR: Intrapericardial approach to the lung route in the treatment of bronchial carcinoma by dissection pneumonectomy. J. Thorac Surg 15:99, 1946.
3. Bergh NP, Schersten T: Bronchogenic carcinoma. A follow up study of a surgically treated series with special reference to the prognostic significance of lymph node metastases. Acta Chir Scand (Suppl) 347:1–41, 1965.
4. Breyer RH, Karstaedt N, Mills SA: Computed tomography for evaluation of mediastinal lymph nodes in lung cancer—correlation with surgical staging. Ann Thorac Surg 38:15–20, 1984.

5. Brock RC: Bronchial carcinoma. Brit. Med. J 2:737, 1948.

6. Caham WG, Watson WL, Pool JL: Radical pneumonectomy. J Thorac Surg 22:449, 1951.

7. Carlens E: Mediastinoscopy: a method for inspection and tissue biopsy in the superior mediastinum. Dis Chest 36:343, 1959.

7a. Fishman NH, Bronstein MH: Is mediastinoscopy necessary in the evaluation of lung cancer? Ann Thor Surg 20:678, 1975.

8. Ginsberg RJ, Nelems JM, Pearson FG, Sanders DE: Mediastinal tomography as an aid in determining operability in carcinoma of the lung. Ann Roy Coll Phys Surg (Canada) 7:45, 1974.

9. Holmes EC, Egan RT: (for the Lung Cancer Study Group): Surgical adjuvant therapy of resectable stage II/III adenocarcinoma and large cell undifferentiated carcinoma of the lung. Proc AASCO C-860:220, 1984.

9a. James EC, Elwood RA: Mediastinoscopy and mediastinal roentgenology. Ann Thor Surg 18:531, 1974.

10. Kirsh MM, Kahn DR, Gago O: Treatment of bronchogenic carcinoma with mediastinal metastases. Ann Thorac Surg 12:11–21, 1971.

11. Konn A, Konn FA, Garvey J: Oblique hilar tomography in mediastinoscopy. Chest 86:424, 1984.

12. Martini N, Flehinger BJ, Zaman MB, Beattie EJ Jr: Prospective study of 445 lung carcinomas with mediastinal lymph node metastases. J Thorac Cardiovasc Surg 80:390–399, 1980.

13. Naruke T, Suemasu K, Ishikawa S: Lymph node mapping and curability at varous levels of metastasis in resected lung cancer. J Thorac Cardiovasc Surg 76:832–839, 1978.

13a. Nieweg OE, Beekhuis H, Piers DA, et al: 57-Cobleomycin and 67-Ga-citrate in the detection and staging of lung cancer. Thorax 38:16, 1983.

14. Paulson DL, Urschel HC Jr: Selectivity in the surgical treatment of bronchogenic carcinoma. J Thorac Cardiovasc Surg 62:554–562, 1971.

15. Pearson FG: Mediastinoscopy: a method for inspection and tissue biopsy in the superior mediastinum. J Thorac Cardiovasc Surg 49:11, 1965.

16. Pearson FG, DeLarue NC, Ilves R, et al: Significance of positive superior mediastinal nodes identified at mediastinoscopy in patients with resectable cancer of the lung. J Thorac Cardiovasc Surg 83:1–11, 1982.

17. Ramsey HE, Cahan WG, Beattie EJ, Humphrey C: The importance of radical lobecomy in lung cancer. J. Thorac Cardiovasc Surg 58:225–230, 1969.

18. Wang KP, Brower R, Haponik EF: Flexible transbronchial needle aspiration for staging of bronchogenic carcinoma. Chest 84:571, 1983.

19. Waxman, AD, Julien PJ, Brachman MB: Gallium scintigraphy in bronchogenic carcinoma. Chest 86:178, 1983.

20. Weisenberger T, Gail M (for the Lung Cancer Study Group): Recurrence patterns in resected stage II/III epidermoid lung cancer. Proc AASCO C-909:232, 1984.

VIII

The Extent of Resection for Localized Lung Cancer

By 1900 there were sporadic attempts at operating for chest problems, chiefly for trauma and suppuration but occasionally for tumor. There had been at least one pneumonectomy done by Macewen in 1895 in a patient who survived. True, it was not a careful dissection as we know this procedure today, but nonetheless the left lung, extensively involved by tuberculosis and pyogenic infection, was removed (Macewen, 1906). This patient effectively demonstrated that a pneumonectomy could be tolerated.

Many years later (1914), in Glasgow, Macewen wrote that he chanced upon a group of Salvation Army workers: "In the middle of the circle stood a man, and he was making an address, unconscious for the moment of the frost and fog and snow. I glanced at him, and I recognized my patient of many years ago—the man with but one lung." Twenty-six years after this meeting, the same patient underwent repair of a hernia (Bowman, 1942)!

Undoubtedly many attempts at lung resection were the result of the farsighted experiments of Block (1881) and Gluck (1881), working independently, who showed that a lung could be excised in dogs and rabbits and the animal could survive. Gluck predicted: "The conditions of the chest for which surgery seems to me to be indicated are as follows: lung abscess, gangrene of the lung, bronchiectasis, phthisical cavities, tumors, and trauma of the lung."

Others were skeptical. In the first text solely devoted to thoracic surgery, *Surgery of the Chest* (Paget, 1896), an address given by Réclus at the French Surgical Congress in 1895 is reproduced. After reviewing the various thoracic operations done to date, Réclus concluded: "Resection of a part of the lung for primary malignant disease is not even worth discussing. An accessible, single, circumscribed growth would be a clinical wonder that would evade our present powers of observation. The utmost that the surgeon can do is, after the example of Krönlein, to follow even into the lung a sarcoma growing from the chest-wall: but this will never be more than one of the brilliant exceptions of surgery." But predictions are often wrong and attitudes do change. Surgical ingenuity, the increasing incidence of bronchogenic carcinoma, and interest in endotracheal and Sauerbruch's negative pressure chamber anesthesia combined to focus on this problem. Successes with pulmonary resection soon followed.

Accounts of pneumonectomy and lobectomy appeared in the medical literature for the next three decades. In the records the first acknowledged and successful pneumonectomy is credited to Nissen in 1931, performed on a patient with bronchiectasis of the left lung using the technique of mass ligation of the hilus. But the operation done two years later by Graham was the fortuitous event that spurred continued efforts to attack bronchogenic carcinoma. Graham intended to do a lobectomy in his 48-year-old physician patient. However, at operation (April, 1933) the location of the tumor was such that the lower lobe could not be saved (Fig. 1); left pneumonectomy was done together with resection of ribs 3 through 9. Radon seeds were implanted into the bronchial stump, which had been closed with a transfixation suture of chromic catgut. An empyema was recognized on the ninth postoperative day and drained. Six weeks after the first operation, the first and second ribs were removed to close the empyema cavity. Recovery was uneventful; the patient lived 30 years after his

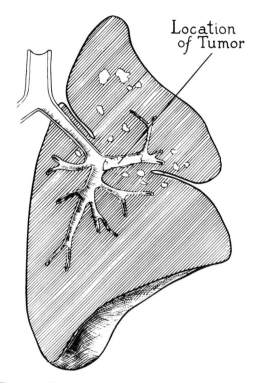

Location of Tumor

Figure 1. Sketch of left lung removed by Graham in 1933. Note location of tumor near bifurcation of left main bronchus and the numerous small abscesses, chiefly in the left upper lobe. (From Graham EA, Singer JJ, and Ballon HC: Surgical Diseases of the Chest. Philadelphia, Lea & Febiger, 1935, p. 840.)

operation and, like Macewen's patient, outlived his surgeon.

Graham's enthusiasm and this patient's continued good health stimulated and encouraged the surgical approach to bronchogenic carcinoma. As Brock so eloquently stated (Brewer, 1984): "Those of us who were struggling with the surgery of bronchial carcinoma in the early 1930's remember only too well the apparent hopelessness of the problem facing the surgeon. Then, like a great light, shone out the report of Graham's success in removing the whole lung in a case of cancer. The news of this travelled rapidly throughout the world. . . . It was not only one case; it was the leaven that stimulated and invigorated the whole field of lung surgery." Three more successful left pneumonectomies were done for tumor in 1933, one by Archibald (1934) and two by Rienhoff (1933).

A dictum for *pneumonectomy* developed. Graham (1933) had written, "Just as experience with carcinoma in other parts of the body has taught that the number of cures is, in general, directly proportional to the extent of

radical removal, so it may be inferred, perhaps, that if the entire lung is removed the patient will have less chance of a recurrence than if only one lobe or a smaller portion is removed." Many others reinforced this advice. Ochsner and DeBakey (1939) declared: "Treatment of pulmonary malignancy consists of total extirpation of the involved lung and removal of the mediastinal lymph nodes. Lobectomy and mass ligation of the hilar structures are condemned . . ." And Rienhoff (1944) was equally emphatic: "Surgical measures short of total pneumonectomy are not efficacious." However, with earlier diagnosis, smaller tumors, and further experience lobectomy did become an acceptable alternative.

Another consideration soon entered the surgical arena. When speed in operating was mandatory, little attention was given to the hilar anatomy, not to mention the detailed arrangement of the bronchi, arteries, and veins distally. Aeby (1880) deserves credit for his pioneer work on bronchial anatomy, but we owe our present knowledge of bronchial and vascular relationships primarily to the efforts of Ewart (1889). He recognized a basic anatomic unit of the lung: "Within each lobe, large groups of lobules being served by separate bronchi are thus kept in practical isolation from each other as regards their air-supply. Each of these sublobar groups may be considered as forming a *separate respiratory district.* . . . Definite support is given to this assumption by the anatomy and the pathology of various morbid processes." Pursuing this concept further, Kramer and Glass (1932) devised the term *bronchopulmonary segment.* And then, instigated by the work of Churchill and Belsey (1939), segmental surgery was applied to various pulmonary problems: "It is suggested that the bronchopulmonary segment may replace the lobe as the surgical unit of the lung." Initially done for tuberculosis and bronchiectasis, segmental resection was soon utilized for bronchogenic carcinoma.

In 1983 Belcher reviewed 8,781 patients with bronchogenic carcinoma operated on by various procedures in England during the years from 1949 to 1980. He noted the decrease in operative mortality in this period but concluded with a discouraging statement: "If the improvement in operative mortality is excluded, there has been no improvement in the survival rates in the last thirty years." The efficacy and feasibility of surgical treatment for lung cancer has been demonstrated, but the question still remains: "*How much* should we take out?"

24

The Extent of Resection for Localized Lung Cancer: Lobectomy*

Nael Martini, M.D.
Brian C. McCaughan, M.B., B.S.
Patricia M. McCormack, M.D.
Manjit S. Bains, M.D.

The three most common cancers in the United States are carcinomas of lung, breast, and colon. Whereas the overall 5-year survival rate is 68% for breast cancer and 50% for colon carcinoma, it is about 13% for lung cancer. The American Cancer Society estimates that 144,000 new cases of lung cancer will be detected in the United States in 1985, and that 125,000 (87%) of those affected will ultimately die of their disease.[1] The poor survival rate is due to the late presentation in many patients and inability to control the tumor when the cancer is advanced or disseminated.

REQUIRED EXTENT OF RESECTION

When the disease is localized, surgical resection is the treatment of choice and offers the best hope for cure. Historically, pneumonectomy was thought necessary for cure regardless of the size or location of the tumor. However, since 1950, several investigators have shown that the same results could be achieved by lobectomy, with fewer complications and with preservation of lung tissue.[2–5]

The extent of resection found to be necessary at the time of thoracotomy depends on the location of the tumor. Lobectomy is the procedure of choice when the disease is limited to a lobe or a lobar bronchus. When the tumor is located in a main bronchus or at the pulmonary hilum or crosses lobar fissures, pneumonectomy is necessary in order to encompass all disease and to obtain clear margins of resection.

---
*Supported in part by the David B. Kaiser Lung Cancer Task Force Fund and the Jesse Philips Fund.

RESULTS WITH CONSERVATIVE RESECTION

An elective segmentectomy or wedge resection has been advocated by some for small peripheral carcinomas of the lung.[6–9] We limit such conservative procedures to patients unable to tolerate more radical operation, such as the elderly or those with limited cardiopulmonary reserve. As reported by McCormack and Martini,[10] 61 patients underwent segmentectomy or wedge resection for carcinoma of the lung at the Memorial Sloan-Kettering Cancer Center between 1949 and 1978. All patients were staged according to the AJCC (American Joint Committee on Cancer) classification,[11] 53 were found to have post-surgical Stage I disease. Of these, 43 had T_1N_0 lesions and 10 had T_2N_0 lesions. No patient undergoing segmentectomy had T_1N_1 disease. The predominant histology was adenocarcinoma.

Pulmonary resection was restricted to these more conservative procedures because of limited pulmonary reserve in 44 patients (due to chronic obstructive pulmonary disease in 42 and a prior pulmonary resection in 2), poor general medical condition in 4 patients, and inaccurate frozen section diagnoses in 5 patients. There were two postoperative deaths following wedge resections (3.7%); both patients had undergone a prior pneumonectomy.

Recurrence was observed within the same lobe in 10 patients, giving a local recurrence rate of 19%. One other patient developed a hilar nodal recurrence invading the main-stem bronchus. Survival was measured by the Kaplan-Meier method, which considers postoperative deaths and deaths from lung cancer.[12] The 5-year actuarial (projected) survival rate for all 53 patients was 33% in 1980 (at 2 years following operation in some patients). Subsequent follow-up now extends for a minimum of 5 years in all patients, and the 5-year survival rate is 50%.

RESULTS WITH LOBECTOMY OR MORE EXTENSIVE RESECTION

In 1977 we reported our results with the surgical treatment of Stage I lung carcinoma.[13] At that time 115 patients had undergone resection, most commonly by lobectomy with mediastinal lymph node dissection. All resections were considered complete and potentially curative. No patients were lost to follow-up, and the actuarial 5-year survival rate at 1 year was 93%, and at 3 years, 85%.

By 1983, follow-up data for 5 or more years were available for 136 consecutive patients with Stage I non–small cell carcinoma of the lung treated by lobectomy (129) or pneumonectomy (7). Eight of the patients had T_1N_1 tumors and were excluded; also excluded from Stage I evaluation were 10 patients with radiologically occult carcinomas of the lung detected on sputum cytology. In most of these patients the central location of the occult tumor precluded a lesser resection than a lobectomy. Of the remaining 128 patients, 50 had T_1N_0 tumors and 78 had T_2N_0 tumors. All 50 patients with T_1 tumors underwent lobectomy, whereas 6 of the 78 patients with T_2 tumors required pneumonectomy. There were two operative deaths (1.5%), and the overall 5-year survival rate was 72% (Fig. 24–1). Within the group of patients with Stage I non–small cell carcinoma treated by lobectomy or pneumo-

nectomy, those with small peripheral tumors (T_1N_0) did better than those with large or more central lesions (T_2N_0). The 5-year survival rate with T_1 disease was 83%, compared with 65% for those with T_2 lesions.

To date, there has been no local recurrence at the resection margin following lobectomy or pneumonectomy. However, three patients developed regional lymph node metastases despite having undergone nodal dissection: one in a contralateral paratracheal lymph node after a right pneumonectomy and two in subcarinal lymph nodes after a right lower and a left lower lobectomy, respectively. Most of the patients for whom treatment failed developed distant metastases.

FACTORS AFFECTING SURVIVAL

Underlying Disease

For Stage I lung cancer, our experience with wedge resection and segmentectomy compares unfavorably with that of pneumonectomy or lobectomy. However, the patients who underwent segmentectomy or wedge resection had underlying medical conditions that precluded a conventional resection. It is not surprising, therefore, that the 5-year survival rate in these patients was less than in those who underwent lobectomy or pneumonectomy. Moreover, the two groups of patients were treated during different periods, and the retrospective TNM staging may be inaccurate in that a formal node dissection was not performed in all those who underwent a conservative resection.

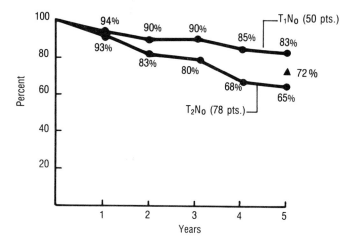
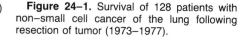

Figure 24–1. Survival of 128 patients with non–small cell cancer of the lung following resection of tumor (1973–1977).

Tumor Stage and Adequacy of Resection

Survival following resection of T_2N_0 tumors has been shown in many reports to be significantly less than for T_1N_0 tumors.[13–15] Despite the greater number of T_2 tumors among the patients who underwent a conventional resection (61%), as compared with those who underwent a conservative resection (19%), there was a significant disease-free survival advantage for those patients in whom a lobectomy or pneumonectomy was performed.

Second Primary Cancers and Local Recurrence

The proponents of conservative resection for small Stage I lung cancer correctly indicate the rather high frequency of the development of a second primary lung cancer in these patients.[6, 9] Of our 136 consecutive patients with Stage I lung cancer treated by lobectomy or pneumonectomy between 1973 and 1977, 44 (32%) have developed a second primary cancer (Table 24–1). In 15 of these patients (34%), this was a second primary lung cancer. Similarly, in a retrospective review of 118 patients with lung cancer surviving 10 or more years, Temeck and colleagues[16] found that 27 had developed a second primary cancer, and that 70% of these were new lung cancers. These findings emphasize two points: first, the need for careful long-term follow-up in all lung cancer patients, and second, the importance of conserving as much lung tissue as possible when resecting "early" lung carcinomas. How-

ever, the chances of curing the first cancer must not be jeopardized by a resection that is less than adequate; preservation of tissue merely to allow for subsequent resection of a second primary tumor is not justified. The high incidence of local recurrence following resections less extensive than lobectomy observed by us and others[6, 9] indicates that the minimal resection for Stage I lung cancer should be lobectomy, provided it is physiologically and technically possible.

CONCLUSIONS

All too few lung cancers are potentially curable. For those patients with Stage I non–small cell carcinoma, however, surgical resection offers a significant chance of cure. Any resection less extensive than lobectomy places the patient at an increased risk of local recurrence and decreases the chances of long-term survival. Only in those patients with compromised cardiopulmonary function do we recommend a conservative resection such as segmentectomy or wedge resection. Regardless of the extent of pulmonary resection, systematic mediastinal lymph node dissection should be routinely performed to ascertain that lymphatic metastases are absent.

Table 24–1. Second Primary Cancers in 136 Patients Following Resection of Stage I Lung Cancer

Site	No. of Patients	
Lung	15	
Breast	9	
Bladder	7	
Head and neck	5	
Larynx		2
Lip		1
Tongue		1
Mouth		1
Gastrointestinal	7	
Colon		4
Pancreas		2
Stomach		1
Total	44 (32%)	

References

1. Cancer Facts and Figures 1985. New York, Am Cancer Society.
2. Beattie EJ Jr: The surgical treatment of lung tumors. Pneumonectomy or lobectomy. Surgery 42:1124, 1957.
3. Churchill ED, Sweet RH, Soutter L, Scannell JG: The surgical management of carcinoma of the lung; a study of the cases treated at the Massachusetts General Hospital from 1930 to 1950. J Thorac Surg 20:349, 1950.
4. Overholt RH: The surgical treatment of bronchogenic carcinoma. Proceedings of the Fourth National Cancer Conference, Minneapolis, MN. Philadelphia, JB Lippincott, 1960. p 309.
5. Paulson DL: Survival rates following resection for bronchogenic carcinoma. Ann Surg 146:997, 1957.
6. Jensik RJ, Faber, LP, Millroy FJ, Monson DO: Segmental resection for lung cancer. A fifteen-year experience. J Thorac Cardiovasc Surg 66:563, 1973.
7. Bonfils-Roberts EA, Clagett OT: Contemporary indications for pulmonary segmental resections. J Thorac Cardiovasc Surg 63:433, 1972.
8. Shields TW, Higgis GA Jr: Minimal pulmonary resection in treatment of carcinoma of the lung. Arch Surg 108:420, 1974.
9. Jensik RJ, Faber LP, Kittle CF: Segmental resection for bronchogenic carcinoma. Ann Thorac Surg 28:475, 1979.

10. McCormack PM, Martini N: Primary lung cancer: results with conservative resection in treatment. NY State Med 80:612, 1980.
11. American Joint Committee on Cancer: Manual for Staging of Cancer, 2nd ed. Philadelphia, JB Lippincott, 1983.
12. Kaplan EL, Meier P: Nonparametric estimation from incomplete observations. J Am Stat Assoc 53:547, 1958.
13. Martini N, Beattie EJ Jr: Results of surgical treatment in Stage I lung cancer. J Thorac Cardiovasc Surg 74:499, 1977.
14. Williams DE, Pairolero PC, Davis CS, et al: Survival of patients surgically treated for Stage I lung cancer. J Thorac Cardiovasc Surg 82:70, 1981.
15. Pairolero PC, Williams DE, Bergstralh EJ, et al: Postsurgical Stage I bronchogenic carcinoma: morbid implications of recurrent disease. Ann Thorac Surg 38:331, 1984.
16. Temeck BK, Flehinger BJ, Martini N: A retrospective analysis of 10 year survivors from carcinoma of the lung. Cancer 53:1405, 1984.

25

The Extent of Resection for Localized Lung Cancer: Segmental Resection

Robert J. Jensik, M.D.

The importance of tissue salvage can have no greater application than in pulmonary surgery. Our particular approach to the surgical management of bronchogenic carcinoma by segmental and subsegmental techniques has been used in 445 patients over the past 25 years.

At the time of thoracotomy the surgeon must resolve the dilemma of the adequacy of the resection versus the excessive loss of uninvolved parenchyma with the possibility of a respiratory deficit. Total lung resection was the predominant thought in the early years of surgical therapy for lung cancer, and no procedure less extensive than pneumonectomy was considered adequate until the mid-1950s, when reported similar survival results with lobectomy established this lesser resection as valid.

OPERATIVE CRITERIA FOR SEGMENTAL RESECTION

In certain clinicopathologic circumstances, a segmental resection is a logical alternative procedure to lobectomy, just as lobectomy was found to be for pneumonectomy. The choice for segmental resection is justified by the following criteria.

Compromised Clinical Status. From the clinical standpoint, significant reduction in respiratory function as a result of chronic obstructive pulmonary disease or other parenchymal fibrotic processes, severe cardiovascular disease, and previous pulmonary resection are the major factors mandating a limited type of resection.

Limited Pathologic Involvement. From the pathologic aspect, most favorable to success are a peripheral location of the tumor in the lobe and the absence of metastatic lymph node involvement at the segmental level, as well as at the lobar or hilar levels and in the mediastinum.

However, even with pathologic involvement beyond the lung, limited resection for debulking of tumor mass is our procedure of choice. Survival following segmentectomy is no worse than that following more extensive resection, and the patient is spared the greater physiologic insult associated with a more radical procedure.

Anatomic Variation: Incomplete Fissure Formation. Extreme variations are seen in degree of completeness and depth of fissure formation between the lobes. On the left side, complete separation of upper and lower lobes is a far less common finding than is some degree of fusion; in some instances, a fissure may be completely absent. On the right side, a completely separate middle lobe is a rare finding, and some degree of fusion of the lower and upper lobes posteriorly is frequently encountered.

There obviously must be vascular and lymphatic channels through this fused parenchyma. Separation of fused middle and upper lobes in performing right upper lobectomy seems no more logical than is separation through the plane between anterior and apical segments in performing a combined apical and posterior segmentectomy for a peripheral tumor other than to provide a "wider margin." If complete lobar fissure formation (three right lobes and two left) were always present, it would be more justifiable to perform lobectomy, since lymphatic and vascular channels would be completely confined within the lobe and crossover lymphatics and vascular channels would not exist.

Another variation is anomalous fissure formation; varying degrees of delineation of the lingula on the left or partial formation of a fissure between basilar and superior segments of the lower lobe on the right may be noted. The latter finding, present in one of the very early cases in our series, encouraged the surgeon to complete this fissure and to remove only the basilar segments of the right lower lobe. The survival time of this patient, the second in our series, was 20 years.

Table 25–1. Classification of Patient Groups in Series of 445 Segmental Resections

Group	No. of Patients
1 Previous resection	65
2 Stage III carcinoma	121
3 Stage I or II carcinoma	259

PATIENT POPULATION

The foregoing operative criteria are derived from our experience at Rush–Presbyterian–St. Luke's Medical Center, where a surgical philosophy of limited resection guides our approach to the management of bronchogenic carcinoma. From 1958 through 1983, 445 patients with carcinoma of the lung were operated upon using segmental or subsegmental procedures. These patients have been divided into three groups, as shown in Table 25–1.

GROUP 1: PATIENTS WITH PREVIOUS PULMONARY SURGERY

Almost all of the 65 patients in the group with previous pulmonary resection had a history of primary or metastatic carcinoma, although there were several instances of resection for tuberculosis or fungal disease. The extent of the initial procedure varied, ranging from segmental operations (26%) to pneumonectomy (18%); the majority of patients (55%) had undergone conventional or sleeve-type lobectomy. A carinal resection had been performed in one patient 2 years prior to sleeve-type resection of the superior segment of the left lower lobe.

Although the loss of parenchyma following initial segmentectomy procedures did not significantly reduce the respiratory reserve, those patients with appreciable compromise in function were far less able to lose even a small proportion of functioning lung than were those patients having minimal impairment in pulmonary function. The greater number of patients (73%), however, who lost at least a lobe or an entire lung initially did sustain significant reduction in lung tissue, indicating the importance of a more conservative resection at the repeat procedure.

Furthermore, there is usually some residual impairment in respiratory mechanics as a result of previous thoracotomy. This factor plays an additional part in reduction of function.

The concept of a repeat operative procedure for carcinoma of the lung, whether it be metastatic, recurrent, or a second primary, has been proposed previously, and the details of this experience, in which segmental resection plays an extremely important part, were reported in 1981.[3] As of December 31, 1983, 92 patients have had sequential procedures, of which 56 (61%) were limited resections. Cumulative survival in patients with metachronous disease is 33% at 5 years and 20% at 10 years; these rates support both the value of a repeat resection and the appropriateness of limited resection.

GROUP 2: PATIENTS WITH STAGE III CARCINOMA

The next largest group in whom limited-type procedures were done were the 121 patients with Stage III carcinoma. The basis for classification of Stage III disease was invasion of the malignancy beyond the lung into the chest wall, mediastinum, or diaphragm. Chest wall invasion was present at the superior sulcus, as is typical of Pancoast's tumor, or in the parietal pleura, the musculature, or rib tissues at a lower site. Mediastinal involvement varied; extension into the esophagus, pericardium or atrium or both, mediastinal pleura, vena cava, or the mediastinal nodes was noted. Extension into the diaphragm from lesions present in basilar portions of the lung likewise constituted a Stage III classification.

With such pathologic involvement beyond the lung, prognosis is unquestionably far worse, with considerably reduced survival time. Although an occasional patient in this group survived over 5 years, survival at 5 years in the entire group by life table analysis was only 9%. Under these circumstances, however, a limited resection provides as long a survival as that following a resection of greater magnitude.

GROUP 3: PATIENTS WITH STAGE I OR II CARCINOMA

The use of limited resection would probably be considered most controversial in patients with Stage I or II bronchogenic carcinoma, who made up our largest group of 259. The presence of metastases in nodal tissues adjacent to the tumor or at the segmental bronchial level determined the classification of disease as Stage II. Only 21 patients (8%) were found to have nodal involvement (N_1), whereas 238 patients (92%) had no evidence of nodal metastases (N_0). The decision for conservative resection in the 21 patients with Stage II disease was made because of clinical circumstan-

Table 25–2. Tumor Size and Nodal Involvement in Stage I or II Carcinoma

Feature	No. of Patients
Tumor Size	
<3 cm: T_1	191 (73.7%)
≥3 cm: T_2	64 (24.7%)
No tumor	4 (1.5%)
Total	259
Nodal Involvement	
Negative: N_0	238 (92%)
Positive: N_1	21 (8%)
Total	259

ces of age, cardiovascular problems, or compromised pulmonary function.

PATHOLOGIC FINDINGS IN STAGE I OR II CARCINOMA

Tumor Size and Nodal Involvement

Important factors determining outcome in our patients with Stage I or II carcinoma (Group 3) were the size of the tumor and metastatic node status. Fortunately, almost three fourths of the patients had T_1 lesions, measuring under 3 cm in diameter. The majority of our patients (92%) were found to be free of nodal involvement. Both metastatic node status and tumor size are shown in Table 25–2.

Cell Type

The various tumors in our Group 3 patients are listed by cell type in Table 25–3. The most common tumor was adenocarcinoma, constituting almost 50% of the cases; this finding is not surprising since the lesions were located mainly in the peripheral portion of the lobe. There was, however, an unexpectedly high proportion—34%—of epidermoid (squamous

Table 25–3. Tumor Cell Type in Stage I or II Carcinoma

Tumor Cell Type	No. of Patients
Adenocarcinoma	126 (49%)
Squamous cell	89 (34%)
Undifferentiated	34 (13%)
Bronchoalveolar	10 (4%)
Total	259

cell) lesions in this location, frequently unrelated to the segmental bronchus.

The third most frequent tumor type was the group listed as undifferentiated, which included both large and small cell types. The latter were indistinguishable from neuroendocrine lesions (small cell carcinoma) except that diffuse nodal involvement was absent.

The bronchoalveolar cell type was the least common, with the nine examples in this group representing slightly less than 4%.

Tumor Site

A variety of procedures were performed in our Group 3 patients as a result of the diverse location of the tumors throughout the lung parenchyma. A slight predominance of left lung involvement was noted; 142 resections were required on the left side, and 117 on the right.

On the left side, resection of the superior division of the left upper lobe was performed most often, followed by removal of the superior segment of the lower lobe. There were eight instances in which tumor extended across the fissure; in these cases, adjacent segmental or subsegmental tissues, or both, of upper and lower lobes were removed.

On the right side, resection of the anterior segment of the upper lobe and of the superior segment of the lower lobe was required most frequently. In one patient 76 years of age who had a middle lobe lesion, lateral segmentectomy was performed, with sparing of the medial segment because of extremely poor pulmonary function; at 3 years postoperatively he was without evidence of recurrence. Six patients had extension of tumor across the fissure, requiring removal of contiguous subsegmental or segmental areas of both lobes. Lateral diagrams of the left and right lungs with the numbers of procedures done in each lobe are shown in Figures 25–1 and 25–2.

TECHNIQUES OF SEGMENTAL SURGERY

Segmental surgery is technically more difficult than lobectomy and may be further complicated by anatomic variations. Lobar patterns are, for the most part, fairly constant as compared with segmental distribution. Probably of most importance in delineating the segment that is to be removed is dissection of the venous pattern distally from the lobar vein,

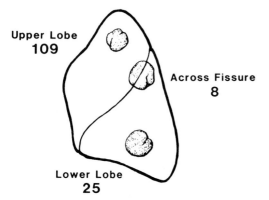

Figure 25–1. Diagram of left lung showing location of 142 segmentectomies for Stage I or II carcinoma.

because the vein branch lies in the intersegmental plane. This branch should be preserved because it drains adjacent segments; either cautery or fine ties can be used to interrupt tributaries from the segment. Another maneuver to facilitate the procedure is to dissect distally on the lobar bronchus and, after its identification, to occlude it with forceps while strong positive pressure is provided by the anesthesiologist. Usually, because of cross-ventilation there will be some expansion of the segment occluded, but significantly less than that occurring with adjacent tissues. Arterial supply always lies adjacent to the segmental bronchus and is interrupted after the appropriate segmental bronchus is identified. It is preferable to interrupt venous branches last, in order to lessen the chance of compromising drainage of the segmental tissues that are salvaged.

Varying degrees of parenchymal fibrosis or bleb or bullous formation may be present,

altering segmental planes. Such abnormalities not only add to the difficulties of resection but increase the number of complications, such as major air leaks and persistent airspace atelectasis, pneumonia, and empyema.

To help control air leak, two techniques have been used. The first of these, reconstituting lung, is shown in Figure 25–3 for apicoposterior segmentectomy of the left upper lobe. After the segment has been removed, the remaining parenchyma of the lobe is rotated in clockwise fashion (as viewed from the lateral aspect), to allow approximation of the anterior segmental surface to the interlobar pleural surface of the lower lobe. Interrupted sutures are placed medially at the apex and laterally; although the approximation is not airtight, the lower lobe pleura helps to seal air leaks more quickly than otherwise. This maneuver can be used to approximate the apical and anterior segments of the right upper to the lower lobe, or if the anterior segment is removed, the middle lobe and anterior aspect of the apical segment are brought together, utilizing the interlobar pleural surface of the middle lobe (Fig. 25–4). However, in many instances, the minor fissure is absent or incomplete, and two raw surfaces result after anterior segmentectomy, similar to the situation in the left upper lobe when the anterior segment is resected. In each instance, the raw surfaces are brought together, suturing along the margins as described previously.

The other technique for control of air leak utilizes parietal pleura mobilized from the anterior, apical, and posterior aspects of the chest; this is placed over large segmental surfaces with sutures to keep the pedicle flap in position. A diagram depicting the suturing parietal pleura to the superior surface of the lingula is shown in Figure 25–5. Although this technique is most commonly used after resection of the superior division of the left upper lobe, large mobilized pleural flaps can be used to cover a segmental surface elsewhere—for example, in an upper lobe with only one remaining segment or in a lower lobe following removal of all basilar segments to cover the undersurface of the remaining superior segment.

Either of these two techniques is preferred over both suturing and folding or stapling of the margins of remaining segments. Since these latter maneuvers reduce segment volume, their use is inconsistent with the objective of tissue salvage.

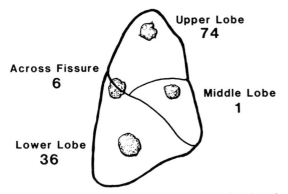

Figure 25–2. Diagram of right lung showing location of 117 segmentectomies for Stage I or II carcinoma.

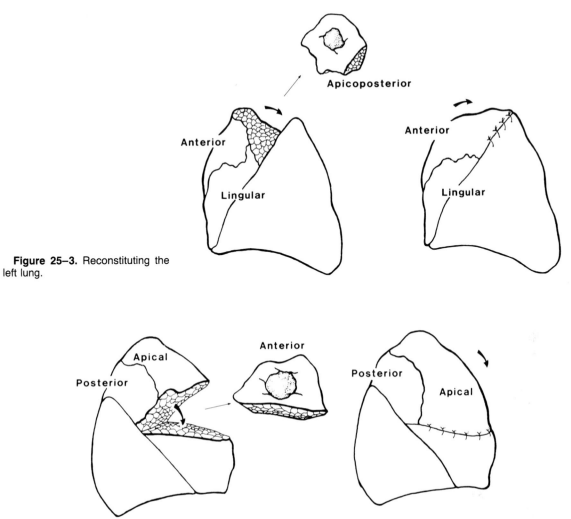

Figure 25–3. Reconstituting the left lung.

Figure 25–4. Reconstituting the right lung.

Figure 25–5. Creation of a parietal pleural flap.

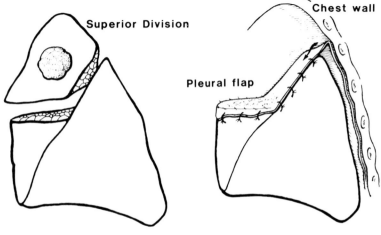

Table 25–4. Frequency of Complications in 259 Segmented Resections for Stage I or II Carcinoma

Complication	No. of Patients	
Postoperative hemorrhage	5	
Persistent air leak	22	
Requiring completion lobectomy		2
Requiring tube thoracostomy		3
Empyema		5
Persistent airspace		2
Protracted air leak		10
Retention of secretions requiring tracheostomy	5	
Cardiac decompensation	3	
Pneumonia	1	
Hemoptysis	1	
Atelectasis	1	
Wound dehiscence	1	

COMPLICATIONS FOLLOWING SEGMENTECTOMY FOR STAGE I OR II CARCINOMA

In spite of precautions taken as described previously, air leak was still the most frequent complication in our patients undergoing segmentectomy for Stage I or II carcinoma, occurring in 22 patients (Table 25–4). Two of these patients required reoperation (completion lobectomy); in three others, replacement of the chest drainage tube was necessary because of the development of significant airspace problems after removal of tubes placed at surgery. In 5 of the patients, empyema developed because of the protracted air leak, but in 10 others, despite this problem, no space infection developed. An occasional patient was discharged from the hospital with tubes in place, but these were usually removed within a 2-week period. In two other patients in whom air leak and persistent airspace were problems, eventually re-expansion of the lung occurred spontaneously without placement of other chest tubes.

Five patients had postoperative bleeding complications; in three, reoperation was required for control. There were two deaths in

Table 25–5. Perioperative Mortality in 445 Segmental Resections

	Patient Group	No. of Patients	No. of Deaths
1	Previous resection	65	4 (6%)
2	Stage III carcinoma	121	5 (4%)
3	Stage I or II carcinoma	259	3 (1%)

the three reoperated, one from respiratory insufficiency and the other from pancreatitis. Retention of secretions was a significant problem in the earlier patients in this series when postoperative suctioning via a flexible bronchoscope was not available. As a result, five patients required tracheostomy.

The remaining complications consisted of cardiac decompensation in three patients and one case each of pneumonia, hemoptysis, atelectasis, and wound dehiscence.

RESULTS

Perioperative Mortality

Perioperative mortality data are shown in Table 25–5. The highest mortality, seen in the patients who had undergone previous resection (Group 1), was related to reduced respiratory function of various degrees, more so if an entire lung had been removed at the first operation. The patients with Stage III cancer (Group 2) had more extensive disease, which probably was a contributing factor to an increase in operative risk in this group.

Group 3, with the most favorable criteria for surgery (Stage I or II disease), also had the lowest mortality: three perioperative deaths, representing slightly more than 1%. There is probably some correlation between this low mortality figure and the greater salvage of lung tissue resulting from resections of limited extent.

Tumor Recurrence

An important consideration in the overall evaluation of segmental surgery for lung cancer is the frequency of recurrence in the same lobe or hilar and mediastinal area, especially in the patients undergoing curative resections. In 31 of the 259 patients in Group 3 "local recur-

Table 25–6. Cumulative Survival Following Segmental Resection for Stage I or II Carcinoma

Survival Period	% Survival in Series		
	1972 (69 Patients)	1978 (168 Patients)	1983 (259 Patients)
5-year	56	53	55
10-year	27	33	32
15-year	27	25	21

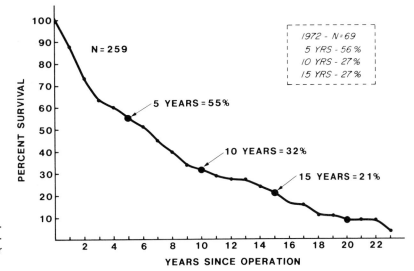

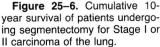

Figure 25–6. Cumulative 10-year survival of patients undergoing segmentectomy for Stage I or II carcinoma of the lung.

rence" developed, representing an incidence of about 12%. More important than the actual percentage, however, is the analysis of the interval between operation and the reappearance of the tumor. In six patients the duration of this period was more than 5 years, with the longest interval being almost 9 years. In all likelihood the "recurrences" represented second primary neoplasms.

Almost a third of the patients were able to undergo a second procedure, especially if the new lesion developed in the same lobe. Completion lobectomy was done in five patients, but the longest period of survival was 3 years and 1 month. One patient in this group underwent a third procedure, completion pneumonectomy, and was alive 1 year later without evidence of a new lesion. The four other

patients had completion pneumonectomies; among these, there was one perioperative mortality. One patient survived an additional 9 years.

The fact that all but one patient survived the second operation suggests that perhaps a more extensive procedure would have been tolerated at the time of the first operation, or that in the patients undergoing completion lobectomies, the second operation would not have been necessary if the entire lobe had been removed initially. However, the 31 patients who required reoperation for recurrence represent a small percentage of the 259 undergoing curative resections; this plus the low perioperative mortality in the Group 3 patients strongly supports the principle of limited resections.

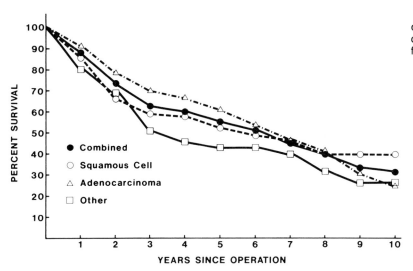

Figure 25–7. Relationships of cell type in Stage I or II carcinoma of the lung and patient survival following segmentectomy.

Survival Rates

Life table analysis of survival has been done periodically at intervals of 5 to 6 years as greater numbers of patients have undergone segmental resections for Stage I or II broncho-genic carcinoma. Table 25–6 lists data for survival in 1972 and 1978, when the series consisted of 69 and 168 patients, respectively.[1, 2] The survival curve as of December 1983 is shown in Figure 25–6; the data are quite similar for all three series. Comparison of survival rates was also made for patients with adenocarcinoma and for those with squamous cell types, as shown in Figure 25–7; no significant statistical differences according to cell type were noted.

In summary, in the treatment of broncho-genic carcinoma the evidence, after consideration of all factors, supports a philosophy of conservative resection.

References

1. Faber LP, Milloy FJ, Monson DO: Segmental resection for lung cancer. A 15-year experience. J Thorac Cardiovasc Surg 66:563–572, 1973.
2. Jensik RJ, Faber LP, Kittle CF: Segmental resection for bronchogenic carcinoma. Ann Thorac Surg 28: 475–483, 1979.
3. Jensik RJ, Faber LP, Kittle CF, Meng RL: Survival following resection for second primary bronchogenic carcinoma. J Thorac Cardiovasc Surg 82:658–668, 1981.

IX

New Anesthetic Techniques for Intrathoracic Operations

The needs of the thoracic surgeon in the operating arena have influenced and spurred the development of new methods of intubation and mechanical ventilation since 1896, when Tuffier and Hallion strongly recommended intubation and insufflation for intrathoracic procedures.

Most experimental studies and clinical applications of high frequency ventilation have occurred during the past 20 years. It is thus more recent and has not received as much attention or use as PEEP/CPAP (positive end-expiratory pressure/continuous positive airway pressure). Many variations in high frequency ventilation have been studied and used clinically. These have resulted in a new group of terms: high frequency positive-pressure ventilation (HFPPV), high frequency oscillation (HFO), high frequency jet ventilation (HFJV), and high frequency chest wall compression (HFCWC). Undoubtedly further modifications and new terms will develop.

High frequency ventilation developed serendipitously as a result of cardiovascular animal experiments by Öberg and Sjöstrand (1969) and Lunkerheimer (1972). In their studies they needed a ventilatory technique that would minimize the intra-arterial pressure fluctuations generally associated with mechanical ventilation. The low tidal volumes and the low peak airway pressures in HFV solved this problem. It is of interest that Emerson (1959) obtained a patent for an "apparatus for vibrating portions of a patient's airway." He stated that "vibrating the column of gas doubtless causes the gas to diffuse more rapidly within the airway and therefore aids in the breathing function by circulating the gas more thoroughly," but apparently he did not test this device or use it clinically (Slutksy et al., 1981).

The increasing variety of operative procedures in thoracic surgery and the application of intrathoracic surgical procedures to individuals with impaired pulmonary function have demanded the development of new anesthetic techniques. As new techniques have developed, the thoracic surgeon has been able to carry out more extensive and more ingenious procedures than previously possible.

The chapters in this section provide information of importance to the practicing thoracic surgeon and others interested in problems of anesthesia and ventilation for intrathoracic operations. High frequency ventilation has excited great interest and enthusiasm, particularly in its application to thoracic surgery, neurosurgery, and laryngeal surgery. Many operations can now be done using HFV more simply and with less morbidity than with standard anesthetic techniques.

However, further studies and modifications are indicated before a definitive place for HFV can be established. More exact knowledge is needed regarding gas exchange at high ventilatory rates, the best method of conditioning the inspired gas, monitoring intra-alveolar pressure, tidal volume and the adequacy of gas exchange, and whether or not reduction in the ventilatory peak pressure is actually beneficial for the patient (Sykes, 1985).

26

New Anesthetic Techniques for Intrathoracic Operations: High-Frequency Low-Compression Ventilation

Ulf H. Sjöstrand, M.D., Ph.D.
Jaime O. Herrera-Hoyos, M.D.
R. Brian Smith, M.D.

The technologic advances in anesthesiology and critical care medicine have been of great importance in the development of modern surgery. In particular, the dramatic improvements in techniques of mechanical ventilation have played a major role.

Conventional types of controlled mechanical ventilation—intermittent positive-pressure ventilation (IPPV) and continuous positive-pressure ventilation (CPPV)—produce rhythmic inflation of the lungs, as described by Björk and Engström in 1955.[1] All ventilator (respirator) systems developed for these modes of ventilation have the same basic functional characteristics: they generally have a large compressible volume and usually operate at frequencies of up to 30 breaths per minute (bpm). The rationale for these design features was that large tidal volumes, with a substantial length of time for both inspiration and expiration, would promote an even intrapulmonary gas distribution.

It is a well-known fact that the undesirable circulatory effects of positive-pressure ventilation are often closely linked to the elevation in mean intrathoracic pressure that it produces. Thus, a controversy arises between physics and physiology in the designing of ventilators to match the breathing pattern with normal pulmonary and cardiocirculatory processes.

In 1967 certain experimental studies required a method of artificial positive-pressure ventilation without circulatory effects synchronous with respiration. For this purpose, high-frequency positive-pressure ventilation (HFPPV) was developed.[2] The original rationale for the HFPPV technique was twofold: (1) the use of endotracheal insufflation, with smaller tidal volumes (V_T) and higher ventilatory frequencies, would reduce ventilatory dead space (V_D), so that adequate ventilation could be obtained at lower maximal and lower mean airway pressures than in IPPV; and (2) with insufflation at a high frequency and with short insufflation periods, the normal resistance of the lungs to inflation would be sufficient to suppress the circulatory effects associated with the ventilatory pattern.[2] In order to compensate for the increased dead space–tidal volume ratio (V_D/V_T) seen in IPPV of high frequency, a ventilator system having negligible compressible volume and internal compliance was required.[2, 3] With conventional ventilators, however, attempts to reduce the circulatory interference—by decreasing the V_T and increasing the ventilatory frequency—have been discouraging, because higher peak and mean airway pressures are required to overcome the large functional dead space characteristics of such systems.[2, 4, 6, 8–10]

TECHNICAL DEVELOPMENTS

Since the clinical introduction of HFPPV in 1971,[2, 3, 5] the development of low-compression ventilator systems has led to an increase in the use of high-frequency insufflation techniques. The design of such systems is based on three principles (Fig. 26–1): that of HFPPV, proposed by Öberg and Sjöstrand in 1967; that of high-frequency oscillation (HFO), by Lunkenheimer and colleagues in 1972; and that of high-frequency jet ventilation (HFJV), by Klain and Smith in 1977.[6] HFPPV initially utilized endotracheal insufflation via an insufflation catheter positioned within the endotracheal tube.[2, 5] Later a pneumatic valve connector was developed (Fig. 26–2A). In this improved system, a conditioned gas mixture is

185

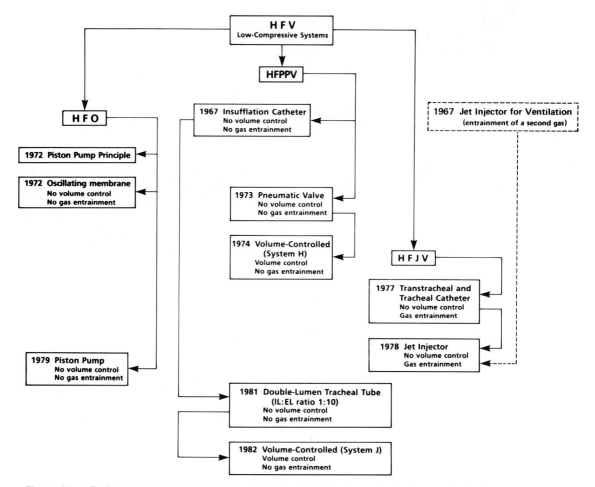

Figure 26–1. Technical development of high-frequency ventilation systems. (From Scheck PA, et al (eds): Perspectives in High Frequency Ventilation. The Hague, Martinus Nijhoff, 1983.)

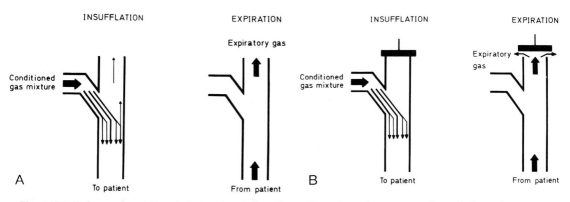

Figure 26–2. Comparison of inspiratory and expiratory flow patterns in an "open system" employing only a pneumatic valve connector (A) with those in system H, "closed" by the addition of an expiratory valve (B). (A, from Sjöstrand UH: Review of the physiological rationale for and development of high-frequency positive-pressure ventilation—HFPPV. Acta Anaesth Scand (Suppl)64:7, 1977. B, From Sjöstrand UH: High-frequency positive pressure ventilation (HFPPV): A review. Crit Care Med 8:345, 1980.)

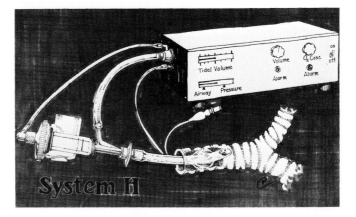

Figure 26–3. System H, with the pneumatic valve connector and an expiratory valve for volume-controlled ventilation. (From Sjöstrand UH et al: Volume-controlled high frequency ventilation as a useful mode of ventilation during open-chest surgery—A report of three cases. Resp Care 27:1380, 1982.)

intermittently delivered via a large-diameter side-arm branching off the main channel of the pneumatic valve connector.[2, 3] This main channel remains open and can be used for insertion of broncho- or laryngoscopic equipment. Even though these two circuits—with or without the valve—are "open" systems, gas entrainment does not occur. This permits airway suctioning during continued ventilation with full control of the gas mixture delivered to the patient.[2, 3, 5, 6]

By addition of a valve to close the outlet port of the main channel of the pneumatic valve connector during insufflation (Fig. 26–2B, *insufflation*), a system with low-compression, volume-controlled ventilation, called system H, is obtained (Figs. 26–2B and 26–3).[6, 7] In this system, at end-inspiration the expiratory valve opens for the expiration phase (Fig. 26–2B, *expiration*).

In 1981 a double-lumen tracheal tube, having an inspiratory/expiratory lumen diameter ratio (IL:EL) of 1:10, was introduced. With this adaptation, the functional and dimensional characteristics of the circuit are similar to those

of the original HFPPV insufflation circuit.[5, 6] The double-lumen tube serves as an integral part of a low-compression system for volume-controlled ventilation called system J (Fig. 26–4). As detailed for system H, with the addition of a valve to the expiratory port or lumen (EL) of the double-lumen tube so that it can be closed during inspiration through the insufflation lumen (IL), pressure/flow-generated volume-controlled ventilation is provided.[6] Owing to the small functional dead space of this system, normocarbia is produced more efficiently.

INTRAPULMONARY GAS DISTRIBUTION DURING LOW-COMPRESSION VENTILATION

The effects of the different high-frequency techniques and ventilatory patterns should be evaluated not only with respect to interference with central and peripheral circulation but also in terms of gas exchange in the lungs. The conventional view of how alveolar ventilation

Figure 26–4. System J, with the double-lumen tube (IL:EL of 1 : 10) and an inspiratory valve for volume-controlled ventilation. (From Scheck PA, et al (eds): Perspectives in High Frequency Ventilation. The Hague, Martinus Nijhoff, 1983.)

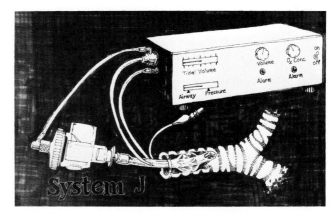

takes place during mechanical ventilation is not applicable to ventilation with low-compression systems at either low or high frequencies.[8, 9] In these systems inspiratory flow has a decelerating character. Volume is the primary, or independent, parameter, and pressure becomes a secondary, or dependent, parameter.[6, 8]

The development of low-compression, small-tidal-volume systems with high and instantaneous inspiratory flow of a true decelerating character has made possible the use of not only *convection*—classical bulk flow with its dependence upon pulmonary time constants—but also *dispersion* to a greater extent than before. Accordingly, high-frequency ventilation with low-compression systems is less affected by inequalities between regional time constants than is conventional low-frequency, large-tidal-volume ventilation. Therefore, the classic concept of a "dead space" in the conducting airways does not apply during high-frequency ventilation.[8, 9]

Comparisons between a conventional ventilator and a low-compression prototype system have demonstrated significant differences in several aspects of function.[10] Both provide adequate ventilation at frequencies between 20 bpm and 60 bpm. There are significant increases in V_D/V_T with increasing frequencies, but this correlation is significantly weaker with the low-compression system. With both systems the functional residual capacity increases with increasing frequencies. With the conventional system, the mean airway pressure increases, whereas with the low-compression system it decreases with normoventilation at increasing frequencies. Substantial differences between the two systems have also been noted in the ventilatory pattern. With the low-compression system, the major fraction of the effective tidal volume is delivered to the lungs during the early phase of inspiration, which gives more time for redistribution of this gas during the rest of the inspiratory period; hence, the intrapulmonary gas distribution (as measured by the N_2 washout technique) is significantly improved when compared with that in conventional ventilation, independent of the ventilatory frequency.[6, 8] Experimental and clinical studies on HFPPV using low-compression ventilators all seem to indicate that gas transfer in conducting airways is enhanced by high inspiratory flow.[6, 9, 10] To generate such high flow with limited tidal volume, low-compression systems and high-frequency ventilation must be used.[6, 8]

CLINICAL APPLICATIONS AND RESEARCH

The initial clinical study on the physiologic effects of HFPPV was performed on a small number of patients during routine surgery.[2, 3] HFPPV was achieved by a system similar to that previously used in animal experiments.[5] In all but 1 of 15 patients with near-normal lungs, adequate alveolar ventilation was obtained with HFPPV, although only minor intrathoracic pressure variations were observed. Arterial oxygen tensions were comparatively high without the need for hyperventilation, indicating that during HFPPV a favorable relation between ventilation and lung perfusion is maintained.[9]

In 1973, HFPPV was applied in clinical practice for bronchoscopy and laryngoscopy under general anesthesia.[2, 3, 11] A ventilator for endoscopic HFPPV (Bronchovent) was also developed.[2]

Bronchoscopy

Bronchoscopy done under local anesthesia requires heavy premedication and greater technical skill than that needed when general anesthesia is used. Even in an uneventful procedure without complications, rigid bronchoscopy may be a frightening experience for the patient. Therefore, general anesthesia is usually required.

Early techniques using a rigid bronchoscope afforded only intermittent access to the airway. Subsequently many bronchoscopic techniques have been developed to provide appropriate ventilation and oxygenation as well as favorable conditions for examination and surgical procedures.[11]

The *injector (Venturi) technique,* introduced by Sanders in 1967,[12] utilizes air entrainment and provides IPPV through an injector nozzle attached to the upper end of the bronchoscope. The injector gas is oxygen, which entrains approximately two to three times its own volume of ambient air via the proximal opening of the bronchoscope. Unless special adjustments are made, this normally provides a maximum of 30% to 35% oxygen. Instrumentation through the bronchoscope interferes with entrainment and thus also with ventilation.

Ventilation via the fixed side-arm of the bronchoscope was first described by Carden and associates[13] and has several advantages over the injector technique. It does not depend on entrainment and allows higher airway pressures during insufflation, thereby providing ventilatory reserve capacity. The side-arm technique also is much more amenable to instrumentation via the bronchoscope. There have been few attempts, however, to optimize or standardize the side-arm technique in order to make ventilation by this means a simple and safe procedure.[11]

High-frequency ventilation for bronchoscopy under general anesthesia was introduced in 1973.[2, 3, 11] In this technique, called *bronchoscopic HFPPV*,[11, 14] the anesthetic gas mixture is intermittently supplied through the fixed side-arm of the bronchoscope (or through the side-arm of a special pneumatic valve adapter) at an insufflation frequency *(f)* of 60 bpm and a relative insufflation time *(t%)* of 22%. No air entrainment occurs through the proximal opening of the bronchoscope, which allows full control of the anesthetic gas mixture delivered to the patient. For bronchoscopic HFPPV, ventilation nomograms have been developed to determine initial ventilator settings for oxygenation and ventilation.[9, 11, 14] Ventilation must then be adjusted on the basis of stethoscopic and clinical evaluation.

With the appropriate ventilator settings, ventilation and oxygenation are not affected following insertion of the bronchoscope in the main bronchus of the diseased lung.[11] Nor do significant changes in ventilation or oxygenation occur when instruments of reasonable relative size are introduced through the bronchoscope. (By contrast, in the injector technique, such instrumentation usually affects air entrainment, thereby reducing ventilatory volume but increasing the inspired oxygen concentration.)

Laryngoscopy and Flexible Fiberoptic Bronchoscopy

The ventilator equipment for bronchoscopic HFPPV[2] was also designed to allow endotracheal insufflation via a nasotracheal catheter for ventilation during laryngoscopy. In order to abolish the injector effect, the insufflation catheter is supplied with side-holes near its tip.[15] It must be emphasized that in *laryngoscopic HFPPV*, expiration must take place through the larynx, outside the insufflation catheter. The continuous, upward-directed flow of gas outside the catheter prevents blood and tissue from being sucked down into the airways.[11, 15] This also prevents admixture of room air, so that despite the apparently "open" system, the supply of oxygen or other gas mixtures can be carefully controlled.

Use of the ventilating laryngoscope with an injector, a modification of Sanders' original technique for ventilation during bronchoscopy, has disadvantages and dangers including paratracheal dissection in the fascial plane. Because of the risks involved,[15] ventilation through a transtracheally introduced catheter has not gained general acceptance. Compared with these techniques, laryngoscopic HFPPV appears to be a superior method that has no injurious effects on the tracheal mucosa.[3, 11, 15]

Flexible fiberoptic bronchoscopy (FFB) has been found to have definite advantages over rigid bronchoscopy. But with FFB carried out under topical anesthesia, episodes of hypoxia and hypercapnia sometimes occur, especially in association with heavy premedication. Bronchoscopic HFPPV allows maintenance of general anesthesia via the rigid scope and simultaneous manipulation of the flexible scope. However, the typical flexible fiberoptic bronchoscope occupies only 10% to 15% of the tracheal cross-sectional area in the adult male; therefore, the use of laryngoscopic HFPPV for general anesthesia may reduce risks of hypoventilation, hypoxia, and barotrauma during FFB.[11] The initial setting of ventilator gas output $(\dot{V}_{vent})$ in FFB should be 10% to 20% above the value given in the ventilation nomogram. Oxygen concentration should not be less than 40%. Ventilation must then be readjusted on the basis of stethoscopic and clinical evaluation.

Since 1973, bronchoscopic HFPPV and laryngoscopic HFPPV have become well-established clinical procedures.[3, 6, 11] In both procedures, *f* is fixed at 60 bpm and inspiratory time *(t%)* at 22% of the ventilatory cycle. Ventilation nomograms are used to determine initial ventilator gas output settings on the special ventilator (Bronchovent). This ventilator has a built-in sensitive airway-pressure-limited safety system.[6, 7] The nomograms were derived from clinical data obtained in 800 bronchoscopies and 500 laryngoscopies. Because no air entrainment occurs, these procedures permit full control of the gas mixture delivered to the patient.

Pediatric Considerations

The rigid bronchoscope is still the instrument of choice in infants and children for detection and removal of foreign bodies within the airways. Ventilation with 100% oxygen in the case of an obstructed airway, or interrupted ventilation for any other reason will make the safety margin comparable to that at the start after an apneic oxygenation procedure. Bronchoscopic HFPPV considerably lessens the anesthetic risks in infants and children.[11]

Tracheal Surgery

HFPPV during resection of tracheal stenosis uses a combination of the techniques for bronchoscopic and laryngoscopic HFPPV.[16] Tracheal stenosis has long been known as a complication of endotracheal intubation or tracheostomy and as a sequela of trauma, infection, and neoplastic changes. The most commonly used reparative procedure is resection of the stenosed area with end-to-end anastomosis.

The methods used for anesthesia vary considerably. The main problem is how to obtain adequate ventilation before and during resection. With conventional techniques, it is often difficult to avoid periods of hypoxia, and critical situations can occur. A radical and drastic solution has been to use the heart-lung machine.[17]

Figure 26–5 illustrates the recommended method of anesthesia for use in repair of tracheal stenosis. With this method, there is no interruption of high-frequency ventilation: the pneumatic valve connector is used during tracheoscopy performed to visualize the affected area; the insufflation catheter (as in laryngoscopic HFPPV) is used during actual resection; and the pneumatic valve connector is used during intraoperative endoscopy performed to evaluate the reconstruction.[16]

Other methods of ventilation using an endotracheal tube are clumsy. The need for alterations of tube position or for exchange of one tube for another increases the risk of hypoxia. Furthermore, a normal-sized tracheal tube hinders the surgeon in suturing the anastomosis.

With HFPPV it is possible to achieve adequate ventilation (Fig. 26–6) without the interference of a bulky endotracheal tube (Fig. 26–5). The trachea can be opened without risk of hypoxia.[16, 18] Because of the continuous positive airway pressure before, during, and after resection, the risk of atelectasis due to the open thorax is reduced. At the same time, lung tissue is easily kept out of the surgical field, permitting free access to the area being resected.[16] Similar advantages have been noted for HFPPV during open-chest surgery.[5, 7]

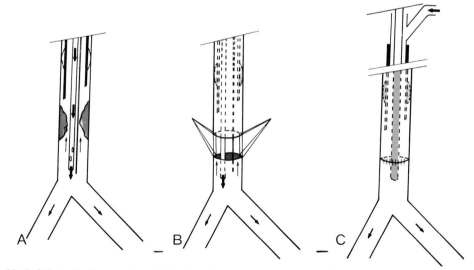

Figure 26–5. Schematic diagram of ventilation techniques and anatomic conditions. *A,* The relation of the endotracheal tube, insufflation catheter, and pressure-measuring catheter to the tracheal stenosis (ventilation type I). *B,* Conditions during the final stage of resection (ventilation type I). *C,* Conditions during the perioperative tracheoscopic examination described in the text (ventilation type II). (From Eriksson I, et al: High-frequency positive-pressure ventilation [HFPPV] during transthoracic resection of tracheal stenosis and during perioperative bronchoscopic examination. Acta Anaesth Scand 19:113, 1975.)

Table 28–8. Arterial Blood Gas Values in Control (IPPV) Group

Patient	Before Chest Opened	30 Min. After Chest Opened	Before Chest Closed	After Chest Closed
PaO_2/FIO_2				
1	449.6	437.2	385.0	432.6
2	260.4	232.8	—	—
3	318.0	340.2	390.4	435.6
4	454.0	354.0	311.4	330.6
5	371.6	231.6	302.8	300.2
6	364.2	346.6	339.6	357.0
Mean ± SD	369.6 ± 75.0	323.7 ± 79.2	345.8 ± 40.6	371.2 ± 60.8
$PaCO_2$				
1	26.4	26.7	27.0	25.9
2	38.2	39.5	—	—
3	29.0	35.0	36.2	29.2
4	29.0	39.2	36.7	38.1
5	28.1	32.1	29.6	49.8
6	32.1	32.7	28.2	27.8
Mean ± SD	30.5 ± 4.2	34.2 ± 4.8	31.5 ± 4.6	34.2 ± 9.9
Arterial pH Estimated from $PaCO_2$				
1	7.51	7.51	7.50	7.51
2	7.41	7.40	—	—
3	7.49	7.45	7.44	7.49
4	7.49	7.41	7.43	7.42
5	7.50	7.46	7.48	7.32
6	7.46	7.46	7.49	7.50
Mean ± SD	7.48 ± 0.04	7.45 ± 0.04	7.47 ± 0.03	7.45 ± 0.08
Measured Arterial pH				
1	7.49	7.50	7.52	7.52
2	7.37	7.37	—	—
3	7.42	7.42	7.38	7.47
4	7.38	7.33	7.36	7.37
5	7.51	7.45	7.46	7.29
6	7.44	7.45	7.46	7.45
Mean ± SD	7.44 ± 0.06	7.42 ± 0.06	7.44 ± 0.07	7.42 ± 0.09

Table 28–9. Arterial Blood Gas Values in HFV Alone Group

Patient	Before Chest Opened		30 Min. After Chest Opened	Before Chest Closed	After Chest Closed
	IPPV	**HFV**			
PaO_2/FIO_2					
1	287.8	334.4	135.6	171.6	225.4
2	396.2	418.2	226.8	206.6	372.4
3	444.4	381.6	279.6	433.0	—
4	484.8	419.4	362.2	374.4	395.4
5	424.8	496.4	225.0	225.2	247.8
6	518.4	414.4	426.4	364.4	336.8
Mean ± SD	426.1 ± 80.4	410.7 ± 53.2	275.9 ± 104.7	295.9 ± 107.8	315.6 ± 75.5
$PaCO_2$					
1	37.1	40.0	40.6	43.6	44.3
2	32.5	26.8	42.3	29.1	30.2
3	22.7	37.5	48.5	32.4	37.2
4	30.6	31.1	38.5	41.3	41.0
5	21.6	51.7	44.0	34.9	33.5
6	34.7	31.4	32.4	45.8	32.6
Mean ± SD	29.9 ± 6.4	36.4[a] ± 8.9	41.1[c] ± 5.4	37.9[a] ± 6.7	36.5 ± 5.4
Arterial pH Estimated from $PaCO_2$					
1	7.42	7.40	7.39	7.37	7.37
2	7.46	7.51	7.38	7.49	7.48
3	7.54	7.42	7.33	7.46	7.42
4	7.48	7.47	7.41	7.39	7.39
5	7.55	7.31	7.34	7.44	7.45
6	7.44	7.47	7.50	7.35	7.46
Mean ± SD	7.48 ± 0.05	7.43[a] ± 0.07	7.39 ± 0.06	7.42[a] ± 0.06	7.43 ± 0.04
Measured Arterial pH					
1	7.44	7.37	7.36	7.35	7.33
2	7.46	7.56	7.43	7.53	7.49
3	7.38	7.46	7.45	—	—
4	7.39	7.35	7.39	7.33	7.31
5	7.44	7.26	7.31	7.37	7.34
6	7.44	7.42	7.40	7.32	7.36
Mean ± SD	7.43 ± 0.03	7.40[b] ± 0.10	7.39 ± 0.05	7.38[b] ± 0.09	7.37 ± 0.07

[a]Significant difference ($p < 0.01$) between HFV alone and HFV on V_D at the same Hz.
[b]Significant difference ($p < 0.05$) between HFV alone and HFV on V_D at the same Hz.
[c]Significant difference ($p < 0.05$) against IPPV.

Table 28–10. Arterial Blood Gas Values in HFV on V_D Group

Patient	Before Chest Opened		30 Min. After Chest Opened	Before Chest Closed	After Chest Closed
	IPPV	HFV			
PaO$_2$/FIO$_2$					
1	384.8	498.6	467.2	385.8	303.8
2	376.4	250.4	315.4	217.6	251.8
3	280.2	396.0	360.2	239.6	215.6
4	546.0	464.2	226.8	416.0	285.4
5	461.8	253.4	250.6	302.2	307.2
6	416.4	330.4	232.0	399.6	—
Mean ± SD	410.9 ± 89.2	365.5 ± 105.3	308.7 ± 93.6	326.8 ± 85.9	272.8 ± 38.8
PaCO$_2$					
1	29.2	46.0	56.5	36.6	35.2
2	38.9	50.0	47.9	49.1	48.3
3	36.5	61.2	47.8	54.8	53.4
4	31.8	40.7	44.2	52.4	44.8
5	34.6	42.1	44.5	53.9	47.0
6	30.2	69.4	40.9	52.6	40.6
Mean ± SD	33.5 ± 3.8	51.6[a, b] ± 11.4	47.0[a] ± 5.3	49.9[a, b] ± 6.8	44.9 ± 6.3
Arterial pH Estimated from PaCO$_2$					
1	7.49	7.35	7.27	7.43	7.44
2	7.41	7.32	7.34	7.33	7.33
3	7.43	7.23	7.34	7.28	7.29
4	7.47	7.39	7.37	7.30	7.36
5	7.44	7.38	7.37	7.29	7.34
6	7.48	7.16	7.39	7.30	7.40
Mean ± SD	7.45 ± 0.03	7.31[a, b] ± 0.09	7.35[a] ± 0.04	7.32[a, b] ± 0.06	7.36 ± 0.05
Measured Arterial pH					
1	7.47	7.37	7.30	7.26	7.35
2	7.42	7.19	7.23	7.18	7.29
3	7.44	7.33	7.36	7.25	7.27
4	7.45	7.36	7.25	7.36	7.39
5	7.37	7.18	7.39	7.29	7.30
6	7.44	7.26	7.38	7.31	7.43
Mean ± SD	7.43 ± 0.03	7.28[a, c] ± 0.08	7.32 ± 0.07	7.28[a, c] ± 0.06	7.34 ± 0.06

[a]Significant difference (p >0.01) against IPPV.
[b]Significant difference (p >0.01) between HFV alone and HFV on V_D.
[c]Significant difference (p >0.05) between HFV alone and HFV on V_D.

in the latter, mild acidosis. All patients had an uneventful postoperative course and were discharged from the recovery room on the operative day.

CONCLUSIONS

In summary HFV alone with a driving pressure of 0.50 kg/cm^2 and at a frequency of 3 Hz (HFV alone group) maintained better pulmonary gas exchange for the entire period of intrathoracic surgery than that achieved with IPPV (control group). CO_2 elimination with HFV alone also was better than with IPPV. With HFV on V_D (6 Hz, 0.50 kg/cm^2), CO_2 elimination was inadequate, leading to respiratory acidosis, although all patients recovered without complications postoperatively. Intrathoracic operations were facilitated by employing either of the two HFV methods.

References

1. Seki S, Fukushima Y, Goto K, et al: Facilitation of intrathoracic operations by means of high-frequency ventilation. J Thorac Cardiovasc Surg 86:388, 1983.
2. Horowitz HH, Carrico CJ, Shires GT: Pulmonary response to major injury. Arch Surg 108:349, 1974.
3. Covelli HD, Nessan VJ, Tuttle WK: Oxygen derived variables in acute respiratory failure. Crit Care Med 11:646, 1983.
4. Narins RG, Emmett M: Simple and mixed acid–base disorder: A practical approach. Medicine 59:161, 1980.
5. Seki S, Kondo T, Konishi H, et al: High frequency ventilation (HFV) as an adjuvant for facilitation of intrathoracic surgery. Kyobu Geka 37:36, 1983. (In Japanese.)
6. Seki S, Goto K, Kondo T, et al: Gas exchange and facilitation of high frequency ventilation in intrathoracic surgery. Ann Thorac Surg 37:491, 1984.

X

Management of Postoperative Thoracotomy Pain

But pain is perfect miserie, the worst
Of evils, and excessive, overturnes
All patience.

JOHN MILTON (1608–1674)

It is the special vocation of the doctor to
grow familiar with suffering.

JOHN GREENLEAF WHITTIER (1807–1892)

The acute pain caused by a thoracotomy incision is of great importance postoperatively. This discomfort is more painful than that caused by the abdominal incision. It frequently interferes with proper ventilation and leads to that circular, vicious pathophysiology of hypoventilation, atelectasis, hypoxia, and hyperpnea, often resulting in pneumonia. As our operative population increases, as more procedures are done in individuals with impaired ventilation, and as our scrutiny continues to make thoracotomy a less morbid procedure, more attention has been devoted to postoperative pain and its relief.

Following the discovery of cocaine by Niemann (1860), numerous efforts were made to explore its clinical effects. Niemann had observed that the cocaine crystal numbed his tongue, but it was not until 1868 that a Peruvian surgeon, Moréno y Maiz, suggested it as a local anesthetic, simultaneously noting that it occasionally produced seizures. Two Viennese physicians, Koller and Freud, popularized cocaine in the 1880's; Koller instituted it as an anesthetic in ophthalmology, and Freud used it as a treatment for morphine addiction! Many others recognized the potential of cocaine as a local anesthetic, Halsted being the first (1885)

to describe its use to produce a nerve conduction block.

The idea of injecting anesthetic solution into the epidural space originated with Corning (1885), who was experimenting with the action of cocaine on the spinal nerves of a dog, although he did not clearly define his site of injection. Presumably because he was a neurologist, his efforts were directed at therapy rather than surgical anesthesia, although in his first article he mentions this latter application.

. . . in order to obtain the most immediate, direct, and powerful effects upon the cord with a minimum quantity of a medicinal substance, it is by no means necessary to bring the substance into direct contact with the cord; it is not necessary to inject the same beneath the membranes, . . . since the effects are entirely due to the absorption of the fluid by the minute vessels. On the other hand, in order to obtain these local effects, it is first necessary to inject the solution in the vicinity of the cord, and, secondly, to select such a spot as will insure the most direct possible entry of the fluid into the circulation about the cord.

From these theoretical considerations I reasoned that it was highly probable that, if the anesthetic was placed between the spinous processes of the vertebrae, it (the anesthetic) would be rapidly absorbed by the minute ramifications of the veins referred to, and being transported by the blood to the substance of the cord, would give rise to anesthesia of the sensory and perhaps also of the motor tracts of the same.

Corning then proceeds to describe the use of this technique in one canine experiment and in one clinical application. At this early time he described his results as "spinal anesthesia," not differentiating between our present terminology of subarachnoid or epidural (extradural, peridural).

The first two articles about spinal (subarachnoid) anesthesia appeared, apparently independently, in 1899 (Bier and Tuffier), both referring to cocaine. The desirable anesthetic effects were noted as well as the complications of headache, nausea, and vomiting.

In 1901, epidural analgesia by the caudal route was recommended by both Sicard and Cathelin as an alternative to subarachnoid injection. During that same year Tuffier reported on his attempts with the lateral lumbar approach for epidural anesthesia.

Concomitantly, the synthesis by Einhorn of the less toxic and better tolerated procaine hydrochloride (Novocain) and its clinical inauguration by Braun (1905) encouraged further development of local and spinal anesthesia, both subarachnoid and epidural.

Epidural anesthesia worked well for the area supplied by the cauda equina (Läwen, 1911), but attempts to use it at higher levels produced variable results (Heile, 1913). Pagés (1921) reawakened interest in the lumbar and thoracic regions, and familiarity with the use of epidural anesthesia in these areas developed. The efforts of Dogliotti (1931, 1933) greatly helped to popularize epidural anesthesia. He thought it superior to local anesthesia, as effective as the usual spinal anesthesia, and without the disadvantages of general anesthesia. As he wrote: ". . . it is a procedure which makes it possible to obtain in the upper parts of the body just as excellent results as may be had in the region of the sacrococcygeal plexus after sacral extradural anesthesia has been performed" (1933).

Although continuous spinal anesthesia was first reported by Dean (1907), its use did not gain wide acceptance until after the articles by Lemmon (1940), who described leaving a malleable needle in place during the operation. Based on experiences with the ureteral catheter to drain the subarachnoid space in meningitis (Love, 1935), others (Manalan, 1942; Irving, 1943; Adams et al., 1943; and Tuohy, 1945) reported passing a fine ureteral catheter through the spinal needle for continuous injection.

The efficacy, benefit, and safety of epidural anesthesia have been well established. Many centers are now using epidural analgesia postoperatively for both thoracic and abdominal procedures. However, investigators employ different substances for epidural injection, continue injections for different time periods, and use other slight modifications. It seems most likely that standardization will occur in the next several years and that epidural anesthesia will become a recognized and generally utilized technique for postoperative analgesia.

29

Management of Postoperative Thoracotomy Pain: Continuous Epidural Infusion of Morphine

Nabil M. El-Baz, M.D.
Anthony D. Ivankovich, M.D.

The discovery in 1973 of opiate receptors in the brain and spinal cord, and in 1975 of their specific mediators, endorphines and enkephalin, marked the beginning of a new era for research on mechanisms of pain and its treatment.[1-3] Highly specific and stereotypic opiate receptors were found at high concentrations in the periaqueductal gray matter of the brain stem, medial thalamus, amygdala, and posterior pituitary, and in the substantia gelatinosa of the posterior spinal gray matter. Numerous physiologic roles of opiate receptors and endorphines have been identified: in pain perception, in control of emotion and behavior, and in neuroendocrinal functions.[4] Because the distribution of opiate receptors in the spinal cord was found to be anatomically related to pain pathways, the antinociceptive effects of intrathecal and epidural injections of narcotics were evaluated.[5, 6]

Intrathecal and epidural administration of narcotics, particularly morphine, has been shown in numerous animal and human studies to provide prolonged, effective, and profound segmental relief of chronic and postoperative pain.[7, 8] The degree and duration of analgesia obtained was found to be dose-dependent. These studies suggested that the probable mechanism of pain relief is a specific blockade of opiate nociceptive pathways in Rexed's laminae 1, 2, and 5 of the posterior spinal gray matter. Epidural administration of narcotics provides effective postoperative analgesia with minimal alteration of neuronal conduction in the sympathetic, sensory, and motor spinal nerves.[9-11] However, in these studies, epidural administration of large doses of morphine (2–10 mg) was associated with a high incidence of nausea, vomiting, pruritus, and urinary retention; in addition, delayed, unexpected, and life-threatening respiratory depression occurred in a small number of patients.[12-14]

In our efforts to minimize the incidence and severity of the systemic side-effects of epidural narcotic analgesia, we developed and evaluated the technique of continuous epidural infusion of morphine (CEpM), 0.1 mg/hour, for pain relief after thoracic surgery.[15, 16] This method was compared with intravenous administration of morphine (our routine method of analgesia), and with intermittent epidural injections of large doses of morphine.

We have evaluated the efficacy of pain relief and the incidence of systemic side-effects of the three methods of morphine analgesia after a variety of intrathoracic surgical procedures (i.e., segmentectomy, lobectomy, pneumonectomy, esophagectomy). Our series comprised 60 patients between 13 and 79 years of age. A standardized nonnarcotic anesthesia technique—employing nitrous oxide, oxygen, and halothane—was used. Our 60 patients were divided at random into three groups of 20 patients each receiving pain treatment over the first three postoperative days, as follows:

Group A: intermittent intravenous (IV) injections of morphine, 2 mg, as necessary for control of pain
Group B: intermittent epidural injections of morphine, 5 mg, as necessary
Group C: continuous epidural infusion of morphine, 0.1 mg/hr

In Group A, intravenous morphine was administered by members of the nursing staff at the request of the patient. In Group B, the epidural catheter was inserted at the end of the surgical procedure and intermittent epidural injections of morphine were given by anesthesia staff members at the request of the patient. In Group C, the epidural catheter was inserted before surgery, and continuous epidural infusion of morphine was started after induction of anesthesia. The solution for epidural infusion was prepared, in the operating room pharmacy, by mixing 10 mg of morphine in 100 ml of normal saline, for a concentration of 0.01% (0.1 mg of morphine in each milliliter). All patients in Group C received continuous epidural infusion of this solution at a rate of 1 ml/hr, delivered through a precalibrated volumetric infusion pump (IMED). Spinal analgesia was supplemented with IV morphine, in doses of 2 mg, as necessary for control of pain, given by the nursing staff at the request of the patient.

In Groups B and C, the epidural catheter was introduced between spinal laminae T3 and T4 through a lateral approach. Accurate placement of the catheter in the epidural space was confirmed by the catheter advancement test (CAT). The CAT (developed by El-Baz) avoids the problems associated with the use of epidural injections of local anesthetics and contrast solution and the use of spinal x-ray films for catheter localization. The test requires thorough knowledge of the anatomic characteristics of the epidural space and surrounding tissue. After the epidural space is identified by loss of resistance to injected air, a soft epidural catheter without stylet is advanced for 20 cm. The lack of resistance to catheter advancement is affirmative of accurate epidural placement; conversely, the presence of resistance to catheter advancement is indicative of inaccurate placement. In our series, use of the CAT allowed accurate placement in all patients. In 10 of our patients, the CAT was followed by catheter localization using a contrast solution (Amipaque) and x-ray films in order to assess the accuracy of placement with the CAT. In this respect, both methods were found to be comparable.

EVALUATION OF ANALGESIA

The three methods of analgesia described previously were used for a period of 72 hours. For the purposes of evaluation, this period was divided into three 24-hour periods, labeled as postoperative days 1, 2, and 3 (see Tables 29–1 and 29–3). Postoperative pain relief was subjectively evaluated by each patient on a visual-analog pain scale ranging from 0 to 10 (0 = no pain, 10 = severe pain). As shown in Figure 29–1, the pain scale used in this study contains five facial expressions of different degrees of pain. The visual-analog scale was designed (by El-Baz) to facilitate and improve the accuracy of subjective pain evaluation by a large number of patients with different socioeconomic backgrounds.

Pain scores were obtained from each patient twice a day at 6:00 AM and 6:00 PM. The pain score was used to evaluate the degree of post-

operative pain and to quantify pain relief obtained. Postoperative pain was graded as severe at a pain score between 8 and 10, fair between 6 and 8, moderate between 4 and 6, slight between 1 and 4, and no pain between 0 and 1. Pain relief was considered poor at a pain score between 6 and 10, fair between 3 and 6, and good between 0 and 3. The pain scores were then compared among the three groups.

The times of injection were recorded for Groups B and C. The number of patients in Group C who requested additional IV morphine supplementation and the dose of morphine given to each patient were recorded. The total dose of morphine used in each group and the number of patients reporting good pain relief in each group were compared and used to evaluate the efficacy of pain relief of these methods of analgesia. The occurrence of side-effects directly related to the method of pain relief was recorded, and the incidence of side effects was compared between groups. Student t-test was used for the statistical analysis of these data; a statistically significant difference was considered at a p value of less than 0.05.

POSTOPERATIVE PAIN RELIEF

For Group A, the mean pain score was 4.1 ± 2.7 for the 72-hour postoperative period, indicating a *moderate* degree of postoperative pain. In Group B, the mean pain score was 2.4 ± 1.8; this was significantly lower than that achieved in Group A ($p < 0.05$). The Group B pain score indicated a *slight* degree of postoperative pain. In Group C, continuous epidural infusion of morphine, 0.1 mg/hr, with occasional IV morphine supplementation, in Group C achieved a mean pain score of 2.6 ± 1.4; this also indicated a *slight* grade of postoperative pain. The mean pain score obtained in Group C was significantly lower than that obtained in Group A ($p < 0.05$) but was not significantly different from that obtained in Group B ($p > 0.05$). Table 29–1 shows the mean pain score achieved in all three groups during the first three postoperative days.

Evaluation of pain relief in these three groups of patients, on the basis of the pain score obtained, showed a progressive improvement of pain relief with time. Pain relief achieved with these methods of morphine analgesia was significantly better on the third postoperative day. The quality of pain relief achieved in Group A was graded as *fair*. Pa-

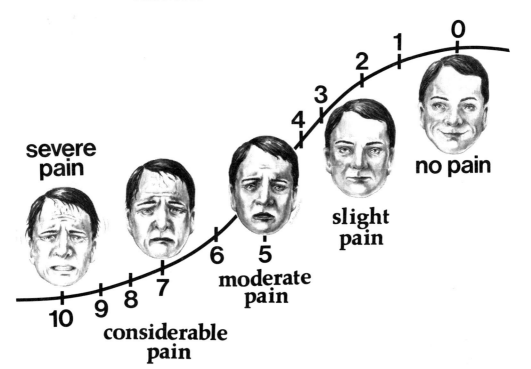

Figure 29–1. Pain scale as determined by facial expression.

tients in Group B achieved better pain relief, graded as *good*. Continuous epidural infusion of morphine, with occasional IV supplementation, also achieved pain relief graded as *good*. Intermittent intravenous administration of morphine achieved *good* pain relief (pain score <3) in nine patients (45%) in Group A; this was significantly lower than that achieved in Group B and in Group C. Intermittent epidural injection of morphine achieved *good* pain relief in 14 patients (70%) in Group B. Continuous epidural infusion of morphine achieved *good* pain relief in 13 patients (65%) in Group C. Table 29–2 shows the degree of pain relief achieved in each group of patients.

The mean IV dose of morphine in Group A was 28.7 ± 7.6 mg/patient/day. The mean dose of morphine administered epidurally in Group B was 18.9 ± 8.7 mg/patient/day. Patients in Group C received continuous epidural infusion of morphine at 2.4 mg/patient/day, which was supplemented occasionally in all patients with IV morphine; the mean dose was 6.6 ± 1.7

mg/patient/day. The mean dose of morphine used in Group A was significantly higher (four times larger) than that given in Group C; the mean dose of morphine used in Group B was also significantly higher (three times larger) than that given in Group C. Table 29–3 shows the doses of morphine administered in each group during the first three postoperative days.

SYSTEMIC SIDE-EFFECTS

The use of intermittent IV morphine in Group A was associated with a low incidence of side-effects. Two patients in this group complained of pruritus, and another three patients developed urinary retention. Intermittent epidural administration of morphine in 5-mg doses as required caused a higher incidence of systemic side-effects; seven patients in this group complained of pruritus, and all patients developed urinary retention. Five patients in Group B developed central narcosis, as evi-

Table 29–1. Pain Scores with Postoperative Morphine Analgesia

| | | Pain Score | |
Patient Group	Day 1	Day 2	Day 3
A: IV morphine 2 mg prn	4.7 ± 1.9	4.1 ± 1.4	3.3 ± 1.7
B: Epidural morphine 5 mg prn	2.7 ± 1.4	2.1 ± 1.7	1.9 ± 1.1
C: Epidural morphine 0.1 mg/hr	2.9 ± 1.4	2.4 ± 0.8	2.1 ± 0.7

Table 29–2. Grading of Pain Relief Obtained

| | No. of Patients | | |
Patient Group	Good (0–3)[a]	Fair (4–6)[a]	Poor (7–10)[a]
A: Intermittent IV morphine	9 (45%)	6 (30%)	5 (25%)
B: Intermittent epidural morphine	14 (70%)	5 (25%)	1 (5%)
C: Continuous epidural morphine	13 (65%)	4 (20%)	3 (15%)

[a]Ranges are pain scores.

denced by loss of consciousness, small (pinpoint) pupils, and slow respiratory rate (below 8 breaths/min). The administration of IV naloxone 0.8 to 1.6 mg in four patients was successful in reversing central narcosis; these four patients required additional IV naloxone in 0.1-mg doses as necessary to maintain consciousness and a respiratory rate above 10 breaths/min. The fifth patient with central narcosis remained semiconscious after IV administration of naloxone, 2 mg, and required intubation with mechanical ventilation overnight. Continuous epidural infusion of morphine, 0.1 mg/hr, supplemented occasionally with IV morphine, was associated with a low incidence of systemic side-effects. One patient in this group complained of pruritus, and another three patients developed urinary retention. Table 29–4 shows the number of patients in each group with side-effects.

RESULTS

Effective pain relief after thoracic surgery, as well as being humanitarian, improves patient's sense of well-being as well as physiologic functions. Adequate postoperative analgesia has been shown to improve pulmonary dynamic spirometry and gas exchange.[17–20] Postoperative analgesia also allows for deep breathing, effective coughing, and efficient chest physiotherapy, causing a significant reduction in the incidence of postoperative pulmonary complications.[18] Adequate postoperative analgesia also causes a minimal increase in sympathetic, hormonal, and metabolic activities, with minimal alteration of cardiovascular functions.[21] Besides the psychological gains of relieving suffering, effective postoperative an-

algesia improves patient movement, allows for early ambulation, and reduces the risk of deep-vein thrombosis.[17–22] Despite these advantages and the availability of a variety of drugs and techniques of analgesia, effective postoperative pain relief remains a major surgical problem and difficult to achieve in the majority of patients.[23, 24]

Systemic administration of narcotics is the most widely used method of analgesia in surgical patients. Intermittent administration of small doses of systemic narcotics (intramuscular, IV, subcutaneous) at fixed intervals has been shown to be an ineffective method of analgesia in surgical patients.[23, 24] In our patients, intermittent IV injections of morphine in 2-mg doses achieved marginal postoperative analgesia, and pain relief was inadequate in a large number of cases. This was the result of difficulty in achieving and maintaining adequate serum drug levels of effective analgesia, owing to individual differences in pharmacodynamics and pharmacokinetics.[25, 26] Although the systemic administration of larger doses of narcotics at short intervals or the use of continuous intravenous infusion of morphine can improve postoperative analgesia, both methods are generally avoided because of the risk of side-effects (hypotension, central narcosis, respiratory depression, drug addiction).[27, 28] Although intermittent systemic administration of small doses of narcotics provides effective analgesia in only a small number of patients, this technique is accepted in surgical practice because of its convenience and high margin of safety. Systemic administration of narcotics can be carried out by the nursing staff, causes a low incidence of mostly benign side-effects, and requires minimal postoperative monitoring and medical supervision.

Table 29–3. Total Morphine Dose (mg/patient/day)

| | Postoperative Day | | |
Patient Group	1	2	3
A: Intermittent IV morphine	34.6 ± 6.7	22.3 ± 8.1	18.2 ± 6.1
B: Intermittent epidural morphine	31.6 ± 7.2	15.9 ± 6.8	13.7 ± 4.1
C: Continuous epidural morphine	8.2 ± 1.4	5.8 ± 1.9	3.9 ± 0.7

Table 29–4. Number of Patients with Systemic Side-effects

Patient Group	Pruritus	Urinary Retention	Central Narcosis
A: Intermittent IV morphine	2 (10%)	3 (15%)	None
B: Intermittent epidural morphine	7 (35%)	20 (100%)	5 (25%)
C: Continuous epidural morphine	1 (5%)	3 (15%)	0

The recent development and evaluation of epidural narcotic analgesia was thought to be an ideal method of pain relief in surgical patients. It was hoped that this method of pain relief would provide selective spinal analgesia and avoid the inconvenience and side-effects associated with epidural injections of local anesthetics.[29-31] The position of the epidural catheter and the site of action of local anesthetics and epidural morphine is shown in Figure 29–2.

Although epidural injection of large doses of morphine has been reported to provide profound and prolonged postoperative analgesia, the duration of analgesia achieved in our patients was short, particularly during the first postoperative day, and frequent injections were required in all patients. The corresponding need for adequate personnel on the anesthesia staff, both to administer the injections and to provide careful observation of the patient, restricts the application of this method of analgesia. Although intermittent epidural injection of morphine in 5-mg doses achieved selective spinal analgesia with minimal alteration of neuronal conduction in sympathetic, sensory, and motor nerves, it caused a high incidence of systemic side-effects and was life-threatening in a few patients. The systemic side-effects observed with the use of epidural morphine were also identical to those described with systemic administration of large doses of morphine indicating a generalized alteration of opiate receptor functions. Morphine given epidurally in large doses has been shown to bind to opiate nociceptive receptors, opiate nonnociceptive receptors, and other nonopiate receptors in the spinal cord and nerves.[32-34] With epidural injection of morphine, serum morphine levels achieved are similar to those with IV and intramuscular (IM) injections.[35-37] We believe that epidural injection of morphine may directly or indirectly alter the functions of the ascending tracts of the spinal cord to increase the sensitivity of higher centers to morphine, so that side-effects

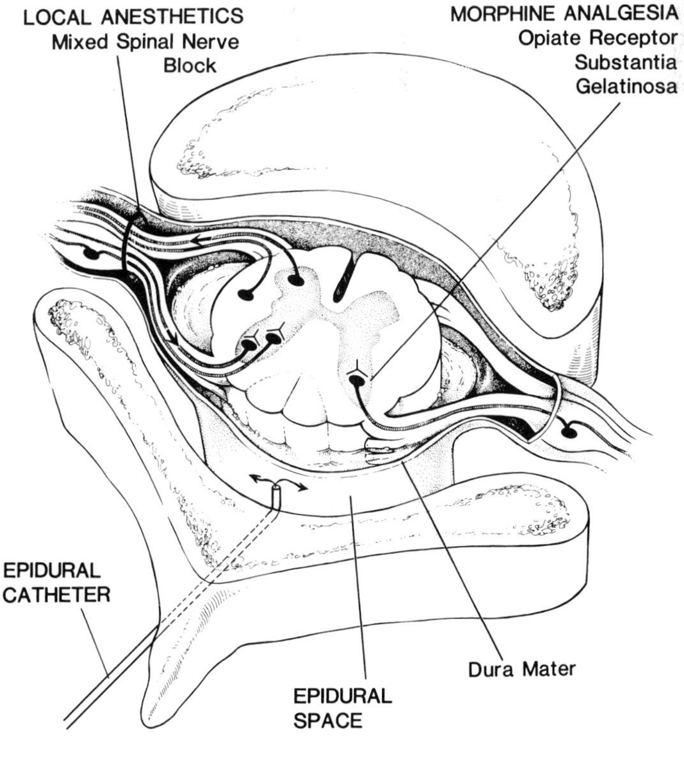

Figure 29–2. Site of action of local anesthetics and of epidural morphine.

LOCAL ANESTHETICS
Mixed Spinal Nerve Block

MORPHINE ANALGESIA
Opiate Receptor
Substantia
Gelatinosa

EPIDURAL
CATHETER

EPIDURAL
SPACE

Dura Mater

can develop even when serum levels are low. This view is supported by reported cases of central narcosis and respiratory depression after systemic administration of small doses of narcotics and sedatives in patients receiving epidural morphine analgesia.[38-40] In spite of the mechanism involved,[41,42] the high incidence of systemic side-effects of epidural injections of large doses of morphine has challenged the safety and value of this approach for postoperative analgesia.

Continuous epidural infusions of small doses of morphine 0.1 mg/hr, with occasional IV morphine supplementation, achieved effective postoperative pain relief. Although continuous infusion of morphine 0.1 mg/hr (1.7 μg/min) achieved progressive selective blockade of opiate nociceptive pathways in posterior spinal gray matter, postoperative analgesia was incomplete and required occasional supplementation with IV morphine. Continuous epidural morphine analgesia was associated with occasional episodes of pain, particularly during an active period of postoperative care (chest physiotherapy and patient ambulation). These painful episodes may be the result of the following factors: (1) occasional increase in pain intensity and neurotransmitters release, which overcomes the competitive blockade of spinal opiate receptors achieved with morphine, (2) the involvement of a large spinal segment in transmission of pain during patient activity, and (3) occasional pain transmission through other nonopiate nociceptive pathways. Partial relief of acute postoperative pain has also been reported after epidural administration of larger doses of morphine and Demerol.[8,37,39] Although supplementation of epidural analgesia, achieved with large doses of narcotics, by systemic narcotics was reported to cause a high incidence of side-effects,[38-40] the concomitant administration of small doses of IV morphine during continuous epidural infusion of morphine at 0.1 mg/hr was associated with minimal systemic side-effects.[15,16] The low incidence of systemic side-effects during continuous epidural infusion of morphine is a major advantage and probably is the result of these factors: (1) slow progressive blockade of opiate and nonopiate receptors in a small segment of spinal cord, (2) low serum morphine levels (undetectable or < 2.5 ng/ml) with continuous epidural infusion of morphine at 0.1 mg/hr,[15] and (3) probably a low concentration of morphine in cerebrospinal fluid.

CONCLUSION

Our evaluation of these three methods of morphine analgesia shows that continuous epidural infusion of morphine at 0.1 mg/hr achieves effective, segmental, and selective postoperative spinal analgesia. Although supplementation of analgesia may occasionally be required, this method of pain relief is associated with minimal systemic side-effects. Furthermore, continuous epidural infusion of morphine is convenient for nursing, surgical, and anesthesia staff and requires only routine postoperative monitoring and medical supervision. This method of analgesia has been used in our practice of thoracic surgery over the last three years and has been found to be a safe, effective, and practical approach to the problems of pain after thoracic surgery.

References

1. Pert CB, Pasternak G, Snyder SH: Opiate antagonists discriminate by receptor binding in brain. Science 82: 1359–1361, 1973.
2. Pert CB, Kuhar MJ, Snyder SH: Opiate receptor: autoradiography localization in rat brain. Proc Natl Acad Sci (USA) 73: 3729–3733, 1976.
3. Cox BM, Goldstein A, Li CH: Opioid activity of a peptide, β-endorphin (61–91), derivative from β-lipotropine. Proc Natl Acad Sci (USA) 73: 1821–1823, 1976.
4. Stoelting RK: Opiate receptors and endorphins: their role in anesthesiology. Anesth Analg (Cleve) 59: 874–880, 1980.
5. Pert A, Yaksh T: Sites of morphine-induced analgesia in the primate brain: relation to pain pathways. Brain Res 80: 135–140, 1974.
6. Kitahata LM, Kasaka Y, Taub A, et al: Lamina-specific suppression of dorsal-horn unit activity by morphine sulfate. Anesthesiology 41: 39–48, 1974.
7. Wang JK, Nauss CA, Thomas JE: Pain relief by intrathecally applied morphine in man. Anesthesiology 50: 149–151, 1979.
8. Behar M, Magora F, Olshwang D, et al: Epidural morphine in treatment of pain. Lancet 1: 527–529, 1979.
9. Magora F, Olshwang D, Eimerl D, et al: Observations on extradural morphine analgesia in various pain conditions. Br J Anaesth 52: 247–251, 1980.
10. Bromage PR, Camporesi E, Chestnut D: Epidural narcotics for postoperative analgesia. Anesth Analg (Cleve) 59: 473–480, 1980.
11. Lanz E, Theiss D, Riess W, et al: Epidural morphine for postoperative analgesia: a double-blind study. Anesth Analg (Cleve) 61: 236–240, 1982.
12. McDonald AM: Complication of epidural morphine. Anaesth Intensive Care 8: 490–491, 1980.
13. Boas RA: Hazards of epidural morphine. Anaesth Intensive Care 8: 377–378, 1980.
14. Bromage PR, Camporesi EM, Durant PAC, Nielsen

CH: Nonrespiratory side effects of epidural morphine. Anesth Analg (Cleve) 61: 490–495, 1982.

15. El-Baz N, et al: Continuous epidural morphine analgesia for pain relief after thoracic surgery. Anesthesiology 57: A205, 1982.

16. El-Baz N, et al: Continuous epidural morphine infusion for postoperative pain relief. Anesth Analg (Cleve) 62: 258, 1983.

17. Bromage PR: Spirometry in assessment of analgesia after abdominal surgery. Br Med J 2: 589–593, 1955.

18. Simpson BP, Parkhouse J, Marshall R, Lambrechts W: Extradural analgesia and the prevention of postoperative respiratory complications. Br J Anaesth 33: 628–641, 1961.

19. Wahba WM, Don HR, Craig DB: Postoperative epidural analgesia: effect on lung volumes. Can Anaesth Soc J 22: 519–527, 1975.

20. Craig DB: Postoperative recovery of pulmonary function. Anesth Analg (Cleve) 60: 46–52, 1981.

21. Kehlet H: Influence of epidural analgesia on the endocrine metabolic response to surgery. Acta Anaesthesiol Scand (Suppl) 70: 39, 1979.

22. Modig J, Malmberg P, Saldeen T: Comparative effects of epidural and general anesthesia on fibrinolysis function, lower limb rheology and thromboembolism after total hip replacement. Anesthesiology 53: 34, 1980.

23. White DC: The relief of postoperative pain. In: Recent Advances in Anaesthesia and Analgesia. Atkinson RS, Hewer CL (eds) New York, Churchill Livingstone, 1982.

24. Scott DB: Postoperative pain relief. Regional Anesthesia (Suppl) 7: S110–S113, 1982.

25. Austin KL, Stapleton JV, Mather LE: Relationships between blood meperidine concentration and analgesic response. Anesthesiology 53: 460–466, 1980.

26. Austin KL, Stapleton JV, Mather LE: Multiple intramuscular injections: a major source of variability in analgesic response to meperidine. Pain 8: 47–62, 1980.

27. Chakravarty K, Tucker W, Rosen M, Vickers MD: Comparison of buprenorphine and pethidine given intravenously on demand to relieve post-operative pain. Br Med J 2: 895–897, 1979.

28. Stapleton JV, Austin KL, Mather LE: A pharmacokinetic approach to postoperative pain: continuous infusion of pethidine. Anaesth Intensive Care 7: 25–32, 1979.

29. Chambers WA, Sinclair CJ, Scott DB: Extradural

morphine for pain after surgery. Br. J Anaesth 53: 921–925, 1981.

30. Rawal N, Sjostrand UH, Dahlstrom B, et al: Epidural morphine for postoperative pain relief: a comparative study with intramuscular narcotic and intercostal nerve block. Anesth Analg (Cleve) 61: 93–98, 1982.

31. Torda TA, Pybus DA, Liberman H, et al: Experimental comparison of extradural and IM morphine. Br J Anaesth 52: 939–942, 1980.

32. Belcher G, Ryall RW: Differential excitatory and inhibitory effect of opiates on non-nociceptive and nociceptive neurons in the spinal cord of the cat. Brain Res 145: 303–314, 1978.

33. Maruyama Y, Shimoji K, Shimizu H, et al: Effect of morphine on human spinal cord and peripheral nervous activities. Pain 8: 63–73, 1980.

34. Tung AS, Yaksh TL: Involvement of multiple opiate receptors in spinally mediated analgesia in the rat. Pain (Suppl) 1: 523, 1981.

35. Weddel SJ, Ritter RR: Serum levels following epidural administration of morphine and correlation with relief of post-surgical pain. Anesthesiology 54: 210–214, 1981.

36. Herz A, Teschemacher H: Activities and site of antinociceptive action of morphine-like analgesics and kinetics of distribution following intravenous, intracerebral, and intraventricular application. Adv Drug Res 6: 70–119, 1971.

37. Glynn CJ, Mather LE, Cousins MJ, et al: Peridural meperidine in humans: analgesic response, pharmacokinetics, and transmission into CSF. Anesthesiology 55: 520–526, 1981.

38. Gustafsson LL, Feychting B, Klingstedt C: Late respiratory depression after concomitant use of morphine epidurally and parenterally. Lancet 1: 892–893, 1981.

39. Gustafsson LL, Schildt B, Jacobsen J: Adverse effects of extradural and intrathecal opiates: report of a nationwide survey in Sweden. Br J Anaesth 54: 479–486, 1982.

40. Cohen ES, Rothblatt AJ, Albright GA: Early respiratory depression with epidural narcotic and intravenous droperidol. Anesthesiology 59: 559, 1983.

41. Bromage PR, Camporsi EM, Durant PAC, Nielson CH: Restoral spread of epidural morphine. Anesthesiology 56: 431–436, 1982.

42. Yaksh TL: Spinal opiate analgesia: Characteristics and principles of action. Pain 11: 293–346, 1981.

30

Management of Postoperative Thoracotomy Pain: Intermittent Epidural Infusion of Morphine

John H. Mehnert, M.D.
Timothy Dupont, M.D.

The pain associated with the posterolateral thoracotomy incision is invariably severe. The resultant splinting has been shown to reduce functional residual capacity of the lungs beyond the restriction observed following abdominal surgery.[1] Several adjunctive techniques for improved postoperative analgesia have been developed, including nerve block, epidural anesthesia, and transcutaneous nerve stimulation, but the majority of surgeons continue to rely on intermittent parenteral narcotic administration, with limited success. The dosage required for therapeutic narcotic levels results in central nervous system depression and a significant incidence of drug reaction. The intermittent intramuscular injection program most commonly employed causes peak blood levels alternating with protracted inadequate concentration. During any surgical procedure, a minimal therapeutic serum level is probably maintained less than 35% of the time.[2] Intravenous narcotic techniques do not reduce the total narcotic dose, and a variability in dose response results in inadequate relief for a significant proportion of patients.[3] The paresis that accompanies analgesia following various regional block techniques, including epidural thoracic anesthesia, produces ventilatory restriction and hypotension.[4, 5]

A relatively new and important method of pain relief, utilizing the epidural administration of a narcotic for direct action on spinal nociceptor (nocioreceptor) sites, appears to supply markedly improved and long-lasting pain relief, with better maintenance of pulmonary function. Epidural narcotics have been used for postoperative analgesia in more than 1000 patients at Mercy Hospital, San Diego, California. Approximately 20% of these have undergone thoracic procedures; the improved analgesic quality has been especially gratifying

in this group. Special problems unique to the postoperative status following cardiac surgery limit the use of the epidural analgesic technique in such patients, as indicated later.

HISTORICAL BACKGROUND

Until recently, the site of action of narcotics was considered to be central, involving a generalized cerebral effect. For this reason, significant cerebral and respiratory depression was accepted as the inevitable cost for achieving adequate analgesia. Recent research has disclosed the presence of centers in the sensory spinal pathways wherein a control mechanism is able to influence the quality of the transmitted nociceptive signal.[6] The perhaps most important of these modulating areas was detected in the dorsal horn of the spinal cord at the synapse of the primary sensory nerve with the ascending tracts. Additional centers for modulation have been discovered in spinal, brain stem, and cortical levels.[7] Concurrently, it was demonstrated that unique opiate receptor sites occur in these pain modulation centers, and that intrinsic opioid substances—enkephalins and endorphins—act to control the modulating effect.[8] Special synapses occur in these modulating centers involving the unmyelinated C and delta (δ) A fibers, which convey deep or true pain sensation. An inhibitory influence is believed to be triggered by the release of enkephalin or endorphin from suppressor nerve endings in these special synapses.

These discoveries lent strong evidence that a significant part of the analgesic effect of exogenous opiates involves a blockade of the pain stimulus by flooding special modulating receptor sites both in the spinal cord and in higher centers. Animal studies were immediately initiated to evaluate the spinal cord role in this modulating influence.[9] These studies were promptly followed by a clinical evaluation in Israel, in 1979, by Behar, who administered morphine epidurally to effect postoperative analgesia.[10] The clinical analgesia obtained was excellent and subsequently clinical investigations of the technique were instituted in many European medical centers. The efficacy of spinal-acting opiates for the relief of postoperative pain is now established in the comprehensive literature, and the technique has been widely utilized clinically. The specificity of the analgesia produced has been especially gratifying. Motor and sensory function is unimpaired, there is no vasomotor blockade, and central depression is minimized because of a smaller total narcotic dose.[11]

METHOD OF ACTION AND TECHNIQUE

The primary centers for pain modulation lie in the substantia gelatinosa of the dorsal horn of the spinal cord. Serendipitously, this site is close to the cord surface and readily reached, through direct absorption, by drugs introduced into the spinal fluid. Intrathecal administration is the most efficient delivery route to the spinal fluid, but the requirement for reintroduction of the narcotic at regular intervals causes this method to be both inconvenient and dangerous.

The intermittent instillation of the narcotic agent through an indwelling epidural catheter has been found to be an ideal means of delivery. Epidural catheterization is widely practiced by anesthesiologists because of its use for administering epidural anesthesia. Proper positioning of the catheter in the epidural space is important, and its correct position is routinely ensured by instillation of 3 cc of 0.5% bupivicaine with 1:200,000 epinephrine. Inadvertent intrathecal positioning is detected by the prompt onset of segmental anesthesia; accidental intravascular injection is detected by significant and immediate tachycardia. If either of these effects occurs, the catheter is repositioned and then retested before instituting morphine analgesia.

The narcotic is usually instilled in sterile preservative-free saline to encourage migration of the drug along the epidural space. Most of the narcotic dose (approximately 90%) is rapidly absorbed by the epidural venous plexus, resulting almost immediately in a serum drug level nearly equivalent to that achieved with an identical intravenous dose.[12] With morphine, the peak serum level occurs approximately 30 minutes following injection, and the narcotic has virtually disappeared from the blood at 4 hours. The analgesic effect of this modicum is modest because of the small total dose.

A more significant analgesia is effected by the remaining 10% of the administered narcotic.[13] This portion diffuses through the dura from the epidural space and enters the spinal fluid, in which it remains for many hours in an unconjugated (active) form. It is gradually absorbed into the adjacent cord substance; here it produces its direct effect on the pain-modulating centers. The spinal fluid circulation causes a gradual rostral spread of the analgesic.[14] In general, manipulation of the spinal level of administration and of the volume of diluent effectively confines the drug to the desired spinal levels. Rarely, spread of the analgesic cephalad can result in central effects, producing complications, described in the following section. For thoracic procedures, a high lumbar or lower thoracic catheterization (L1–2 to T10) has been favored. For pain relief following abdominal surgery, insertion of the catheter at the L2–3 or L3–4 level has been most effective.

The spinal-acting analgesic requires time for initial spinal fluid loading; with morphine, this period is usually 20 to 40 minutes. A significant analgesia is thereafter produced, which, once established, persists for a mean of 12 to 14 hours. Morphine has been the narcotic most frequently used to accomplish epidural analgesia, although many other narcotic agents, especially fentanyl, have been found to be effective.[11] Morphine is widely available in a vehicle that is preservative-free,* its pharmacology is familiar, and it is relatively lipophobic, which results in slower absorption into the cord for a more prolonged action.

CLINICAL DATA

We have recently reported our experiences with the use of intermittent epidural morphine instillation for postoperative pain relief.[15] Our series consisted of a group of 268 patients

---

*Preservative-free morphine sulfate is available as Duramorph PF. Each milliliter contains morphine sulfate 0.5 mg or 1.0 mg and sodium chloride 9 mg in water for injection. Available in single dose ampules of 5 mg/10 ml or 10 mg/10 ml. Manufactured by Elkins-Sinn, Inc., Cherry Hill, N.J. 08034.

Table 30–1. Surgical Procedures for Which Epidural Analgesia Was Used Postoperatively in 40 Patients

Procedure	No. of Patients
Posterolateral thoracotomy	
Removal of pleural tumor	1
Biopsy of lesion in lung	5
Wedge resection of lung	2
Lobectomy	20
Pneumonectomy	2
Vagotomy and transdiaphragmatic pyloroplasty	1
Mediastinal cyst excision	1
Thoracoabdominal incision	
Esophagectomy	1
Gastroesophagectomy	5
Median sternotomy	
Mediastinal tumor	1
Coronary artery by-pass graft	1

whose clinical course could be properly evaluated retrospectively. Of these patients, 40 (15%) had undergone major thoracic surgical procedures. Table 30–1 lists the operations performed in this group.

An important benefit of epidural spinal analgesia is the small total narcotic dose required. The range of dosage used in this group of thoracic patients was 2 to 6 mg, with the great preponderance of doses at 3 to 5 mg (Table 30–2).

Figure 30–1 plots the intervals between instillations administered as required for satisfactory analgesia. As depicted, the median interval between narcotic instillations was 12 hours. Our analysis of each 24-hour period revealed that 52% of the patients required only one instillation, and 36%, two instillations; only 12% required three instillations of narcotic for adequate pain relief. Of the total number of instillations, 21 (13%) were fol-

Table 30–2. Morphine Doses for Epidural Analgesia Following Thoracic Surgery in 40 Patients

Dose (mg)	No. of Instillations	
2	18	10%
2.5	1	
3	36	23%
3.5	8	
4	71	38%
5	47	25%
6	4	2%

lowed by more than 24 hours of analgesia. The average dose of morphine was 4 mg, and two injections over 24 hours was the usual frequency; it is apparent that an average total dosage of 8 mg of morphine instilled epidurally was able to produce effective pain relief for 24 hours in patients who underwent major thoracic surgery. This quantity of narcotic agent is approximately one sixth that required for parenteral administration. Because of the reduced total narcotic dose, the patients were found to be more alert and cooperative, with an improved sense of well-being.

Evaluation of Pain Relief

A retrospective analysis of the degree of analgesia obtained is difficult, but the following observations, made just prior to a narcotic instillation, are relevant. Of the patients receiving an instillation, 13% stated that they were experiencing no pain at that time. Nevertheless, analgesic was given prophylactically by the house staff, in anticipation of a possible subsequent need for instillation at a less convenient time. We believe that injections can be given in this manner if at least 6 hours have ensued since the last administration, but we prefer to await the return of pain. The pain was mild at the time of reinstillation for 50% of the patients. Mild pain was defined as distress occurring only with motion or with cough. Constant but moderate pain was reported by 28%; only 8% described the pain as severe or intense. A further indication of the quality of pain relief was the absence of respiratory complications during the postoperative course. Atelectasis was detected radiographically in only 2 of the 40 patients.

Ineffective analgesia was not a problem in this thoracic surgery group but was experienced initially in six patients within our larger series. When the epidural catheter was reinserted at a different spinal level in four of these six, satisfactory analgesia followed in each instance. For this reason, we believe that a lack of effective analgesia can, in large part, be considered to be due to improper positioning of the epidural catheter.

Complications

The complications that occurred following epidural administration of morphine in this small group of thoracic patients are listed in Table 30–3. Urinary retention due to complex

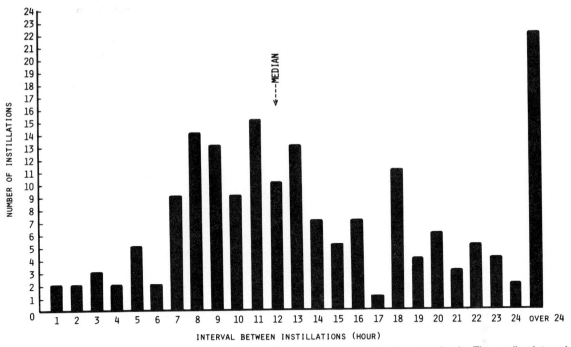

Figure 30–1. The time interval between morphine instillations given as required to control pain. The median interval is 12 hours. Analgesia extended beyond 24 hours following 13% of the instillations.

spinal action is the most common side-effect,[11] with a reported incidence of as high as 35%. Because of its frequency, we usually insert urinary catheters during the period of epidural analgesia. Since most of the patients have indwelling urinary catheters placed during the immediate postoperative course for other reasons, this has not been a significant problem. Pruritus was the second most prevalent complication, occurring in 10% of our patients, and has been reported in from 16% to 30% in larger series.[11] This itching paresthesia is not an allergic phenomenon, and its effect is countered by the administration of naloxone. The complaint is ordinarily mild, and usually no specific therapy is necessary. Nausea and/or vomiting, side-effects common to all forms of

narcotic therapy, occurred in 6% of our patients. Hypoventilation (<12 breaths/min) was observed in one patient, but this was reversed immediately following a single injection of naloxone.

Infection at the catheter site did not occur in our thoracic surgery patients, but in our total experience one patient has developed fever and meningismus 48 hours after removal of an epidural catheter that had been used over a 4-day period. Cultures of the spinal fluid showed the presence of α-hemolytic streptococci, and appropriate antibiotic therapy resulted in complete and prompt recovery. This instance of intrathecal infection emphasizes the need for asepsis, and our sterile technique with these catheters is identical to that for central venous lines. We have usually limited the use of the catheter to 4 days for this reason.

As previously reported in the literature,[15] one patient in our total experience has suffered paresis during epidural therapy. Other investigators who have reviewed this case believe that the paresis was unrelated to the analgesic method. We have uncovered no other report of this complication.

The abrupt onset of apnea during therapy, although rare, can be life-threatening and must be constantly anticipated.[16] This apnea may develop abruptly several hours following instillation of the narcotic, with no prodromal

Table 30–3. Complications Following Epidural Morphine in 40 Thoracic Surgery Patients

Complication	No. of Cases
Itching	4 (10%)
Nausea and/or vomiting	3 (7.5%)
Urinary retention	2 (5%)
Hypotension	1 (2.5%)
Backache	1 (2.5%)
Headache	1 (2.5%)
None	28 (70%)

symptoms. Apnea is believed to be due to rostral spread of the intrathecal narcotic, which reaches and depresses central respiratory centers. If it occurs, apnea will respond promptly and reliably to intravenous naloxone administration.[11] Interestingly, pain relief is not inhibited by naloxone. The respiratory status of all patients in whom epidural narcotic analgesia is used must be followed carefully, preferably in a monitored area such as the intensive care unit or a progressive care area. Respiratory monitors are available but as yet are not completely reliable.

Postoperative Care

As previously noted, we ordinarily discontinue epidural narcotic therapy on the fourth day postoperatively. The analgesic effect persists for an additional 12 to 24 hours, and most patients find that oral analgesics are sufficient to control the pain thereafter. Only 5 of the 40 patients in our group required parenteral narcotic administration subsequent to removal of the catheter, and only three of these required more than three doses.

In our hospital, the supervision of pain control with the epidural technique has been delegated to the anesthesiologist, who has the responsibility not only for inserting the epidural catheter and ascertaining its initial effectiveness but also for managing the continuing instillations. The anesthesiologist or a member of the anesthesia resident staff administers the narcotic. We believe that proper evaluation of the condition of the patient and the requirement for a sterile technique for administration make this preferable. We do not presently recommend administration of the drug by nurses. This makes the use of the procedure difficult in hospitals lacking a resident physician staff.

INDICATIONS AND CONTRAINDICATIONS

The goal of postoperative analgesia is to provide effective pain relief accompanied by minimal central nervous system depression. With intermittent parenteral narcotic therapy, staff inattentiveness and a fear of possible patient overutilization frequently result in undertreatment.[17] In addition, differences in age, weight, and pharmacologic variability require adjustments in dosage and frequency of injection. For these reasons, the intermittent intramuscular administration of a narcotic is frequently incapable of providing satisfactory analgesia.

Continuous or intermittent small-dose intravenous infusion has become popular, especially in critical care units, in which close attendance is possible. Since peak-trough problems are lessened, the total narcotic dose is usually less, but the subjective response to pain is variable, requiring the constant attendance of competent professional personnel who can evaluate the patient's status and respond appropriately. Self-administration intravenous and intramuscular injection techniques have been developed,[18, 19] but their cumbersomeness and the contraints just noted limit their applicability.

The virtues of the epidural technique become apparent. Once inserted, the epidural catheter provides an easy, painless means for administration of the agent. The analgesic response is prolonged and the total dose of the narcotic is a fraction of the parenteral requirement. Central depression is therefore minimized.

The most gratifying effect of epidural analgesia is the improvement in patient alertness and cooperation due to an improved quality of pain relief. We previously evaluated the required postoperative hospital stay in a matched group of patients who had undergone knee replacement: we found a two-day reduction in hospitalization (12.4 days reduced to 10.3 days) when epidural analgesia was used as compared with routine intermittent intramuscular treatment. This improvement was believed due to earlier mobility of the patient and more cooperation during physiotherapy.

Although it provides excellent analgesia for thoracic procedures, a major limitation of the epidural technique is its proscription following surgery of the head, neck, or upper extremities. The risk of apnea is believed to be increased when the narcotic is instilled at the cervical levels, and no author advocates the use of the technique for these regions.

There is also a constraint to the use of epidural analgesia following cardiac surgery. Because of the requirement for heparinization, the frequent need for significant blood replacement, and the use of the pump oxygenator, cardiac surgery patients represent a group with increased risk of bleeding diathesis. The fear of the development of an epidural hematoma, with possible cord compression, has resulted in our decision to withhold epidural catheterization immediately postoperatively and for 24 hours thereafter. Additionally, the pain following median sternotomy is not as intense as that experienced after posterolateral thoracotomy.

Having used the method following pulmonary procedures, our cardiac surgeons are increasingly turning to epidural analgesia when a patient complains of inordinate pain or threatens atelectasis owing to poor cough when the first 24 hours have passed.

The specter of lethal apnea has been a major deterrent to the widespread use of epidural narcotics. In our total experience involving approximately 1000 patients, only two (one reported in this cardiothoracic series) required naloxone as an antidote to hypoventilation during the administration of epidural morphine; a similar low incidence reported by Reiz,[20] Gustafsson,[21] and others put the problem in a proper perspective. Many of the effective drugs and techniques employed in medical care imply the principle of small risk for significant gain.

Indwelling epidural infusion units are being used for the control of pain in terminally ill patients, especially those with far advanced carcinoma. By this means, effective analgesia can be provided for many weeks.

CONCLUSION

Because pain is usually more intense following cardiothoracic surgical procedures, and since the consequence of pain is frequently a pulmonary complication, the development of a more effective means for postoperative analgesia should be of interest to the cardiothoracic surgeon. A new analgesic technique utilizing the epidural administration of morphine for direct spinal effect can result in improved analgesia with a small total narcotic dose. The only significant complication to be anticipated is the possible occurrence of apnea, for which reason the respiratory status of these patients must be closely monitored.

References

1. Spence AA, Smith G: Postoperative analgesia and lung function. A comparison of morphine with epidural block. Br J of Anaesthes 43:144–148, 1971.

2. Austin KL, Stapleton JV, Mather LE: Relationship between blood meperidine concentrations and analgesic response: a preliminary report. Anesthesiology 53:460–466, 1980.

3. Tamsen A, Hartvig P, Dahlstrom B, et al: Patient controlled analgesic therapy in the earlier postoperative period. Acta Anaesthesiol Scand 23:462–470, 1979.

4. Cory TC, Mulroyd MF: Postoperative respiratory failure following intercostal block. Anesthesiology 54:418–419, 1981.

5. Conecher ID, Payes ML, Jacobson L, et al: Epidural analgesia following thoracic surgery. Anaesthesia, 38:546–551, 1983.

6. Melzak R, Wal PD: Pain mechanisms, a new theory. Science 150:971–979, 1968.

7. Bowsher D: Pain pathways and mechanisms. Anaesthesia 33:935–944, 1978.

8. Snyder SH: Opiate receptor and internal opiates. Sci Am 236:44–56, 1977.

9. Yaksh TL, Rudy TA: Studies on the direct spinal action of narcotics in the production of analgesia in the rat. Pharmacol Exp Ther 202:411–428, 1977.

10. Behar M, Margora F, Olshwang D, Davidson JT: Epidural morphine in the treatment of pain. Lancet 1:527–528, 1979.

11. Yaksh TL: Spinal opiate analgesia: characteristics and principles of action. Pain 11:293–346, 1981.

12. Weddel SH, Ritter RI: Serum levels following epidural administration of morphine and the correlation with postoperative pain. Anesthesiology 54:210–214, 1981.

13. Asari H, Inouye K, Shibota T, Soga T: Segmental effect of morphine injected into the epidural space in man. Anesthesiology 56:75–77, 1981.

14. Bromage PR, Comparesi EM, Durant PAC, Nielsen CH: Rostral spread of epidural morphine. Anesthesiology 56:431–436, 1982.

15. Mehnert JH, Dupont TJ, Rose DH: Intermittent epidural morphine instillation for control of postoperative pain. Ann Surg, 146:145–151, 1983.

16. McCaughey W, Graham JC: The respiratory depression of epidural morphine. Anaesthesia 37:990–995, 1982.

17. Sriwatanakul K, Weis O, Alloza JL, et al: Analysis of narcotic analgesia usage in the treatment of postoperative pain. JAMA 250:926–929, 1983.

18. Welchow EA: On demand analgesia. Anaesthesia 38:19–25, 1983.

19. Tamesen A, Hartvig P, Dahlstrom B, et al: Patient controlled analgesic therapy in the early postoperative period. Acta Anaesthesiol Scand 23:462–470, 1979.

20. Reiz S, Westberg M: Side-effects of epidural morphine. Lancet, 1:203–204, 1980.

21. Gustafsson LL, Schildt B, Jacobsen K: Adverse effects of extradural and intrathecal opiates: report of a nation-wide survey in Sweden. Br J Anaesth 54:479–485, 1982.

31

Management of Postoperative Thoracotomy Pain: Lumbar Epidural Narcotics

Jay B. Brodsky, M.D.
Mark S. Shulman, M.D.
James B. D. Mark, M.D.

One of the most challenging problems in the postoperative care of the thoracic surgical patient is the treatment of incisional pain. Analgesia is important: a comfortable, cooperative patient will breathe deeply, cough, and ambulate, and the incidence of pulmonary complications will be reduced.

In most centers, parenterally administered narcotics are given for postoperative analgesia, but intravenous and intramuscular narcotics can have deleterious effects. These side-effects include obtundation, nausea, vomiting, respiratory depression, and suppression of cough. We believe that the use of parenteral narcotics alone is not the ideal way to treat post-thoracotomy incisional pain.

Intraoperatively, the surgeon can easily perform direct intercostal nerve blocks using local anesthetics just prior to reinflating the collapsed lung during operations utilizing one-lung anesthesia. Such nerve blocks provide less than ideal relief of incisional pain and they are occasionally associated with marked hypotension.[1] Several explanations have been postulated for this phenomenon. Unrecognized dural puncture or perineural spread of the anesthetic with subsequent spinal block can occur. Because subarachnoid space can extend up to 8 cm past the intervertebral foramen along the nerve roots, the dura can be accidentally entered during the intercostal nerve block. Inadvertent intravascular injection, alone or combined with systemic absorption of the local anesthetic, can also cause hypotension. Finally, paralysis of the thoracic vasomotor nerves (a marked unilateral "sympathectomy") is still another possible cause of the hypotension seen with intraoperative intercostal nerve blocks.

More recently, intercostal nerve cryoanalgesia (the freezing of a nerve in order to produce decreased neuronal activity) has been shown to give excellent post-thoracotomy incisional pain relief. The analgesia often lasts for as long as 4 weeks. Some but not all investigators have reported improved postoperative ventilatory parameters in patients receiving cryoanalgesia compared with those in patients receiving parenteral narcotics. All investigators have noted that narcotic requirements are markedly reduced in patients receiving cryoanalgesia. To date, there have not been any complications reported with this technique.

Local anesthetic drugs given through a catheter placed in the epidural space at either a lumbar or a thoracic level are also effective in treating postoperative pain. However, the motor block that often accompanies the desired sensory block prevents immediate postoperative ambulation and may even limit the use of intercostal muscles for deep breathing and coughing. Postural hypotension can result from the associated "sympathectomy." The duration of pain relief with even the longest-acting local anesthetics is relatively short. The need for frequent "refills" every 1 to 2 hours makes this technique impractical in most hospital settings.

Presently, we believe that the "ideal" treatment of post-thoracotomy incisional pain is by epidurally administered narcotics given through a thoracic[2] or lumbar epidural catheter.[3-5] We use only lumbar epidurals for our thoracotomy patients. We avoid thoracic epidurals because of technical difficulties with this approach. Most anesthesiologists have experience with placing lumbar epidurals, and this technique offers all the advantages for treating post-thoracotomy incisional pain without the possibility of spinal cord trauma from attempted epidural placement at a thoracic spinal cord level.[4, 5]

We prefer to place the epidural catheter prior to the start of the operation. Therefore, if an epidural is planned, cooperation between the surgeon and anesthesiologist is essential since the operation will be delayed 15 to 20 minutes while the catheter is placed and tested. We feel this brief delay is a small price to pay for the considerable benefits obtained in both intra- and postoperative care of the patient.

In the operating room prior to induction of general anesthesia, the L2–3 epidural space is identified, and a catheter is placed into it. The patient is given 500 ml of either Ringer's lactate or normal saline intravenously as a volume load prior to injection of any local anesthetic. A test dose of 3 to 5 ml of lidocaine, 1.5%, with epinephrine, is given through the catheter. If there are no signs of intravascular or subarachnoid injection from this test dose, then 5 minutes later an additional dose of 18 to 20 ml of either lidocaine, 1.5%, or bupivacaine, 0.75%, is administered. We proceed with induction of general anesthesia once we are certain that the catheter is in the epidural space—that is, once a definite anesthetic level is confirmed by pinprick testing.

General anesthesia is induced with sodium thiopental. A short-acting muscle relaxant (succinylcholine or atracurium) is used to facilitate tracheal intubation with a double-lumen endobronchial tube. For maintenance of general anesthesia we use one of the potent inhalational anesthetic agents (halothane, enflurane, or isoflurane) and 100% oxygen. Nitrous oxide is not used at all during the operation. Parenteral narcotics are completely avoided, both preoperatively and during the procedure, for reasons explained later in this discussion.

We use epidurally administered local anesthetics throughout the operation in order to supplement the general anesthetics; thus the required amounts of inhalational agents are minimized. However, the local anesthetics can cause hypotension. Therefore, we use this technique of intraoperative epidural anesthesia only in normotensive patients with no history of coronary artery disease. Since infusion of large amounts of intravenous fluid can have a deleterious effect on the postoperative course in patients undergoing pneumonectomy or those with severe chronic pulmonary disease, we treat any hypotension from the epidural block with an intravenous vasopressor, usually ephedrine. These patients are frequently sensitive to this drug and usually respond to small amounts (5 mg). The motor block from the same local anesthetic decreases or eliminates the need to use muscle relaxants intraoperatively.

Depending on which local anesthetic is used, if the patient is hemodynamically stable, the catheter is refilled approximately every hour with lidocaine, or every 2 hours with bupivacaine. The volume of each "top-up" dose, 15 to 18 ml, is less than the initial dose. If a refill is needed within an hour of the anticipated completion of surgery, we lower the concentration of the local anesthetic to lidocaine, 0.5%, or bupivacaine, 0.25%, in order to reduce the chance of intercostal motor block, which can affect postoperative ventilation. In these low doses, the local anesthetic still provides satisfactory analgesia without motor block.

The epidural narcotic may be administered at any time after the correct position of the catheter is determined. The epidural narcotic should not be given less than 45 minutes before the anticipated completion of surgery in order to allow the narcotic sufficient time to work. Almost all of our patients are extubated in the operating room at the end of the operation. They usually awaken free of incisional pain. If the epidural narcotic has been given late in the operation, 1 to 3 mg of intravenous morphine is also given at this time. The patients are comfortable and are able to respond to commands to breathe deeply and to cough.

Pain relief is rated excellent in almost all patients, and satisfactory in most of the others. After thoracotomy the analgesia obtained with lumbar epidural narcotics is indistinguishable from that obtained with injection of the same drug into a thoracic epidural space.[4, 5]

Narcotics given at the lumbar epidural level improve post-thoracotomy ventilatory parameters when compared with those of patients receiving conventional intravenous morphine for analgesia. However, the measured ventilatory functions are still markedly reduced from preoperative values.[5]

For clinical research studies, we have used preservative-free morphine. The dose of morphine is 5 to 10 mg in 10 to 15 ml of saline. The analgesia obtained is profound. Because the site of action of epidurally administered narcotics is on the opiate receptors in the spinal cord, the disadvantages of epidurally administered local anesthetics (motor block, hypotension) and parenteral narcotics (nausea, obtundation) are usually not seen.

Preservative-free morphine (Duramorph) has only recently become commercially available. For several years we have used hydromorphone (Dilaudid) in a dose of 1.25 to 1.5 mg in 10 to 20 ml of saline, given through a catheter placed at a lumbar level, for our patients undergoing thoracotomy. Hydromorphone contains no preservatives nor added chemical stabilizers. For this reason we feel it is ideal for epidural administration since we are concerned about the possibility of neurotoxicity from the preservatives present in other available narcotic solutions such as morphine. To date there have been *no* reports associating neurologic damage with the use of epidural narcotics containing preservatives, so our concerns about this potential problem may be unwarranted.

Very rarely, the analgesia from the epidural narcotic is incomplete or unsatisfactory. Frequently, the complaint of discomfort has been not incisional pain but rather shoulder or back ache. This may represent referred pain from diaphragmatic irritation. The central diaphragm is innervated by nerve fibers originating at C3–5, a spinal cord level not usually reached with the volume of hydromorphone solution we routinely use. By increasing the volume and enabling more of the narcotic to reach higher levels before diffusing out of the epidural space, we have on occasion successfully treated complaints of shoulder pain following thoracotomy.[6] In such cases, the patient must be closely observed postoperatively because the larger volume of narcotic solution used may also allow more narcotic to reach the brain stem, causing respiratory depression.

Delayed respiratory depression, the most serious side-effect of epidural narcotics, is extremely uncommon. Most reports of clinically significant respiratory depression have been in patients given epidural narcotics and parenteral narcotics concomitantly. In a nationwide survey in Sweden of 6000 patients receiving epidural narcotics, only 3 who received epidural narcotics alone without parenteral narcotics had signs of respiratory depression.[7] Therefore, we avoid parenteral narcotics, either as a premedication or intraoperatively, when we plan to use epidural narcotics. Occasionally, we give very small amounts of parenteral morphine or Demerol postoperatively to supplement the epidural narcotic, but in these cases the patient is monitored even more carefully than usual for signs of respiratory problems.

Even though respiratory depression after epidural narcotics is infrequent, most clinicians who use this technique, including us, recommend that the patient be closely monitored in an intensive care unit (ICU) setting for at least 12 hours (and usually 24 hours) after receiving the epidural narcotic. If available, an apnea monitor should be used.

The lipid solubility of the narcotic used is important. For a poorly soluble drug such as morphine, a significant amount of the drug is not immediately bound to the spinal cord receptors and is free to diffuse through the cerebrospinal fluid.[8] This may account for the cases of delayed respiratory depression reported with the use of epidural morphine. This complication presumably occurs when the narcotic reaches the respiratory control center located in the brain stem. Hydromorphone is more highly lipid soluble than is morphine. Like the local anesthetics, the epidural effect of hydromorphone appears to be segmental—that is, most of the drug is bound to the spinal cord near the level of injection, and less drug is free in the cerebrospinal fluid.

We believe the complication of delayed respiratory depression, rare with epidural morphine, is still rarer when a highly lipid-soluble narcotic like hydromorphone is used. We have not yet observed any instance of delayed respiratory depression in the several hundred patients to whom we have given this drug. However, since there have not been any large series published on the use of epidural hydromorphone, the incidence of respiratory complications with the use of this agent is still unknown.

Unfortunately, the more lipid-soluble the narcotic, the shorter its length of action. A single dose of epidural morphine will provide 18 to 24 hours of analgesia. Epidural hydromorphone will provide 8 to 12 hours of relief of incisional pain. Normally, we readminister the hydromorphone at least once overnight before discharging our patients from the ICU to the ward the day after surgery.

Since we believe that patients receiving epidural narcotics should be monitored in an ICU setting, and since such care is extremely expensive, we usually limit our use of epidural narcotics to the first 24 hours following operation. We normally prefer to switch to parenteral narcotics at that time, rather than to keep the patient in the ICU for epidural narcotic administration alone. For the patients requiring a longer ICU stay, the epidural catheter is kept in place, and narcotics are given as needed for as long as the patient is in the ICU. We have treated pain for up to 3 days with intermittent injections of hydromorphone administered approximately every 8 to 12 hours as needed.

We and others have found that the total narcotic requirement for surgical patients who have received epidural narcotics is much less after they are discharged to the ward and treated conventionally with parenteral narcotics than for patients not given epidural narcotics from the start.[9] The reasons for this diminished requirement are unknown.

Not all discomfort following thoracic operations is from the wound itself. Since epidural narcotics are effective in treating incisional pain, the patient often may focus attention on other unpleasant sensations. The nursing personnel caring for the patient receiving epidural narcotics must be instructed *not* to give additional parenteral narcotics to treat these other complaints.

All narcotics administered by the epidural route can have side-effects. Urinary retention and generalized pruritus are the most common complications. Urinary retention is reported to occur in as many as 20% of patients receiving epidural narcotics. All of our thoracotomy patients have an indwelling urinary catheter placed at the time of operation; therefore, the incidence of urinary retention in our patients who have been given epidural hydromorphone is unknown. Pruritus of varying degree, usually mild, occurs in 20% to 30% of our patients.

In conclusion, we use a combined technique of epidural and general anesthesia for thoracotomy. Epidural anesthesia with local anesthetics has certain advantages in the intraoperative management of thoracic surgery patients. The use of local anesthetics for sensory and motor blockade during surgery minimizes the required amounts of general anesthetics and muscle relaxants. Since muscle relaxants are frequently not used at all, the potential problem of inadequate reversal of the muscle relaxants at the end of the procedure is avoided.

Narcotics given through the same epidural catheter provide excellent postoperative relief of pain, with a minimum of side-effects. Our patients are comfortable; they are sitting and out of bed sooner than similar patients given only parenteral narcotics for analgesia. Early ambulation and the ability to cough and to carry out deep-breathing exercises reduce the potential for serious respiratory complications. The need for postoperative endotracheal suction or bronchoscopy is rare.

The thoracic epidural route for narcotics offers no advantages over the lumbar route for post-thoracotomy pain relief and in fact has certain disadvantages, as noted previously. Therefore, we place all our epidural catheters at the lumbar level. We prefer hydromorphone or preservative-free morphine (Duramorph). The risk of neurotoxicity from preservatives and stabilizers such as sodium bisulfite is not present when either of these two preparations is used. We believe that the greater lipid-solubility of hydromorphone also reduces the possibility of delayed respiratory depression, since the effects of this agent are more segmental than morphine.

We monitor all of our patients receiving epidural narcotics in an ICU; so far there have been no clinically significant delayed respiratory problems associated with epidural hydromorphone. Even so, because of economic considerations, we prefer to change to parenteral narcotics for analgesia once the patient is stable enough to be transferred out of the ICU. Patients receiving epidural narcotics seem to have fewer complications than those seen in conventionally treated patients, and can be discharged earlier from the hospital.

References

1. Brodsky JB, Mark JBD: Hypotension from intraoperative intercostal nerve blocks. Regional Anesthesia 4:17–18, 1979.
2. El-Baz NM, Ganzouri AR, Gottschalk W, et al: Thoracic epidural morphine analgesia for pain relief after thoracic surgery. Anesthesiology 57:A205, 1982.
3. Welch DB, Hrynaszkiewicz A: Postoperative analgesia using epidural methadone. Administration by the lumbar route for thoracic pain relief. Anaesthesia 36:1051–1054, 1981.
4. Steidl LJ, Fromme GA, Danielson DR: Lumbar versus thoracic epidural morphine for post-thoracotomy pain. Anesth Anal (Cleve) 63:A277, 1984.
5. Shulman MS, Sandler AN, Bradley JW, et al: Post-thoracotomy pain and pulmonary function following epidural and systemic morphine. Anesthesiology 61:569–575, 1984.
6. Horan CT, Beeby DG, Brodsky JB, Oberhelman HA: Segmental effect of lumbar epidural hydromorphone: a case report. Anesthesiology 62:84–85, 1985.
7. Gustafsson LL, Schildt B, Jacobsen K: Adverse effects of extradural and intrathecal opiates: Report of a nationwide study. Br J Anaesth 54:479–485, 1982.
8. Bromage PR, Camporesi EM, Durant PAC, Nielsen CH: Rostral spread of epidural morphine. Anesthesiology 56:431–436, 1982.
9. Brodsky JB, Merrell RC: Epidural administration of morphine postoperatively for morbidly obese patients. West J Med 140:750–753, 1984.

XI
Muscle Flaps and Thoracic Problems

Early surgeons who resected the chest wall gave little consideration to chest wall reconstruction; with the problems of anesthesia, pneumothorax, and hemorrhage, it was a victory if the patient survived. The first recorded resections of the chest wall *that entered into the pleural space* were by the French surgeon Richérand in 1818 and by the American Antony in 1823. Richérand removed segments of the sixth and seventh ribs and part of the pleura in a patient with recurrent carcinoma. The wound was packed and healed sufficiently so that the patient left the hospital on the 27th day with a defect in which ". . . the pericardium and the lungs had contracted adherence with the contour of the quadrilateral aperture, a kind of window made in front of the heart." In his patient Antony resected most of the fifth and sixth ribs together with a portion of the right lung ". . . judged to be between one and two pounds in weight." The wound was allowed to granulate. (See Figure 1.) In this 17-year-old patient, the "tumor" was a pyogenic or tuberculous osteomyelitis of the rib with underlying pneumonia. Richérand's patient soon died from recurrence of the cancer but Antony's patient survived.

With the increasingly frequent use of thoracic procedures and the advent of radiation, which often created injuries of the chest wall, numerous efforts to develop means of closing chest wall defects were made during the early part of the 20th century.

The concept of flaps for soft tissue coverage has been present for several thousand years, initiated by the practice in India of cutting off noses (and ears) to punish criminals, as a form of brutality, and in ordinary physical encounters. The need for correction of these problems encouraged the growth of surgery, established many basic principles of wound healing, and began the specialty of plastic surgery.

The procedure for rotating a cheek flap to form a new nose is described first in the Sushruta Samhitá, ca. 600 B.C. Thus, Sushruta has been termed the "father of plastic surgery." Although it was practiced for many years in India, the forehead flap procedure, or "Indian rhinoplasty," was not reported to the Western world until almost 1800.

As written in 1795 by 'B.L.': "The Hindoos certainly deserve the praise of making artificial noses in a superior way to any people in the world; an art, unfortunately for them, the more necessary, as in no part of the world is the practice of cutting off noses so common. The process of repairing them was recommended in Europe about three hundred years ago, and was said to have originated with the Calabrians, from whom it was received by the surgeons of Bologna."

The violent way of life in medieval Europe, the cosmetic deformities produced by the widespread disease of syphilis, and the penal custom of cutting off prisoners' noses and ears often resulted in facial mutilations.

Tagliacozzi, following the lead of Antonio Branca, established plastic surgery in the Western world with his magnificent opus of 1597. He perfected and described in this work in great detail reconstructive techniques for the nose, ear, and lips by a pedicle flap from the arm, now known as the "Italian operation."

Abrashanoff (1911) reported the use of a pedicled muscle flap to solve the difficult problem of chronic bronchial fistula. Subsequently this has been utilized with minor variations by many others (e.g., Eggers, 1920; Kanavel, 1921; Halsted and Thurston, 1927). Pool and Garlock (1929) recommended using a muscle flap from neighboring muscle tissue and inserting this flap into the bronchus as one "inserts a cork into the neck of a bottle." Wangensteen (1935), in his paper on bronchopleural fistula closure with a pedicled muscle flap in seven patients, stated: ". . . the pedicled muscle flap is an agency which has a wide field of application in general surgery."

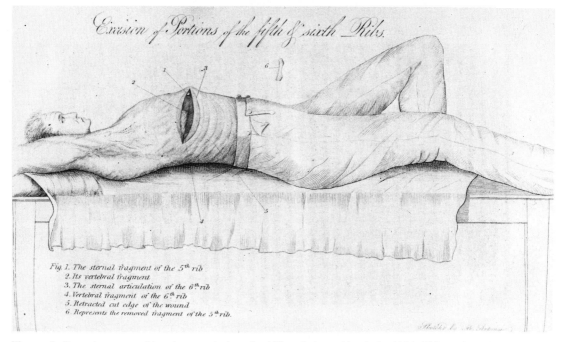

Figure 1. Seventeen-year-old male operated on by Milton Antony, March 3, 1821. This patient developed pain, swelling, erythema, and intermittent ("hectic") fever after falling from a horse and injuring his chest two or three years previously. The diagnosis was "extensive abscess . . . about this carious bone." The operation was apparently done in the patient's home; no anesthesia is described. No attempt at reconstruction of the chest wall was made.

Use of the greater omentum is less frequent and more recent than muscle flaps. The numerous and varied applications of omentum are well described by Kiricuta, its chief proponent (1980).

There are many situations in thoracic surgery where new or additional blood supply, coverage, and obliteration of a space are needed. The following chapters ably illustrate different ways in which some of these problems have been solved.

32

Muscle Flaps and Thoracic Problems: Applicability and Utilization for Various Conditions

Joseph I. Miller, M.D.

Recent progress in the field of plastic surgery, with increased use of muscular and myocutaneous flaps, has opened a new era in the management of complex thoracic problems. The understanding of flap physiology and of the ready availability of tissue for flap transposition has greatly enhanced the management of primary complex thoracic operations by preventing certain complications and has also aided in the management of complications once they occur.

Muscle flaps permit the transfer of healthy vascular tissue into contaminated or otherwise compromised areas and the obliteration of a potentially large dead space,[1] with obvious benefits. In primary reconstruction procedures, transposing healthy muscle into wounds with good blood supply significantly improves the probability of uneventful healing at the outset.

From July 1, 1979, to July 1, 1983, 98 patients on the Cardio-Thoracic Surgical Service of Emory University Affiliated Hospitals underwent an extrathoracic muscle flap procedure for the management of a cardiothoracic problem (Table 32–1). In this series, extrathoracic muscle flaps were utilized successfully to manage a variety of problems: post-pneumonectomy empyema; bronchopleural fistula following lobectomy; fistula with localized rupture following gastrointestinal procedures; infection of an ascending aortic replacement; and mediastinitis following open surgery. Muscle flaps were also used for anastomotic reinforcement in tracheal resection, and in primary reconstruction of the sternum and of the chest wall.

PRINCIPLES OF COMPLETE FLAP CLOSURE

The principles of complete flap closure presented here are those we employ in the management of post-pneumonectomy empyema. Various technical aspects and related physiologic considerations, however, are applicable in flap procedures used in the management of other thoracic lesions as well.

Our basic approach to complete flap closure is outlined in Table 32–2.

ROUTE OF FLAP ENTRY

All extrathoracic muscle flaps require a route of entry into the chest. The location of the opening is generally determined by the muscle's blood supply, and should be placed so that the blood vessels are under no tension after transposition. Generally, resection of 2 inches of the appropriate rib is all that is required to allow flap entry. Figure 32–1 shows the typical sites of entry for the pectoralis major and latissimus dorsi flaps.

CLOSURE OF RESIDUAL SPACE

The predominant points in the surgical technique are as follows: (1) No residual space

Table 32–1. Indications for Extrathoracic Muscle Flap Procedures in 98 Patients with Thoracic Disease

Indication	No. of Patients
Post-pneumonectomy empyema	5
Bronchopleural fistula following lobectomy	7
Anastomotic reinforcement in tracheal resection	4
Postoperative gastrointestinal tract fistula with localized rupture	2
Postoperative complications involving heart and great vessels	1
Total sternal reconstruction	1
Chest wall reconstruction	4
Mediastinitis following open heart surgery	74

Table 32–2. Summary of Principles of
Complete Flap Closure

1. Preoperative antibiotics based on sensitivity studies
2. Reopen original incision
3. Debride cavity widely
4. Identify fistula, if present
5. Swing flaps
6. Routine tube drainage for 7 to 10 days
7. Entire space must be filled

must remain; and (2) there must be a sufficient amount of transposed tissue that any intrathoracic space can be filled. If a space is left, it will generally be just beneath the fifth or sixth rib in the mid-axillary line; this can be closed by a short 3-inch resection of the ribs over the space without cosmetic deformity. The filling of an entire pleural space with flaps is shown diagrammatically in Figure 32–2.

POSTOPERATIVE MANAGEMENT

Following transposition of the muscle flap, the wound is closed primarily, and chest tubes are left to Pleurovac suction for 7 to 10 days. Appropriate antibiotics are given according to results of sensitivity studies.

SPECIFIC MUSCLE FLAPS

The techniques of flap mobilization have been described in detail by Mathes and Nahai.[2]

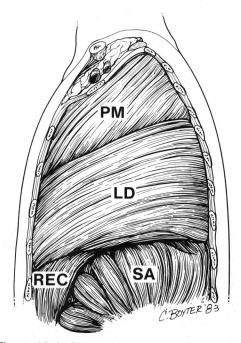

Figure 32–2. Diagram showing filling of an entire pleural space with muscle flaps and their anatomic location. *PM* = pectoralis major; *LD* = latissimus dorsi; *SA* = serratus anterior; *REC* = rectus abdominis.

The extrathoracic muscle flaps utilized in our post-pneumonectomy patients were, in order of frequency, the latissimus dorsi, serratus anterior, pectoralis major, omentum, and rectus abdominis, in various combinations (Fig. 32–3). The percent flap coverage of the usual

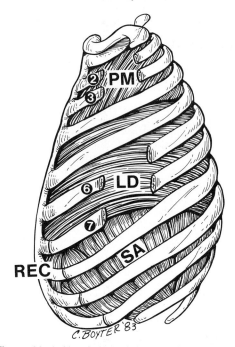

Figure 32–1. Usual sites of rib resection for entrance of the pectoralis major and latissimus dorsi flaps into the pleural space. *PM* = pectoralis major; *LD* = latissimus dorsi; *SA* = serratus anterior; *REC* = rectus abdominis.

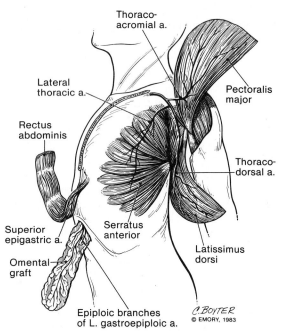

Figure 32–3. Extrathoracic muscle flaps that can be utilized in closure of a post-pneumonectomy empyema cavity.

adult pneumonectomy space by each flap is given in Table 32–3; these figures are based upon clinical estimation of coverage at the time of surgery and in cadaver studies.

Omentum. The omentum can be brought into the pleural space as a flap or a free graft. It is the flap of choice to cover an open bronchial stump because of its excellent blood supply. It has been shown that neovascularity is evident in the stump within 48 hours after placement of an omental flap around a closed stump. The omental flap is generally brought up through a separate anterior opening in the diaphragm and laid over the bronchial stump, with tacking sutures around this, as shown in Figure 32–4. We generally do not use this flap unless an open bronchial stump is present, or unless there is not enough muscle present to fill the space.

Pectoralis Major. The pectoralis major flap is one of the two most commonly utilized extrathoracic muscle flaps. It has a dual blood supply: from the predominant thoracoacromial artery to the major pedicle, and from the internal mammary artery to the major pedicle and the secondary pedicles. It may be used as a reverse turn-over flap or be placed directly into the wound. Entry of the flap into the chest requires a 2-inch rib resection. The pectoralis major is the flap of choice for sternal infections, but is utilized after the latissimus dorsi and serratus anterior for the pleural space.

Latissimus Dorsi. The latissimus dorsi muscle flap is our most commonly utilized flap for thoracic defects. Its predominant blood supply is from the thoracodorsal artery. It may be used as a turn-over flap or placed directly into the wound. It may be brought directly through the incision or through a separate small rib resection.

Serratus Anterior. The serratus anterior is our second-choice flap for filling a pneumonectomy space. It is particularly good for filling a smaller space. Its entrance into the chest is through the primary chest incision.

Rectus Abdominis. The rectus abdominis flap is used predominantly in closure of the sternal wound in postoperative mediastinitis.

Table 32–3. Percent Flap Coverage of Pneumonectomy Space

Flap	% Coverage
Latissimus dorsi	30–40
Serratus anterior	10–15
Pectoralis major	20–30
Pectoralis minor	0–2
Omentum	5–15
Rectus abdominis	5–15

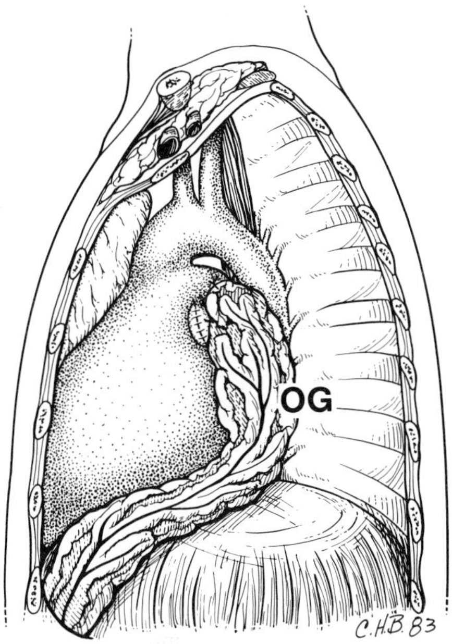

Figure 32–4. The omental graft or flap (*OG*) is brought through an anterior opening in the diaphragm and placed over the bronchial stump.

In post-pneumonectomy problems, this flap is held in reserve, in case some part of the flap should not "take" and a subsequent flap should become necessary; to date, this has not been necessary in our patients.

Combination Flaps. If a pleural cavity is small to moderate in size, it can be filled with a latissimus dorsi and serratus anterior flap. A larger cavity will require rise of the latissimus dorsi, the serratus anterior, and the pectoralis major and pectoralis minor, as well as the omentum.

THORACIC LESIONS MANAGED BY EXTRATHORACIC MUSCLE FLAP PROCEDURES

The following discussion describes our experience with the use of extrathoracic muscle flaps in thoracic disease, with particular emphasis on postoperative pneumonectomy empyema and on mediastinitis following open heart surgery.

Post-pneumonectomy Empyema

Post-pneumonectomy empyema, with or without bronchopleural fistula, is one of the most serious complications that can occur following pneumonectomy. Numerous methods have been used to deal with this complication, ranging from complete 12-rib thoracoplasty to varying degrees of rib resection combined with irrigating techniques, as originally described by Claggett and Geraci[3] and later by Stafford and Claggett.[4] Each method has met with varying degrees of success. A success rate of 65% to 70% was initially reported for the latter method (the "Claggett procedure"); in a more recent report, however, this method was successful in only 25% to 35% of cases.[5]

At the present time, single-stage complete flap closure, with primary closure of the wound, is our method of choice in dealing with post-pneumonectomy empyema, with or without bronchopleural fistula. During the past 3 years, we have used this procedure in five patients with post-pneumonectomy empyema, with a successful outcome in all patients.[6] The time period from the original operation to the flap procedure ranged from 3 to 18 months. Two patients had benign disease, and three patients had malignant disease.

The empyema, with or without bronchopleural fistula, is managed initially by closed-chest drainage in the acute stage. Use of a chest tube may be sufficient, or the drainage incision may require conversion to an Eloesser flap, pending the patient's comfort and adequacy of drainage. At the appropriate time interval (3 months for benign disease and approximately 1 year for malignant disease), single-stage complete muscle flap closure is performed (Table 32–2). The original incision is reopened, and the cavity debrided so that good granulation tissue is present. If a bronchopleural fistula is present, an attempt is made at identification. Its edges are freshened, and the fistula is closed if technically possible. An omental flap is brought up through an anterior diaphragmatic incision (Fig. 32–4) and tacked around the fistula with 3–0 sutures. Appropriate flaps are then swung to fill the pleural space; we begin with a latissimus dorsi and follow with whatever flaps are necessary to fill the space, depending upon anatomic location and size of the space (Fig. 32–2).

All patients were discharged within 19 days and had no further problems. In two patients, it was necessary to resect 2 inches of two separate ribs to allow the chest wall musculature to come in at the area of the previous incision.

Bronchopleural Fistula Secondary to Lobectomy

In the patient who develops a bronchopleural fistula secondary to lobectomy, with no associated cavity, the fistula will generally close with conservative management. However, when a cavity is present, surgical intervention often becomes necessary. Methods of management have included the Claggett procedure, completion pneumonectomy, or thoracoplasty. We have utilized extrathoracic muscle flaps, predominantly the pectoralis major or latissimus dorsi, to close the bronchopleural fistula and fill the empyema space in seven patients, with a successful outcome in five patients. One patient required an additional rectus abdominis flap because of a persistent drainage tract from an open bronchus, though no space remained. The surgical technique is similar to that described for flap closure of the post-pneumonectomy empyema space.

Anastomotic Reinforcement in Tracheal Resection and Sleeve Pneumonectomy

Two of the most serious complications following tracheal resection or sleeve pneumonectomy are tracheo–innominate artery fistula or breakdown of the anastomotic resection. Both of these complications can generally be prevented by the application of a pedicled muscle flap at the completion of the procedure. In two of our patients undergoing primary tracheal resection, one by a cervical approach and the other by a cervicomediastinal approach, pedicled muscle flaps (a sternothyroid flap and a sternohyoid flap, respectively) were used to reinforce the tracheal anastomosis by a circumferential wrap and to separate the anastomosis from the innominate artery. In two other patients undergoing sleeve tracheobronchial resection, we have utilized a pedicled reverse pectoralis major flap to reinforce the anastomosis and prevent leakage into the mediastinum. Jensik and colleagues[7] reported a 30% mortality with sleeve pneumonectomy; in the majority of cases, death was secondary to anastomotic breakdown. We believe that this complication can be largely avoided by careful surgical technique and application of a pedicled pectoralis major flap to wrap the anastomosis completely. Our experience in this area is limited, but the early results are encouraging.

Postoperative Gastrointestinal Tract Fistula with Localized Rupture

Two of our patients had developed esophagogastric bronchial fistula following esophagogastrectomy with local rupture into the tracheobronchial tree without free rupture into the pleural space. In each of these patients, primary repair was performed, closing the defect in the tracheobronchial tree primarily and wrapping it with a pedicled pectoralis major flap, thus separating it from the primary esophagogastric anastomosis. In one patient, the stomach was returned to the abdomen, and a colon interposition was subsequently performed to restore gastrointestinal continuity.

Postoperative Complications Involving the Heart and Great Vessels

Our application of muscle flaps in the management of problems involving the heart and great vessels has included only one case, but our experience suggests that the potential for future use is excellent.

A patient who had previously undergone aortic valve replacement for calcific aortic stenosis presented 1½ years after the original aortic valve surgery with subacute bacterial endocarditis, an ascending arch aneurysm, and valve ring abscess. He underwent replacement of the aortic root and ascending aorta with a composite graft and transposition of the coronary arteries. Postoperatively, he developed purulent drainage from the superior mediastinum. He was returned to the operating room, where pectoralis major muscle flaps were placed completely around the composite graft, and the sternum was closed over tube drainage. His subsequent postoperative course was uneventful.

If a synthetic graft must be placed into an infected field, it is easy to wrap the graft with a pedicled pectoralis major flap, thereby walling off the graft from potential mediastinal infection.

Sternal Reconstruction

One patient underwent resection and reconstruction of the entire sternum for a benign form of end-stage chondromalacia with severe sternal and skeletal deformities and marked limitation of respiration. The sternum was reconstructed utilizing a pectoralis major and rectus abdominis flap for a sternal floor over the pericardium. Block-wire rib struts were placed over this to the severed rib ends. A turn-over pectoralis major muscle flap was then placed over the newly constructed rib struts of the sternum to form an "outer table." This is a new application of muscle flaps for total sternal reconstruction.

Mediastinitis Following Open Heart Surgery

Postoperative sternal wound infection with dehiscence, mediastinitis, or both is one of the most serious complications that can result following median sternotomy for open heart surgery. Although the incidence is low, ranging from 0.5% to 1.5% in various series, this complication is associated with significant morbidity and mortality. Prior to 1978, our approach to postoperative open heart mediastinitis was establishment of an inflow–outflow mediastinal drainage system, with primary closure of the sternum over these tubes; however, the success rate with this approach was only 50%. Beginning in 1978, we used debridement with muscle flap closure as a primary means of treating this problem. During nine months in 1979, 1052 patients underwent open heart surgery, with 10 patients developing a median sternotomy infection. This complication was treated successfully by muscle flap closure, with no mortality.

At present there are three methods of treating open heart sternal wound problems:

1. *The open method.* This is of historical significance only and is rarely used today. The sternum is opened, debrided, and left open to heal by secondary intention. This is time-consuming and not well tolerated by the patient.

2. *The closed technique.* This consists of debridement and closure over an irrigating system. The chest tubes are generally left in place for 7 to 14 days, with the mediastinum irrigated with an appropriate antibiotic solution, depending upon results of sensitivity studies, as well as systemic antibiotics. This method is effective in those cases with limited sternal or mediastinal involvement but rarely effective when the infection is significant or there is more advanced involvement.

3. *Muscle flap coverage.* This method is indicated when the closed method has failed, or when the extent of the sternal infection is significant, requiring extensive debridement of the sternum and costal cartilages.

Details of the surgical technique of muscle flap closure of the infected median sternotomy wound have been previously reported.[8, 9] The pectoralis major muscle and rectus abdominis muscle provide excellent coverage of the entire sternal wound: The pectoralis major covers the upper two thirds of the wound, and the rectus abdominis covers the lower third.

From June 1, 1979 to June 1, 1982, 5480 patients underwent open heart surgery on the Cardio-Thoracic Surgical Service of Emory

University Affiliated Hospitals; of these, 64 patients developed wound infections. There were five deaths in this group from generalized sepsis or multiple organ failure, rather than from vascular rupture, as they occurred before muscle flaps were widely used for this purpose.[10] The mean hospitalization period was 29 days, which represents a significant decrease from that normally required for such patients.

At the present time, we utilize muscle flap closure as the primary means of treatment when the closed method has failed, or when the magnitude of the initial infection indicated a poor prognosis. The rationale of therapy for this method dictates debridement of the infected sternotomy wound, and the wound is closed with transposed, well-vascularized pectoralis major muscle flaps.

The technique of muscle flap closure should be available to all surgeons involved in the devastating complications of mediastinal wound infection following open heart surgery.

CONCLUSIONS

The advancement of muscle flap techniques has greatly enhanced the care of the cardiothoracic surgical patient. Previously common complications of surgical procedures or primary problems in thoracic disease are now handled easily using these management concepts.

With utilization of the pectoralis major and latissimus dorsi muscle flaps, more than 75% of cardiothoracic problems can be successfully managed. Tracheobronchial and gastrointestinal anastomoses may be wrapped or reinforced; large chest wall defects and cavities may be filled.

Credit must be given to Dr. Maurice Jurkiewicz and his associates in the Division of Plastic Surgery of Emory University School of Medicine for their pioneering work in this field. Their work has made the management of our surgical patients much easier.

The technique of muscle flap closure should be in the armamentarium of all practicing cardiothoracic surgeons.

References

1. Fisher J, Bone DK, Nahai F: Reconstruction of the sternum. In Mathes SJ, Nahai F (eds): Clinical Applications for Muscle and Musculocutaneous Flaps. St. Louis, CV Mosby, 1982.
2. Mathes SJ, Nahai F: Clinical Applications for Muscle and Musculocutaneous Flaps. St. Louis, CV Mosby, 1982.
3. Claggett OT, Geraci JE: A procedure for the management of pneumonectomy empyema. J Thorac Cardiovasc Surg 45:141, 1963.
4. Stafford EG, Claggett OT: Post-pneumonectomy empyema: neomycin instillation and definite closure. J Thorac Cardiovasc Surg 63:771, 1972.
5. Claggett OT: Personal communication, 1983.
6. Miller JI, Mansour KA, Nahai F, et al: Single stage complete muscle flap closure of the post-pneumonectomy empyema space: a new method and possible solution to a disturbing complication. Ann Thorac Surg 38:227, 1984.
7. Jensik RJ, Faber LP, Kittle CF, et al: Survival in patients undergoing tracheal sleeve pneumonectomy for bronchogenic carcinoma. J Thorac Cardiovasc Surg 84:489, 1982.
8. Jurkiewicz MJ, Bostwick J, Hester RT, et al: Infected median sternotomy wound—successful treatment by muscle flaps. Ann Surg 191:738, 1980.
9. Nahai F, Morales L, Bone DK, et al: Pectoralis major muscle turn-over flaps for closure of the infected sternotomy wound with preservation of form and function. Plast Reconstr Surg 70:471, 1982.
10. Bostwick J, Hester RT, Craver JM, et al: Median sternotomy infections—management with muscle flaps. Unpublished paper, 1983.

33

Muscle Flaps and Thoracic Problems: Chest Wall Defects: Reconstruction with Autogenous Tissue

Peter C. Pairolero, M.D.
Philip G. Arnold, M.D.

HISTORICAL CONSIDERATIONS

Reconstruction of chest wall defects has been a constant challenge to the surgeon for the past several decades. Parham in 1898 described his experience with surgical management of chest wall tumors.[1] He pointed out the significant earlier contributions of Fell and O'Dwyer in control of ventilation.[2-4] During the next 50 years, advances in thoracic surgery occurred rapidly. Tumors of the chest wall were classified further by Lund,[5] Hedblom,[6] Harrington,[7] and Zinninger,[8] and the first successful pneumonectomy for lung cancer was performed by Graham and Singer in 1933.[9] During this period, advances in endotracheal ventilation and closed-chest drainage allowed thoracic surgery to reach a sophisticated level. Management of chest wall defects, however, remained difficult and controversial.

In 1947, Watson and James[10] described the use of fascia lata grafts for closure of the chest wall. During that same year, Maier[11] reported the use of large cutaneous flaps, which frequently included the opposite breast, to close defects of the anterior chest wall occurring secondary to resection for carcinoma of the breast. The following year, Bisgard and Swenson[12] utilized free rib grafts as horizontal stents to reconstruct the resected sternum. Finally, the surgical treatment of recurrent breast carcinoma involving the chest wall was advocated by Pickrell and colleagues.[13]

In 1950, Campbell[14] described transposition of the latissimus dorsi muscle followed immediately by skin grafting for reconstruction of full-thickness defects of the anterior thorax. Unfortunately, this excellent method of reconstruction went unnoticed for the next 20 years, until interest in muscle transposition was revived and the technique refined. Also in the 1950s, workers such as Blades and Paul,[15]

Converse and colleagues,[16] and Myre and Kirklin[17] continued to advance the art and science of chest wall reconstruction.

The 1960s brought further refinements of the general reconstructive techniques and principles by Rees and Converse,[18] Starzynski and coworkers,[19] Martini and coworkers,[20] and Le Roux.[21] Many of these procedures, however, still required multiple stages and long periods of hospitalization. In 1963, Kiricuta[22] of Rumania described transposition of the greater omentum for reconstruction of chest wall defects.

During the past 15 years, numerous surgeons have made significant contributions to the technique of reconstruction of the thorax.[23-41] Muscle and musculocutaneous flaps using the latissimus dorsi, pectoralis major, serratus anterior, rectus abdominis, and external oblique muscles have been used most frequently in reconstruction of the chest wall. The clarification of related functional anatomy and blood supply has resulted in more aggressive resections in the treatment of chest wall tumors and in the surgical amelioration of the ravages of radiation therapy. Recent reports by McCormack and colleagues[42] and later by Larson and McMurtrey[43] have confirmed that aggressive resection of the chest wall with immediate dependable reconstruction is reasonable for managing these problems.

ETIOLOGY

Defects of the chest wall occur almost always as a result of neoplasm, radiation, or infection (Table 33–1). The chest wall defect produced by resection of most neoplasms involves loss of the skeleton and frequently the overlying soft tissues. Infection, radiation necrosis, and trauma produce partial- or full-thickness defects, depending upon their severity.

Table 33–1. Etiology of Chest Wall Defects

Neoplasm
    Primary chest wall
    Metastatic chest wall
    Contiguous lung cancer
Infected median sternotomy or
    lateral thoracotomy wounds
Radiation necrosis
Trauma

PREOPERATIVE CONSIDERATIONS

The ability to close large chest wall defects is the main consideration in the surgical treatment of most chest wall afflictions. Excision should not be undertaken if the surgeon does not have the confidence and ability to close the defect. The critical questions of whether or not the reconstructed thorax will support respiration and protect the underlying organs must be answered when considering both the extent of resection and the method of reconstruction of the chest wall. This is true whether the thoracic lesion is a neoplasm, an infection, or radiation necrosis. Adequate resection and dependable reconstruction are the mandatory ingredients for successful treatment. It is our strong belief that these two important facets of surgical management are accomplished most safely by the joint efforts of a thoracic surgeon and a plastic surgeon.

Reconstruction of chest wall defects involves consideration of several specific factors (Table 33–2): The location and size of the defect are of utmost importance, but the patient's past medical history and local conditions of the wound may drastically alter a reconstructive choice. Primary closure, when possible, remains the best option available. If the defect is only partial-thickness and the surrounding tissue will accept and support a skin graft, reconstruction in this manner is quite reasonable. If the tissue surrounding a partial-thickness defect will not reliably accept a skin graft,

Table 33–2. Considerations in Reconstruction of Chest Wall Defects

Location of defect
Size of defect
Full-thickness versus partial-thickness defect
General condition of the patient (e.g., effects of ongoing chemotherapy, steroid therapy)
Condition of the local tissues (e.g., previous irradiation, localized infection, inflammation, scarring)
Duration of the defect
Lifestyle and occupation of the patient
Prognosis with underlying disease

a situation that frequently occurs with radiation necrosis, omental transposition with skin grafting is utilized. If full-thickness reconstruction is required, consideration must be given to both structural stability of the thorax and soft-tissue coverage. Reconstruction with synthetic mesh and muscle transposition remains our treatment of choice for a noninfected full-thickness defect.

SKELETAL RECONSTRUCTION

Reconstruction of full-thickness defects of the bony thorax is controversial. In some defects, usually small, the skeletal component can be ignored and the defect closed with only soft tissues. If, however, structural stability is required, either autogenous tissue, such as fascia lata or ribs, or prosthetic material, such as the various meshes, metals, or methylmethacrylate, may be used.

It is our opinion that full-thickness skeletal defects resulting from excision of tumors in both the sternum and the lateral chest wall are best reconstructed with autogenous rib or with synthetic mesh if the wound is not contaminated. We routinely use Prolene mesh or more recently a Goretex soft tissue patch in closing skeletal defects resulting from chest wall involvement of underlying lung cancer or recurrent breast cancer. If the wound is contaminated owing to previous radiation necrosis or necrotic neoplasm, reconstruction with prosthetic material is not advised because the prosthesis may subsequently become infected, resulting in obligatory removal. In such cases, reconstruction with a musculocutaneous flap alone is preferred. Our experience with the methylmethacrylate mesh "sandwich" is limited.

SOFT-TISSUE RECONSTRUCTION

Both muscle and omental transposition can be utilized in the reconstruction of soft-tissue chest wall defects. Muscle can be transposed as muscle alone or as a musculocutaneous flap.

MUSCLE TRANSPOSITION

Latissimus Dorsi. The latissimus dorsi muscle is the largest flat muscle in the thorax. Its dominant thoracodorsal neurovascular leash has an arc of rotation that allows coverage of the lateral and central back as well as of the anterolateral and central front of the thorax.[14, 44] Its dependable musculocutaneous vascular connections permit its use also as a reliable musculocutaneous flap. This muscle flap can cover huge chest wall defects; virtually one half of the overlying tissue on the back can be elevated on the blood supply of a single latissimus dorsi muscle in the uninjured, non-irradiated patient. The donor site may require a skin graft when large musculocutaneous flaps are elevated, but this disadvantage is small when considered in light of the benefits of transposing large, robust flaps to either the anterior or posterior thorax for full-thickness reconstruction. If the dominant blood supply is compromised owing to previous trauma or surgery, the muscle can still dependably be transposed on the branch of the adjacent serratus anterior muscle.[32]

Pectoralis Major. The pectoralis major muscle is the second largest flat muscle on the chest wall and in many respects is the mirror image of the latissimus dorsi muscle. Its dominant thoracoacromial neurovascular leash, which enters posteriorly at about the level of the mid-clavicle, allows both elevation of the muscle, as either a muscle flap or a musculocutaneous flap,[24] and its rotation centrally for chest wall reconstruction. The pectoralis major muscle is as reliable as the latissimus dorsi flap. It is of major benefit in reconstruction of anterior chest wall defects such as those resulting from sternal tumor excisions and infected median sternotomy wounds.[25] Generally, in chest wall reconstruction only the muscle is transposed, and the skin is closed primarily, thereby avoiding the distortion created by centralizing the breast. Reconstruction in this manner is more symmetrical and aesthetically acceptable. If central skin must be excised, symmetry of the breast can still be maintained, since the transposed muscle readily accepts and supports an overlying skin graft. If necessary, the muscle may also be transposed on its secondary blood supply via the perforators from the internal mammary vessels.

Rectus Abdominis. The internal mammary neurovascular leash allows utilization of the rectus abdominis muscle for chest wall reconstruction. The inferior epigastric vessels must be divided to allow rotation to the chest wall. This muscle can be mobilized and moved either as a muscle flap or as a musculocutaneous flap, with the skin component oriented either horizontally or vertically, or at some point between. The vertical skin flap, however, is more reliable since it is oriented along the long axis of the muscle and thus maintains more musculocutaneous perforators. The donor site is usually closed primarily.

The rectus abdominis muscle is most useful in reconstruction of lower sternal wounds.[25] Either muscle can be utilized because their arcs of rotation are identical. Care must be taken to choose the muscle that has patent and uninjured internal mammary vessels. Angiographic demonstration of vessel patency may be helpful in determining which musculocutaneous unit would be most reliable, particularly in previously irradiated patients.

Serratus Anterior. The serratus anterior muscle is a small flat muscle that is located in the mid-axillary line between the latissimus dorsi and pectoralis major muscles. Its blood supply comes from the serratus branch of the thoracodorsal vessels and from the long thoracic artery and vein. This muscle can be utilized alone or as an adjunctive flap in tandem with the pectoralis major or the latissimus dorsi flap; it also augments the skin-carrying ability of either of its neighbors. In our experience, the serratus anterior muscle has been particularly useful as an intrathoracic muscle flap.[26, 27]

External Oblique. The external oblique muscle may also be transposed as a muscle flap or a musculocutaneous flap, and it is most useful in closing defects of the upper abdomen and lower thorax. It reaches the inframammary fold without tension, but does not readily extend higher. The primary blood supply is from the lower thoracic intercostal vessels.[6–12] The advantage of the use of this muscle is that lower chest wall defects can be closed without distortion of the breast.

Trapezius Muscle. The trapezius muscle has been useful to close defects at the base of the neck or the thoracic outlet, but it is not a consistently useful muscle in reconstruction of the remainder of the chest wall. Its primary blood supply is the dorsal scapular vessels.

OMENTAL TRANSPOSITION

Omental transposition has been most useful in reconstruction of partial-thickness chest wall defects.[36] This is particularly true with radiation necrosis that does not involve tumor. In this situation, the skin and soft tissues are debrided down to what remains of the thoracic skeleton, which may be either bone or cartilage but frequently is only irradiated ischemic scar. The transposed omentum, with its excellent blood supply from the gastroepiploic vessels, adheres to the irradiated wound and readily accepts and supports an overlying skin graft. Because the omentum has no structural stability of its own, it is not particularly useful in full-thickness defects; in such cases, additional support, such as fascia lata, bone, or prosthetic material, is necessary.

Omental transposition is exceedingly helpful when planned muscle flaps have been utilized but have failed with partial necrosis. Generally, this results in only a soft-tissue defect, and pleural seal with respiratory stability is not required, thus allowing a most threatening situation to be salvaged.

CLINICAL EXPERIENCE

We performed 100 consecutive chest wall reconstructions during a recent 7-year period.[45] There were 52 females and 48 males in our series; age ranged from 13 to 78 years, with an average of 53 years. Forty-two patients had tumors involving the chest wall, 24 had infected median sternotomy wounds, 19 had radiation necrosis, and 15 had combinations of the three.

Of the 100 patients, 76 required skeletal resection of the chest wall. An average of 5.7 ribs were resected. Total or partial sternectomies were performed in 29 patients.

Ninety-two of the 100 patients underwent 142 muscle transpositions: In 77 of these procedures, the pectoralis major was used; in 29, the latissimus dorsi; and in 36, other muscles, including serratus anterior, rectus abdominis, and external oblique muscles. The omentum was transposed in 10 patients. Chest wall skeletal defects were closed with Prolene mesh in 29 patients and with autogenous ribs in 11. Eighty-nine patients underwent primary closure of the skin.

The 100 patients underwent an average of 2.1 operations. Hospitalization averaged 17.5 days. There was one perioperative death, and two patients required tracheostomy. Follow-up averaged 21.6 months. There were 24 late deaths, predominantly from pulmonary or distant metastases; there were no late deaths related to either resection or reconstruction of the chest wall. All 99 patients who were alive 30 days after operation had excellent results at the time of last follow-up evaluation, or at death occurring later from other causes.

Not all of our patients had reconstruction of the missing bony thorax. We believe that each situation should be analyzed separately. For example, the full-thickness defect created following a resection of a large segment of the chest wall for neoplasm is best reconstructed by replacing the skeletal layer of the thorax, if possible. In contrast, resection of the bony thorax in a patient who has previously received radiation therapy, and who now presents with an open, fungating recurrent breast carcinoma or a radiation ulcer, frequently does not result in a pneumothorax. In this situation, the lung is often adherent to the chest wall, and the omentum can be utilized for reconstruction. Nevertheless, we generally use the omentum only for partial-thickness injuries in which remaining fibrous tissue or ribs are present to provide support, or for secondary procedures after reconstructive efforts have failed. Our first choice for management of full-thickness defects is always muscle or musculocutaneous transposition.

CONCLUSIONS

Reconstruction of large chest wall defects can be performed safely and with lasting long-term benefits. It is our strong belief that the two key elements of successful surgical management—namely, adequate and accurate resection of the chest wall lesion and dependable reconstruction—are accomplished most effectively by the joint efforts of a thoracic surgeon and a plastic surgeon.

References

1. Parham FW: Thoracic resection for tumors growing from the bony wall of the chest. Trans South Surg Gynecol Assoc 11:223–363, 1898.
2. Fell GE: Forced respiration. JAMA 16:325–330, 1891.
3. O'Dwyer J: Fifty cases of croup in private practice treated by intubation of the larynx with a description of the method and of the dangers incident thereto. Med Rec 32:557–571, 1887.
4. O'Dwyer J: His methods of work on intubation; the measure of his success; the interest of both to young graduates. NY Med Rec 65:561–564, 1904.
5. Lund FB: Sarcoma of the chest wall. Ann Surg 58:206–217, 1913.
6. Hedblom CA: Tumors of the bony chest wall. Arch Surg 3:56–85, 1921.
7. Harrington SW: Surgical treatment of intrathoracic tumors and tumors of the chest wall. Arch Surg 14:406–429, 1927.
8. Zinninger MM: Tumors of the wall of the thorax. Ann Surg 92:1043–1058, 1930.
9. Graham EA, Singer JJ: Successful removal of an entire lung for carcinoma of the bronchus. JAMA 101:1371–1374, 1933.
10. Watson WL, James AG: Fascia lata grafts for chest wall defects. J Thorac Surg 16:399–406, 1947.
11. Maier HC: Surgical management of large defects of the thoracic wall. Surgery 22:169–178, 1947.
12. Bisgard JD, Swenson SA Jr: Tumors of the sternum:

report of a case with special operative technic. Arch Surg 56:570–577, 1948.

13. Pickrell KL, Kelley JW, Marzoni FA: The surgical treatment of recurrent carcinoma of the breast and chest wall. Plast Reconstr Surg 3:156–172, 1948.
14. Campbell DA: Reconstruction of the anterior thoracic wall. J Thorac Surg 19:456–461, 1950.
15. Blades B, Paul JS: Chest wall tumors. Ann Surg 131:976–983, 1950.
16. Converse JM, Campbell RM, Watson WL: Repair of large radiation ulcers situated over the heart and the brain. Ann Surg 133:95–103, 1951.
17. Myre TT, Kirklin JW: Resection of tumors of the sternum. Ann Surg 144:1023–1028, 1956.
18. Rees TD, Converse JM: Surgical reconstruction of defects of the thoracic wall. Surg Gynecol Obstet 121:1066–1072, 1965.
19. Starzynski TE, Snyderman RK, Beattie EJ Jr: Problems of major chest wall reconstruction. Plast Reconstr Surg 44:525–535, 1969.
20. Martini N, Starzynski TE, Beattie EJ Jr: Problems in chest wall resection. Surg Clin North Am 49:313–322, 1969.
21. Le Roux BT: Maintenance of chest wall stability. Thorax 19:397–405, 1964.
22. Kiricuta I: L'emploi du grand epiploon dans la chirugie du sein cancereux. Presse Med 71:15–17, 1963.
23. Alonso-Lej F, de Linera FA: Resection of the entire sternum and replacement with acrylic resin: report of a case of giant chondromyxoid fibroma. J Thorac Cardiovasc Surg 62:271–280, 1971.
24. Arnold PG, Pairolero PC: Use of pectoralis major muscle flaps to repair defects of the anterior chest wall. Plast Reconstr Surg 63:205–213, 1979.
25. Pairolero PC, Arnold PG: Management of recalcitrant median sternotomy wounds. J Thorac Cardiovasc Surg 88:357–364, 1984.
26. Arnold PG, Pairolero PC, Waldorf JC: The serratus anterior muscle: intrathoracic and extrathoracic utilization. Plast Reconstr Surg 73:240–248, 1984.
27. Pairolero PC, Arnold PG, Piehler JM: Intrathoracic transposition of extrathoracic skeletal muscle. J Thorac Cardiovasc Surg 86:809–817, 1983.
28. Irons GB, Witzke DJ, Arnold PG, Woods MB: Use of the omental free flap for soft-tissue reconstruction. Ann Plast Surg 11:501–507, 1983.
29. Boyd AD, Shaw WW, McCarthy JG, et al: Immediate reconstruction of full-thickness chest wall defects. Ann Thorac Surg 32:337–346, 1981.
30. Brown RG, Fleming WH, Jurkiewicz MJ: An island flap of the pectoralis major muscle. Br J Plast Surg 30:161–165, 1977.
31. Burnard RJ, Martini N, Beattie EJ Jr: The value of

resection in tumors involving the chest wall. J Thorac Cardiovasc Surg 68:530–535, 1974.
32. Eschapasse H, Gaillard J, Fournial G, et al: Utilisation de prostheses en resine acrylique pour la reparation des vastes pertes de substance de la paroi thoracique. Acta Chir Belg 76:281–285, 1977.
33. Fisher J, Bostwick J, Powell RW: Latissimus dorsi blood supply after thoracodorsal vessel division: the serratus collateral. Plast Reconstr Surg 72:502–509, 1983.
34. Graham J, Usher FC, Perry JL, Barkley HT: Marlex mesh as a prosthesis in the repair of thoracic wall defects. Ann Surg 151:469–479, 1960.
35. Hodgkinson DJ, Arnold PG: Chest-wall reconstruction using the external oblique muscle. Br J Plast Surg 33:216–220, 1980.
36. Jurkiewicz MJ, Arnold PG: The omentum: an account of its use in the reconstruction of the chest wall. Ann Surg 185:548–554, 1977.
37. Jurkiewicz MJ, Bostwick J III, Hester TR, et al: Infected median sternotomy wound: successful treatment by muscle flaps. Ann Surg 191:738–743, 1980.
38. Longacre JJ, Maurer EP, Keirle AM: Immediate skeletal reconstruction of an extensive bilateral defect of the anterior chest wall: case report. Plast Reconstr Surg 53:593–595, 1974.
39. McGraw JB, Penix JO, Baker JW: Repair of major defects of the chest wall and spine with the latissimus dorsi myocutaneous flap. Plast Reconstr Surg 62:197–206, 1978.
40. Neale HW, Kreilein JG, Schreiber JT, Gregory RO: Complete sternectomy for chronic osteomyelitis with reconstruction using a rectus abdominis myocutaneous island flap. Ann Plast Surg 6:305–314, 1981.
41. Ramming KP, Holmes EC, Zarem HA, et al: Surgical management and reconstruction of extensive chest wall malignancies. Am J Surg 144:146–151, 1982.
42. McCormack P, Bains MS, Beattie EJ Jr, Martini N: New trends in skeletal reconstruction after resection of chest wall tumors. Ann Thorac Surg 31:45–52, 1981.
43. Larson DL, McMurtrey MJ, Howe HJ, Irish CE: Major chest wall reconstruction after chest wall irradiation. Cancer 49:1286–1293, 1982.
44. Bostwick J III, Nahai F, Wallace JG, Vasconez LO: Sixty latissimus dorsi flaps. Plast Reconstr Surg 63:31–41, 1979.
45. Arnold PG, Pairolero PC: Chest wall reconstruction: Experience with 100 consecutive patients. Ann Surg 199:725–732, 1984.

34

Muscle Flaps and Thoracic Problems: Coverage of A Chronic and Infected Mediastinal Wound

Stephen J. Mathes, M.D.

Despite the frequency of open heart procedures, mediastinal wound complications are uncommon. In a review of results of such procedures performed in 3239 patients over a period of 3 years, the incidence of infection was only 1.54%.[1] When infection does occur, a complex wound, with exposure of mediastinal contents to bacterial invasion, may result. Progressive bacterial involvement of sternal and costal cartilage is common. Suture line invasion into major vascular prosthesis and coronary artery vein graft may also occur, with subsequent thrombosis or suture line rupture with life-threatening hemorrhage.[2-4] Recent advances in reconstructive surgery using muscle flaps have been effective in management of the chronic infected mediastinal wound when used in conjunction with aggressive wound debridement. Since the immediate coverage of an infected wound seems contrary to established surgical principles, current controversies in management of this difficult wound are reviewed in the following discussion, which presents the physiologic basis for and clinical experience with use of muscle flaps for mediastinal wound closure.

FACTORS PREDISPOSING TO INFECTION

The sternal splitting incision offers direct exposure to the mediastinum and is now the preferred incision for the majority of myocardial revascularization and open heart procedures. However, the sternum is poorly vascularized through its perichondrical circulation, especially when compared with ribs and intercostal muscles, which are endowed with excellent blood supply through intercostal vessels, with both endosteal and periosteal circulation. Operative measures such as cauterization and bone wax damage perichondrial circulation, and sternal wires may further interrupt the internal mammary arteries during wound clo-

sure. Urgent reoperation for bleeding or sternal dehiscence obviously increases risk of further sternal devascularization and bacterial contamination. Prior mediastinal radiation therapy results in chronic vascular insufficiency and predisposes to susceptibility to infection and wound necrosis. Similarly, diabetes and autoimmune disease (e.g., scleroderma) may impair sternal circulation. These predisposing factors are frequently observed in patients presenting with chronic infected mediastinal wounds after mid-sternotomy incisions.

MANAGEMENT OF THE CHRONIC INFECTED WOUND

Conventional Management

Immediate use of culture-specific antibiotic therapy and wound debridement will generally control wound sepsis. However, resolution of chronic infection is not readily achieved without removal of all infected cartilage and chronic granulation tissue. Without reliable tissue to cover the debridement defect, the surgeon is naturally reluctant to proceed with such an aggressive approach. Consequently, minimal debridement of necrotic tissue, topical and systemic antibiotic therapy, and wound packing with frequent changes have become standard methods of care.[5-7] Wound closure by secondary contracture is generally achieved only after prolonged therapy and significant patient morbidity. Even with wound closure, intermittent episodes of recurrent cellulitis and spontaneous wound drainage from the prior sternal wound are observed.

Management by Muscle Flap Transposition

The transposition of muscle as a flap based on its major or dominant vascular pedicle is

246

now well established as a reliable technique for management of the chronic infected wound.[8, 9] Two large muscle units, the *pectoralis major*[10] and *rectus abdominis*,[11] lie close to the anterior mediastinum. These muscles elevated as flaps will cover extensive mediastinal defects. The *latissimus dorsi* muscle unit[12] from the posterior thorax will also cover anterior chest and mediastinal defects after mobilization as a flap. Use of these muscle flaps for immediate wound coverage allows removal of all infected sternum and costal cartilages. Immediate coverage of the mediastinal debridement site allows single-stage chest wall reconstruction for the chronic wound.

SELECTION OF MUSCLE FLAPS

The selection of a muscle flap or flaps must take into consideration not only the amount of coverage required but the availability and integrity of the blood supply to each. Case reports describing the rise of the various flaps and results in each case are presented under Clinical Experience later in this chapter.

Pectoralis Major. The major vascular pedicle to the pectoralis major muscle, the thoracoacromial artery, is located beneath the clavicle at the medial edge of the pectoralis minor. Since this vascular pedicle is located distant to the mediastinum, it is rarely involved in prior operative trauma, infection, or radiation injury. After release of both origin and insertion, this muscle will cover the mediastinal defect based on this vascular pedicle. For large defects, bilateral pectoralis major muscle flaps are frequently used to both fill the anterior mediastinal defect and cover the site of sternal and costal cartilage debridement.

The pectoralis major may also be transposed based on its secondary vascular pedicles, segmental branches of the internal mammary artery. However, in extensive wounds in which the entire sternum is necrotic or has been debrided, the internal mammary artery may be occluded or may have been previously ligated. If there is doubt regarding the status of this artery, a selective arteriogram will determine whether it is patent. In well-localized chronic infections, the medially based pectoralis major muscle is preferred since the flap dissection is easily performed through the sternal debridement wound and the flap covers the mediastinal area.

Rectus Abdominis. The rectus abdominis muscle will survive transposition as a flap based on superior epigastric artery, a continuation of the internal mammary artery. Similar precautions regarding patency of the internal mammary artery also apply to selection of this muscle as a flap for mediastinal reconstruction. However, retrograde arterial flow via the intercostal arteries into the superior epigastric artery will often support this muscle even when the proximal internal mammary artery is no longer patent. After release of the muscle's origin and division of its inferior source of circulation, the inferior epigastric artery, the muscle is transposed superiorly to cover the anterior mediastinum. This muscle is used in conjunction with both pectoralis major muscles when these do not provide adequate mediastinal coverage. Also, the rectus abdominis muscle is frequently utilized for small inferior mediastinal wounds.

MUSCLE FLAP SAFETY

The safety of these flaps is confirmed in a recent survey of results reported by 105 surgeons who used these muscles in 244 patients for chest wall and mediastinal reconstruction. The pectoralis major failed to provide stable wound coverage in only 3% of patients.[13] Likewise, recipient site complications due to flap loss occurred in only 7% of 133 patients in whom rectus abdominis flaps were used. Thus, wound coverage by muscle flaps has provided a reliable technique for immediate coverage of the mediastinal wound after aggressive wound debridement.

CLINICAL EXPERIENCE

Wound Criteria

In a recent review of 54 consecutive patients with infected wounds, specific wound criteria were identified in which coverage of the infected wound represented the most effective method for wound management:[14] (1) established infection for 6 months, (2) exposure of bone, mediastinum, or other vital structures, (3) mechanical or vascular limitations to delayed closure techniques, and (4) no response to wound debridement and prolonged antibiotic therapy. Wound treatment included debridement, muscle flap closure, and culture-specific antibiotic therapy. Antibiotic selection was initially based on preoperative sinus tract cultures and altered as required after culture of bone and cartilage debridement specimens. Of the 54 patients, 93% demonstrated stable wound coverage without recurrent infection over follow-up periods ranging from 1 to 4.6 years.

Physiologic Benefits of Flap Coverage

It is not surprising that the mediastinum and pelvis are two common areas in which chronically infected wounds are resistant to standard methods of local wound care. In both areas, a poorly vascularized cavity prevents wound contracture, and debridement is often timid owing to lack of local tissue for wound coverage. The muscle flap both fills this cavity with living tissue and simultaneously provides stable coverage.

The addition of vascularized tissue such as muscle within the site of wound debridement provides direct delivery of the components of the host defense mechanism (phagocytic leukocytes), oxygen, and systemic antibiotics to the wound.[15] Laboratory studies have demonstrated these unique properties of muscle, not present in random-pattern skin flaps. When the random-pattern flap is compared with the musculocutaneous flap using paired flaps in the canine experimental model, the musculocutaneous flap demonstrates superior resistance to bacterial inoculation on both its deep and skin surfaces.[16] Studies evaluating tissue oxygen delivery within these flaps demonstrate significantly greater oxygen delivery in the musculocutaneous flap.[17] After bacterial inoculation within both the random-pattern skin and the musculocutaneous flaps, a significant increase in blood flow is noted only in musculocutaneous flap. Although leukocyte mobilization is greater in the random-pattern flap, leukocytes in the musculocutaneous flap are well localized at the site of bacterial inoculation.[18] It appears that the rapid delivery of oxygen and leukocytes within the muscle flap to the wound both correct local wound ischemia and improve the environment for leukocyte function. Thus, a muscle flap not only provides wound coverage but also corrects local wound ischemia and hypoxia, thereby allowing wound healing without recurrent infection.

Case Reports

The following personal cases illustrate use of muscle transposition for coverage in chronic and infected mediastinal wounds. In each instance specific modifications of muscle flaps have been done to accomplish reconstruction.

Patient 1 (Fig. 34–1). A 50-year-old man's coronary artery revascularization procedure was complicated initially by wound dehiscence and later by wound infection. Thrombosis of vein grafts resulted in myocardial infarction 3 months after the revascularization procedure. Over the next 14 months, frequent sternal debridements, antibiotic therapy, and open wound management were utilized for management of the mediastinal infection. Owing to persistence of this difficult wound, the patient was referred for surgical management. The reconstructive procedure utilized included debridement of all costal cartilages and the medial third of both clavicles. Bilateral pectoralis major muscle flaps were elevated based on the muscles' major vascular pedicle, the thoracoacromial artery (Fig. 34–1*B*). The muscles covered the entire mediastinal defect (Fig. 34–1*C*). The anterior chest wall skin was mobilized and closed directly over the muscle flaps. Despite extensive chest wall debridement, extubation was possible at 5 days following surgery, and the patient was discharged at 3 weeks. Culture-specific antibiotic therapy was given for 10 days postoperatively. At 2 years after chest wall reconstruction, the patient was without evidence of recurrent infection (Fig. 34–1*D*). The pectoralis major muscles continued to maintain chest wall stability despite absence of sternum and costal cartilages.

Patient 2 (Fig. 34–2). A 29-year-old male medical student underwent mitral valve replacement in 1976 to correct valvular damage following bacterial endocarditis. The postoperative course was complicated by bleeding. After re-exploration, the patient developed a wound infection, which was treated with open drainage and packing. Wound closure was eventually accomplished. However, frequent recurrent infections occurred over the ensuing 8 years, requiring intermittent hospitalization, antibiotic therapy, and sinus tract irrigation. This patient (now a 38-year-old physician-lawyer) was referred for treatment of his chronic infected mediastinal wound (Fig. 34–2, *A* and *B*). Initial evaluation at referral included selective arteriography to confirm the patency of the right internal mammary artery. The arteriogram indicated this was sufficient to allow management by wound debridement and use of a medially based pectoralis major muscle flap for mediastinal reconstruction. After the central sternum and anterior mediastinum were debrided, the right pectoralis major muscle flap was elevated based on its secondary vascular pedicles, the medial segmental branches of the internal mammary artery. The muscle was split so that the inferior half of the muscle could be used to fill the inferior mediastinal wound, the site of chronic infection (Fig. 34–2*C*). The superior half of the muscle was then utilized to cover the sternal defect. The patient received culture-specific antibiotic therapy for 10 days after surgery, at which time he was discharged from the hospital. At 2 years following surgery, the patient had stable chest wall reconstruction and was without evidence of recurrent infection (Fig. 34–2*E*).

Patient 3 (Fig. 34–3). A 54-year-old woman underwent staging laparotomy and mediastinal radiation therapy for Hodgkin's disease in 1974. In 1978, she underwent pericardiectomy for constric-

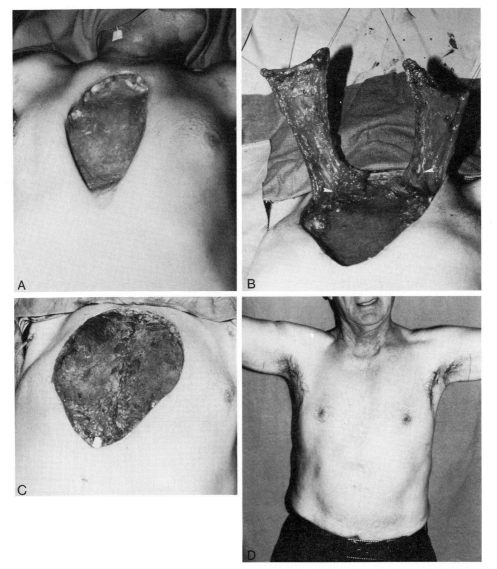

Figure 34–1. Bilateral pectoralis major muscle flaps for mediastinal reconstruction in a 50-year-old man. *A*, Chronic mediastinal wound infection 14 months following a myocardial revascularization procedure. *B*, Wound debridement included removal of bilateral costal cartilages and the medial third of both clavicles. The bilateral pectoralis major muscle was elevated for wound coverage. Note site of muscle vascular pedicle (*left arrowhead*) and the thoracoacromial artery (*right arrowhead*). *C*, Bilateral pectoralis major muscle coverage site of mediastinum and cartilage debridement. *D*, Results of mediastinal reconstruction at 2 years postoperatively. The patient has stable chest wall coverage without recurrent infection.

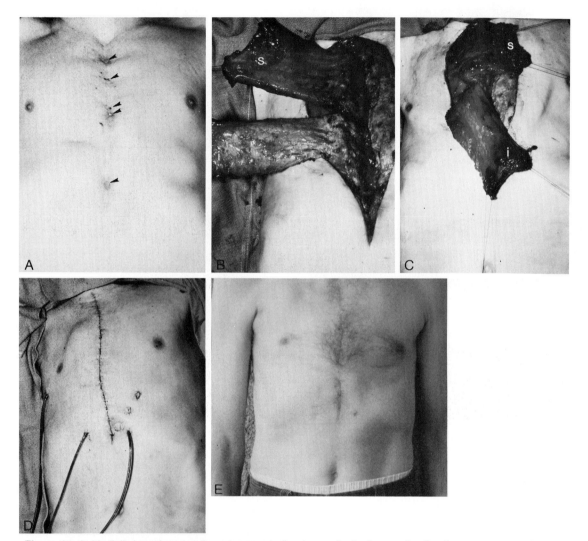

Figure 34–2. Medially based pectoralis major muscle flap for mediastinal reconstruction in a young man with an 8-year history of recurrent mediastinal infections following mitral valve replacement surgery. *A,* Sites of chronic draining sinus tracts (*arrowheads*). *B,* Following debridement of infected sternal cartilages and the posterior inferior mediastinal wound, a right pectoralis major muscle flap was elevated based on secondary segmental vascular pedicles from the internal mammary artery. The muscle was split into superior (*s*) and inferior (*i*) halves. *C,* The inferior half of muscle (*i*) was placed into the posterior inferior mediastinum; the superior half (*s*) was placed over the site of sternal debridement. *D,* The skin was closed directly over the muscle flaps. A suction catheter was utilized during the initial postoperative period. *E,* At 2 years following mediastinal reconstruction, the patient has stable chest wall coverage without evidence of recurrent infection.

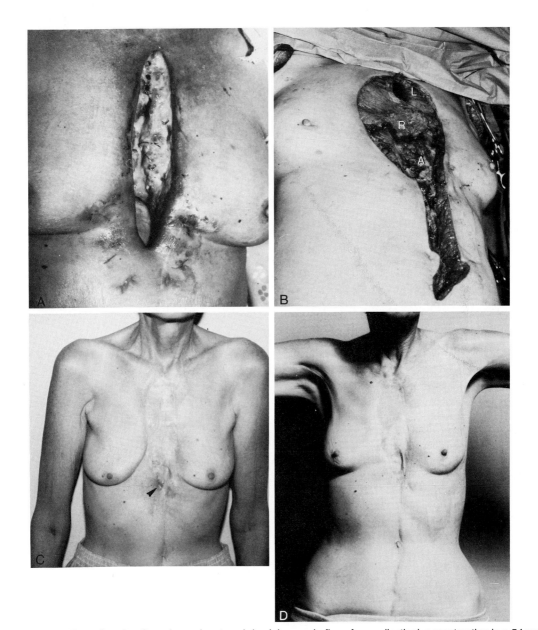

Figure 34–3. Bilateral pectoralis major and rectus abdominis muscle flaps for mediastinal reconstruction in a 54-year-old woman.

A, Anterior mediastinal infection involving the sternum and costal cartilages. (From Mathes SJ, et al: Ann Surg 198:427, 1983. Reproduced with permission.)

B, Wound debridement included the removal of sternum and superior costal cartilages. Bilateral pectoralis major muscles (*L, R*) were used to cover the site of sternal debridement. The left rectus abdominis muscle (*A*) was placed into the posterior mediastinal wound.

C, At 3.5 years after mediastinal reconstruction, the patient developed recurrent infection in a retained right inferior costal cartilage (*arrowhead*). (From Mathes SJ, et al: Ann Surg 198:427, 1983. Reproduced with permission.)

D, Results at 4.5 years after the initial mediastinal reconstruction and at 1 year after treatment of the recurrent infection using a right rectus abdominis flap. She has stable chest wall reconstruction and, at 2 years after the second muscle flap procedure, is without recurrent infection.

tive pericarditis. Her postoperative course was complicated by development of chronic infection of sternum, costal cartilages, and anterior mediastinum. In 1979, the patient was referred for treatment of her acutely infected mediastinal wound (Fig. 34–3A). She underwent debridement of the entire sternum and upper costal cartilages. Immediate reconstruction required use of both pectoralis major muscle flaps based on the muscle's major vascular pedicle, the thoracoacromial artery; the left rectus abdominis muscle also was elevated based on its superior vascular pedicle, the superior epigastric artery, and used to fill the inferior mediastinal wound (Fig. 34–3B). Despite local wound sepsis and poor myocardial function at the time of this procedure, the patient's condition immediately improved following wound closure, with resolution of infection and stable wound coverage. At 3 years after the initial wound closure, the patient developed a small area of recurrent infection in a retained right inferior costal cartilage (Fig. 34–3C). The wound debridement site was closed with a right rectus abdominis muscle transposition flap. At 2 years following the second procedure for treatment of recurrent infection, the patient was asymptomatic, without evidence of further infection and with stable wound coverage (Fig. 34–3D).

CONCLUSIONS

Although midsternotomy wound complications are rarely observed following cardiovascular surgery, chronic infection may not respond to standard wound care and antibiotic therapy. The use of muscle flaps in conjunction with thorough wound debridement represents a safe method to accomplish both stable wound coverage and infection control in a single-stage procedure. Muscle flap coverage should be considered in the patient who develops this complex wound.

References

1. Jurkiewicz MJ, Bostwick J III, Hester TR, et al: Infected median sternotomy wound: successful treatment by muscle flaps. Ann Surg 191:738–744, 1980.
2. Macmanus Q, Okies JE: Mediastinal wound infection and aorta coronary graft patency. Am J Surg 132:558, 1976.
3. Sanfelippo PM, Danielson GK: Complications associated with median sternotomy. J Thorac Cardiovasc Surg 63:419, 1972.
4. Culliford AT, Cunningham JN, Zeff RH, et al: Sternal and costochondral infections following open-heart surgery. J Thorac Cardiovasc Surg 72:714, 1976.
5. Shumacker HB Jr, Mandelbaum I: Continuous antibiotic irrigation in the treatment of infection. Arch Surg 86:384, 1963.
6. Bryant LR, Spencer FC, Trinkle JK: Treatment of median sternotomy infection by mediastinal irrigation with an antibiotic solution. Am Surg 169:914, 1969.
7. Ochsner JL, Mills NL, Woolverton WC: Disruption and infection of the median sternotomy incision. J Cardiovasc Surg 13:394, 1972.
8. McCraw, JB, Dibbell DG, Carraway JH: Clinical definition of independent myocutaneous vascular territories. Plast Reconstr Surg 60:341–352, 1977.
9. Mathes SJ, Nahai F: Classification of the vascular anatomy of muscles: experimental and clinical correlation. Plast Reconstr Surg 67:177, 1981.
10. Brown RG, Fleming WH, Jurkiewicz MJ: An island flap of the pectoralis major muscle. Brit J Plast Surg 30:161, 1977.
11. Mathes SJ, Bostwick J: A rectus abdominis myocutaneous flap to reconstruct abdominal wall defects. Brit J Plast Surg 30:282, 1977.
12. Campbell DA: Reconstruction of the anterior thoracic wall. J Thorac Surg 19:456, 1950.
13. Mathes SJ, Nahai F: Muscle and musculocutaneous flaps. In Goldwyn R (ed.): The Unfavorable Result in Plastic Surgery. Boston, Little, Brown & Co, 1984, p 91.
14. Mathes SJ, Feng LJ, Hunt TK: Coverage of the infected wound. Ann Surg 198:420, 1983.
15. Mathes SJ: The muscle flap for management of osteomyelitis. N Engl J Med 306:294–295, 1982.
16. Chang N, Mathes SJ: A comparison of the effect of bacterial inoculation in musculocutaneous and random pattern flaps. Plast Reconstr Surg 70:1–9, 1982.
17. Gottrup F, Firmin, R, Hunt TK, Mathes SJ: The dynamics of tissue oxygen in healing flaps. Surgery 95:527, 1984.
18. Feng LJ, Price D, Hohn D, Mathes SJ: Blood flow changes and leukocyte mobilization in infection: A comparison between ischemic and well perfused skin. Surg Forum 33:603, 1983.

XII

The Management of Massive Hemoptysis

Severe and continued hemoptysis is terrifying, both for the patient and for those near him. Accounts of this symptom are familiar and dramatic—the musical brilliance of Frederic Chopin interrupted frequently by his "frightful spitting of blood" and coughing up of "basins of blood," and the death of Molière from uncontrollable hemorrhage shortly after acting the part of Argan, the hypochondriac, in the fourth performance of his comedy, "The Imaginary Invalid."

The exact source of pulmonary hemorrhage was commented on by Fearn (1841). He described the autopsy findings in a tuberculous patient who died from massive hemoptysis: ". . . an evacuated cavity, two inches in diameter, and into it was seen jutting a distinctly defined *aneurismal sac,* as large as a nutmeg, which had burst by a clefty-like opening." Fearn believed this was ". . . a well-marked example of aneurism of a branch of the pulmonary artery." Because of his more detailed description, however, this phenomenon was named after Rasmussen (1868). For many years the *aneurysm of Rasmussen* was thought to be a dilated portion of the pulmonary artery. Study of the vascular pattern in diseased lungs has shown that the bleeding is not from the pulmonary artery, but from either hypertrophied bronchial arteries or pulmonary arteries supplied by the bronchial circulation.

After injecting them with contrast medium, Cudkowicz (1952) examined the bronchial arteries of patients who died of pulmonary tuberculosis. He demonstrated that thrombosis of the pulmonary artery had occurred, with marked proliferation and gross dilatation of the bronchial arteries. "The walls of tuberculous cavities were found to have only a bronchial arterial blood supply" he wrote, noting that this had been suggested previously by Calmette (1923), and Wood and Miller (1938). The clinical implications are obvious: patent bronchial arteries to the diseased areas allow antituberculous drugs to reach the tuberculous foci and ". . . surgical measures to combat profuse haemoptysis are unlikely to be successful if they are concentrated upon the pulmonary arteries alone." Comparable changes, hypertrophy and proliferation of the bronchial arteries, were found by Liebow and associates (1949) in bronchiectasis.

The management of massive and uncontrollable hemorrhage has always challenged the surgeon. Because tuberculosis was the chief cause of severe hemoptysis for many years, artificial pneumothorax became its recommended treatment. It was supplemented by additional measures such as phrenicotomy, pneumoperitoneum, thoracoplasty, plombage, or extrapleural pneumolysis, according to how easily the lung collapsed (i.e., the extensiveness of the disease). If intrapleural adhesions were present and prevented collapse, the Jacobeus technique of intrapleural pneumolysis could be used (Alexander, 1925). These maneuvers attempted to compress the lung and empty cavities of their content, thus reducing the granulation tissue that might erode blood vessels. With the acceptance of thoracotomy, such procedures were soon discarded.

Efforts to stop massive pulmonary hemorrhage in seven patients by mass ligation of the hilus, a technique promoted by Sauerbruch, were described by Eloesser (1938). The method was successful in only two of the seven. Eloesser expressed discouragement with mass ligation, emphasized that "pulmonary hemorrhage may originate in the bronchial circulation," and suggested that "it may prove less dangerous not to stop with ligation, but to remove the lobe from which the hemorrhage comes."

Successful pneumonectomy for massive bleeding in a tuberculous patient was initially reported by Pitkin (1941), and subsequently by Ryan and Lineberry (1950) and Ross (1953). Bronchiectasis, carcinoma of the lung, and broncholithiasis were soon recognized as important and often frequent causes of severe hemoptysis. One episode of massive hemoptysis was considered a ". . . definite indication for exploratory thoracotomy" by Ehrenhaft and Taber (1955), who operated on 12 patients with severe hemorrhage not caused by either pulmonary tuberculosis or bronchogenic carcinoma.

Most recently, pulmonary aspergilloma has become a not uncommon cause of severe hemoptysis (Jewkes and coworkers, 1983; Rafferty and coworkers, 1983). Resection of the lung for aspergilloma was first done by Gerstl (1948) and later by Yesner and Hurwitz (1950). In many patients the aspergilloma infection is superimposed on severe cavitary or cystic disease, extensive enough to preclude thoracotomy.

Resection is accepted as the preferred treatment for severe hemoptysis. The problem of the best management for massive pulmonary hemorrhage in patients unable to withstand thoracotomy continues.

35

The Management of Massive Hemoptysis: Control by Angiographic Methods

Marlene R. Eckstein, M.D.
Arthur C. Waltman, M.D.
Christos A. Athanasoulis, M.D.

Massive hemoptysis is defined as bleeding 500 to 600 ml in a 24-hour period.[1, 2] Uflacker and colleagues[3] consider massive hemoptysis to represent any amount of bleeding that fills the anatomic dead space of the lungs and causes asphyxiation. Among the many causes, the most common include pulmonary tuberculosis, abscess, bronchiectasis, cystic fibrosis, aspergilloma, pneumoconiosis, bronchial carcinoma, and Hodgkin's disease.[2] On a rare occasion massive hemoptysis may be secondary to pulmonary arterial bleeding due to Rasmussen's aneurysms of cavitary tuberculosis or arteriovenous fistulae.[4]

The treatment of choice in massive hemoptysis has been surgical resection of the involved lung segment.[5–7] Mortality from massive hemoptysis ranges from 50% to 100%.[6–8] Although aggressive surgery has reduced mortality to about 17%,[6–8] when the patient is actively bleeding at the time of surgery, the mortality reaches as high as 35%.[7, 9] In addition, some patients also have diffuse and severe pulmonary disease in which surgery is contraindicated or must be temporarily postponed until the clinical condition becomes more stable.[10] Mortality from massive hemoptysis in these patients is approximately 70%.[6, 7, 9]

Contraindications to surgery include diffuse and bilateral chronic pulmonary disease, an occult bleeding site, nonresectability due to metastatic bronchogenic carcinoma, a low vital capacity of 40% or less of the predicted normal volume, recurrent hemoptysis following surgery, and cystic fibrosis with diffuse involvement of the lung fields.[1, 7] In these instances, most surgeons welcome preoperative help in stopping the hemorrhage and in improving the patient's condition. Bronchial arteriography may help to localize the bleeding site by demonstrating a variety of angiographic characteristics, discussed in a subsequent section, whether or not actual extravasation of contrast is seen. Bronchial arteriography with embolization is a method of treatment now gaining more and more acceptance as an effective procedure to control massive and/or recurrent hemoptysis in such patients with diffuse lung pathology or in whom surgery is contraindicated.

Bronchial arteriography was performed for the first time in 1963 by Nordenström.[11] Since then the technique and related anatomy have been described in detail by both Reuter[12] and Viamonte[13] and their colleagues. Catheterization of the bronchial arteries may be relatively easy owing to hypertrophy of these vessels secondary to the underlying pathologic condition. Embolization of these arteries for control of massive or recurrent hemoptysis was reported first by Rémy and coworkers in 1974.[14] Since then these workers have reported 104 cases, the largest series to date.[2] Smaller series reported by others[1, 3, 7, 10, 15–17] have also demonstrated that bronchial artery embolization is effective in the management of massive and/or recurrent hemoptysis.

PATIENT PREPARATION

Prior to bronchial arteriography, informed consent is obtained from the patient or family members after full explanation of the procedure and its potential risks, complications, and alternatives. Prior to angiography, findings on the physical examination, including neurologic evaluation, are reviewed by the vascular radiologist. An assessment of cardiopulmonary status is very important. If the patient is critically ill, as are many with massive hemoptysis, adequate ventilatory support and blood volume replacement, cardiac and blood pressure monitoring, and arterial blood gas determinations are necessary.

PREANGIOGRAPHIC LOCALIZATION OF BLEEDING SITES

If the bleeding site in the lung can be localized to a particular segment, bronchial arteriography can be performed more quickly and selectively. A chest radiograph may help if any definite lesions are seen. Whenever possible, bronchoscopy should be performed with the hope of identifying the bleeding site to aid in the angiographic catheterization and possible embolization. Unfortunately, in many cases, the bleeding is so massive that the site of hemorrhage is obscured.

Nuclear scintigraphic localization using Tc[99m] sulfur colloid[18, 19] also may be helpful in precisely localizing the site of pulmonary hemorrhage. It should be used as a complement to rather than as a replacement for more invasive procedures such as bronchoscopy and selective bronchial arteriography. Using scintigraphy, Winzelberg and colleagues[19] accurately determined the pulmonary bleeding source in 4 of 11 patients with a bleeding rate of 50 to 200 ml in 24 hours and demonstrated indirect evidence of the bleeding site in another patient. This technique may be helpful in determining the site of hemorrhage in patients who are bleeding too much for accurate bronchoscopy.

Scintigraphy using Tc[99m]-labeled red blood cells may prove to aid in localization of the bleeding site in patients with intermittent bleeding.[19] Unfortunately, in those patients who are massively hemorrhaging, detection of the bleeding site by scintigraphy may not be possible, or the patient may be too unstable to delay the angiographic procedure.

Localization of the bleeding site by use of any or all of the aforementioned modalities optimizes the success and efficacy of selective arterial catheterization and possible embolization. This is true except in those instances of diffuse bilateral pulmonary involvement, such as in cystic fibrosis, where bilateral embolization is performed regardless of the site of hemorrhage.[1, 10]

TECHNIQUE

Bronchial Arteriography

Once a decision has been made to perform arteriography in order to localize the bleeding site for potential control of the massive hemoptysis, a transfemoral arterial approach is made, and the angiographic catheter is placed selectively into the bronchial artery on the suspected side first, if known. If preangiographic localization of the bleeding was not possible or if bilateral pulmonary disease is present, then both the right and left bronchial arteries are catheterized. Knowledge of the anatomy of the bronchial arteries is necessary for efficacious catheterization. Variations in the bronchial anatomy do occur; however, the usual anatomic distribution consists of one bronchial artery on the right side with two on the left side in 40% of patients, one bronchial artery on each side in 21%, two bronchial arteries on each side in 20%, and two bronchial arteries on the right side with one on the left side in 10% (Fig. 35–1).[1, 11, 20]

The bronchial arteries usually originate from the thoracic aorta slightly above the left mainstem bronchus at the level of T5 or T6. The

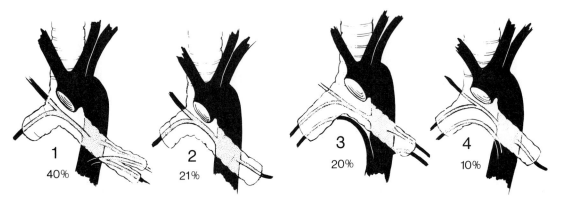

Figure 35–1. Origin of the bronchial arteries from the thoracic aorta. The four patterns shown are found in approximately 90% of patients. *1,* One bronchial artery arising on the right and two on the left (40%). *2,* One bronchial artery arising on the right and one on the left (21%). *3,* Two bronchial arteries arising on the right and two on the left (20%). *4,* Two bronchial arteries arising on the right and one on the left (10%). (From Olson RR, Athanasoulis CA: Hemoptysis: Treatment with transcatheter embolization of the bronchial arteries. In Athanasoulis CA et al (eds): Interventional Radiology. Philadelphia, WB Saunders, 1982.)

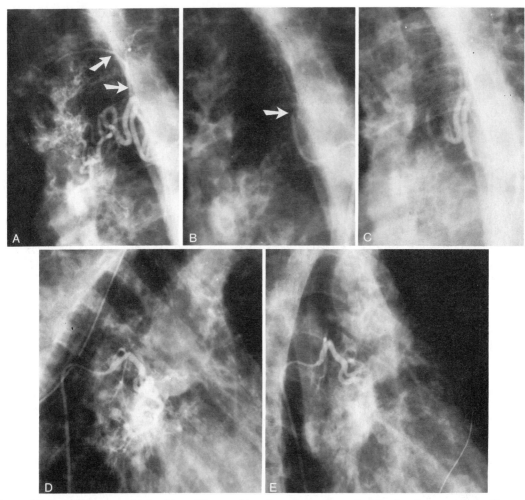

Figure 35–2. Arteriograms obtained in a 20-year-old male patient with cystic fibrosis who presented with massive hemoptysis. *A,* Right bronchial arteriogram obtained on admission shows hypertrophy of the bronchial artery and branches but no extravasation. Note origin of supreme intercostal (*arrows*) from bronchial artery. *B,* Catheter position prior to embolization. Note position of catheter tip well past the origin of the right supreme intercostal (*arrow*) seen in *A. C,* Bronchial arteriogram after embolization. *D, E,* Left bronchial arteriogram prior to (*D*) and after (*E*) embolization with surgical gelatin. The patient had no recurrent bleeding for 10 months. (From Olson RR, Athanasoulis CA: Hemoptysis: Treatment with transcatheter embolization of the bronchial arteries. In Athanasoulis CA et al (eds): Interventional Radiology. Philadelphia, WB Saunders, 1982.)

right bronchial artery usually presents as the first branch of the right second or third intercostal artery, although in some cases it may originate directly from the descending aorta. On occasion it may form a common branch with the right supreme intercostal artery (Fig. 35–2*A*). The left bronchial artery arises from the aorta. Other sites of bronchial origins include the subclavian, internal mammary, or thyrocervical arteries.[1] Bronchial blood supply may develop as well through pleural adhesions due to the underlying pathologic process, and this supply may be the cause of recurrent hemorrhage in some patients despite initial embolization success.

After the appropriate bronchial artery is catheterized, small test injections with a meg-

lumine iothalamate contrast medium are performed to confirm the catheter location. Angiographic serial filming is then obtained using magnification technique (1.5–2×) with coned-down images to the field of interest. Injection rate and filming sequence are determined by the flow characteristics of the vessel being studied at the time of the test injection. Subtraction films that remove the superimposed bone and lung structures in order to see better the opacified vessels are obtained to look for the presence of a spinal radicular artery. This artery originates from intercostal arteries and occasionally shares a common origin with the right bronchomediastinal artery. Many investigators consider the presence of a spinal radicular artery on arteriography of a bronchial artery to be an absolute contraindication to embolization because of the risk of spinal cord injury.[1, 2, 10, 16, 21, 22] Others believe that the high mortality in nonsurgical patients with massive hemoptysis offsets this risk and makes it a relative contraindication; in such cases, they proceed with embolization, using extreme care.[3, 15]

Transcatheter Embolization

If selective bronchial arteriography with or without additional vessel catheterizations demonstrates evidence of the source of the pulmonary hemorrhage, embolization is performed. The bleeding site is determined definitely if active extravasation of contrast medium is seen angiographically. However, extravasation is rarely demonstrated (Fig. 35–2A). Therefore, other angiographic characteristics are used to establish the area of pathology and cause of the hemoptysis. These include the presence of an increased number and caliber of the bronchial arterial branches with evidence of increased vascularity of each injected vessel supplying the area of interest, evidence of systemic-to-pulmonary shunting, and aneurysmal vascular structures.[17] Several arteries may have to be injected with contrast since nonbronchial systemic arteries may penetrate the lung via the triangular ligament as well as through pleural adhesions.[2, 23–25] Therefore, injection of one or more bronchial, intercostal, subclavian, internal mammary, and pulmonary arteries may be required to demonstrate any or all the angiographic features described previously. In this way, transcatheter embolization of the appropriate feeding vessels is performed even though active extravasation is not seen. Since systemic arterial–to–pulmonary arterial shunts occur with inflammatory diseases of the lung, sometimes it is necessary to occlude a bleeding branch of the pulmonary artery as well.[3, 26] Of course, the greater the

number of feeding systemic arteries, the less are the chances for success of embolization. In conditions such as cystic fibrosis where involvement of the lung is diffuse and bilateral, transcatheter embolization on both sides is recommended.[10]

The goal of bronchial artery embolization is to provide immediate control of the hemorrhage. In addition, the aim is to achieve lasting hemostatic control in those patients who do not proceed to surgery and to improve the clinical conditions in those patients who will undergo subsequent surgical intervention.[1–3] The most frequently used embolic agent for bronchial artery embolization is surgical gelatin (Gelfoam). Isobutyl-2-cyanoacrylate has been used once,[1] and the future role of cyanoacrylate or of absolute ethanol has not been defined as yet.

During the procedure, extreme care must be taken to prevent reflux of the embolic agent. Reflux can be avoided by several steps, including gently wedging the catheter into the vessel with care not to cause spasm; using small surgical gelatin fragments to occlude the smaller branches first, followed by larger occluding fragments; monitoring fluoroscopically the progression of embolization; terminating the procedure when 70% to 80% of the vessel is occluded;[1] and using whenever possible balloon occlusion catheters.[27]

RESULTS

The results of bronchial artery embolization by several investigators are summarized in Table 35–1. The two largest series were reported by Rémy[2] and Uflacker[3] and their coworkers. Rémy's group performed bronchial artery embolization in 104 patients. Of these, 49 were embolized acutely for hemoptysis; the remaining 55 were embolized electively after the acute episode had resolved. In 41 of the 49 acutely embolized patients, immediate con-

Table 35–1. Summary of Clinical Studies on Use of Bronchial Artery Embolization in Massive Hemoptysis

Study	Total in Series	Results (No. of Patients) Acute Bleeding Controlled	Recurrence (at 1–24 mo)	Major Complications
Wholey et al[15]	5	4/5	0/4	0/4
Harley et al[16]	1	1/1	1/1	0/1
Rémy et al[2]	104	41/49	6/41	11/104
Fellows et al[10]	13	12/13	0/12	0/13
Magilligan et al[7]	7	7/7	2/7	0/7
Vujic et al[17]	5	5/5	0/5	1/5
Uflacker et al[3]	33	26/33	4/26	0/33
Eckstein et al (unpublished 1985)	7	7/7	5/7	0/7

trol of the bleeding was achieved, with only 6 patients experiencing recurrent hemoptysis 2 to 7 months later. Rémy and colleagues reported one complication of small bowel necrosis out of 104 embolizations performed.[2] This complication was treated by segmental resection. These workers also stated that 10 patients experienced dysphagia of 2 to 3 days' duration.

Uflacker and coworkers[3] reported 33 cases of bronchial arterial embolization. Of these, 26 were controlled by embolization alone; in the remaining 7 cases, bronchial artery embolization followed by surgery was required. Of 26 patients embolized, 22 had lasting control, with recurrence of bleeding reported in only 4 patients within 1 to 24 months. There were no major complications reported. In this series, Uflacker's group found that there was a high rebleed rate (43%) and a high mortality rate among patients with mycetoma and residual pulmonary disease. This was due to revascularization and recanalization of vessels with the resorption of the embolic agent and formation of collaterals. Therefore, in these cases, bronchial artery embolization only temporized the acute bleeding episode to ready the patient for more permanent control with surgical resection of the involved area.

In a smaller series reported by Vujic and coworkers,[17] one patient was embolized twice, and one patient was studied angiographically but was not embolized. A complication of spinal cord infarction was encountered in one patient as the only complication in the series. This occurred despite the fact that no spinal cord branches were seen on the arteriogram prior to embolization.

When massive hemoptysis is treated by clinical modalities alone, the mortality is approximately 75%. This mortality rate decreases to between 21% and 23% when the patients are treated solely by surgery.[5, 8] The use of bronchial artery embolization alone or followed electively by surgery has reduced the mortality to between 7% and 9%.[3]

COMPLICATIONS

Occlusion of the bronchial arteries in experimental animals and in humans has not caused any clinical or radiologically detectable pulmonary ischemia.[2, 28, 29] It is expected that transient chest pain and fever may be experienced by the patient in the 48 to 72 hours following embolization. These side effects are not considered complications. Retrosternal burning with dysphagia has been reported in 10 patients by Rémy and colleagues,[2] and there

has been one reported case of an esophagobronchial fistula following embolization of the bronchial artery.[30] The most feared potential complications that may result at the time of or after transcatheter embolization for control of hemoptysis are spinal cord injury and occlusion of other vessels by reflux.

Spinal cord injury as a result of bronchial arteriography alone was described in earlier reports;[21, 22] however, recovery was complete in days or months. The neurotoxic effects in these cases were attributed to transverse myelitis and Brown-Séquard syndrome secondary to contrast agent toxicity. It is now believed that the use of a low-neurotoxic contrast medium (iothalamate) in small quantities has reduced the incidence of this complication.

To decrease the risk of spinal cord injury, a very diligent search of the bronchial arteriogram for the presence of spinal radicular arteries is carried out. Subtraction films and magnification views are necessary to identify these vessels; if spinal branches are seen, most angiographers would not proceed with embolization.[1, 2, 10, 16, 21, 22] Some workers consider the presence of the spinal radicular artery to be only a relative contraindication,[3, 15] and Uflacker and coworkers[3] proceeded to embolize nine patients in this category but used larger pledgets of embolic material so that peripheral vessel occlusion and spinal cord injury were prevented. Vujic and colleagues[17] reported one incidence of spinal cord infarction despite the fact that no spinal artery branches were seen on the pre-embolization arteriogram.

Occlusion of other vessels by reflux is another possible complication that must be considered whenever embolization of any vessel is undertaken. Rémy and coworkers[2] reported one case of small bowel infarction and another of severe epigastric pain, which resolved in a few hours. These complications were caused by reflux of the embolic material at the time of administration and can be avoided by proper catheter positioning, gentle injections of the contrast and embolic agents, use of a balloon catheter, and termination of the embolization procedure before the entire vessel is occluded.

CONCLUSIONS

Because massive hemoptysis often can be fatal, some means of intervention is crucial. Bronchial arteriography and embolization usually offer a safe and effective nonoperative method of control of hemorrhage. These procedures may be indicated in those patients who are not surgical candidates or in those who require immediate stabilization so that they can undergo surgical resection at some later date. In some cases, bronchial artery embolization is an alternative method when conservative modalities fail and when the only recourse is pulmonary resection; bronchial arteriography followed by transcatheter embolization may temporarily control the bleeding so that the patient may be prepared for a more elective surgical procedure. In other cases, these procedures obviate the need for surgery altogether. The use of bronchial artery embolization for the control of massive hemoptysis with or without surgery has reduced a mortality rate of 75% with medical treatment alone, or of 21% to 23% with surgery alone,[5, 8] to 7% to 9%.[3]

Although serious potential complications of spinal cord injury and unintentional embolization of other vessels may be caused by bronchial artery embolization, their incidence can be reduced and possibly avoided completely by the techniques already described. It is also necessary to weigh the low incidence of these complications against the life-threatening situation presented by massive hemoptysis. In the severely ill patient with hemoptysis, therefore, bronchial artery embolization should be a method of choice for the control of bleeding.

References

1. Olson RR, Athanasoulis CA: Hemoptysis: Treatment with transcatheter embolization of the bronchial arteries. In Athanasoulis CA, Greene RE, Pfister RC, Roberson GH (eds): Interventional Radiology. Chap 12, p 196. Philadelphia. WB Saunders, 1982.
2. Rémy J, Arnaud A, Fardou H, et al: Treatment of hemoptysis by embolization of bronchial arteries. Radiology 122:33, 1977.
3. Uflacker R, Kaemmerer A, Neves C, Picon PD: Management of massive hemoptysis by bronchial artery embolization. Radiology 146:627, 1983.
4. Wagner RB, Baeza OR, Stewart JE: Active pulmonary hemorrhage localized by selective pulmonary angiography. Chest 67:121, 1975.
5. Garzon AA, Cerruti M, Govrin A, Karlson KE: Pulmonary resection for massive hemoptysis. Surgery 67:633, 1970.
6. Sehhat S, Oreizie M, Moinedine K: Massive pulmonary hemorrhage: Surgical approach as choice of treatment. Ann Thorac Surg 25:12, 1978.
7. Magilligan DJ Jr, Ravipati S, Zayat P, et al: Massive hemoptysis: Control by transcatheter bronchial artery embolization. Ann Thorac Surg 32:392, 1981.
8. Crocco JA, Rooney JJ, Fankishen DS, et al: Massive hemoptysis. Arch Intern Med 121:495, 1968.
9. Garzon AA, Govrin A: Surgical management of massive hemoptysis: A ten-year experience. Ann Surg 187:267, 1978.
10. Fellows KE, Khaw KT, Schuster S, Shwachman HO: Bronchial artery embolization in cystic fibrosis; technique and long-term results. J Pediatr 95:959, 1979.
11. Nordenström B: Selective catheterization and angiography of bronchial and mediastinal arteries in man. Acta Radiol [Diagn] (Stockh) 6:13, 1963.
12. Reuter SR, Tord O, Abrams HL: Selective bronchial arteriography. AJR 84:87, 1965.
13. Viamonte M Jr, Parks RE, Smoak WM III: Guided catheterization of the bronchial arteries. Parts I, II, III. Radiology 85:205, 1965.
14. Rémy J, Voisin C, Dupuis C, et al.: Traitement des hémoptysies par embolisation de la circulation systémique. Ann Radiol 17:5, 1974.
15. Wholey MH, Chamorro HA, Rao G, et al: Bronchial artery embolization for massive hemoptysis. JAMA 236:2501, 1976.
16. Harley JD, Killien FC, Peck AG: Massive hemoptysis controlled by transcatheter embolization of the bronchial arteries. AJR 128:302, 1977.
17. Vujic I, Pyle R, Hungerford GD, Griffin CN: Angiography and therapeutic blockade in the control of hemoptysis. Radiology 143:19, 1982.
18. Winzelberg GG, Wholey MH: Scintigraphic detection of pulmonary hemorrhage using Tc-99m-sulfur colloid. Clin Nucl Med 6:537, 1981.
19. Winzelberg GG, Wholey MH, Sachs M: Scintigraphic localization of pulmonary bleeding using technetium Tc 99m sulfur colloid: A preliminary report. Radiology 143:757, 1982.
20. Cauldwell EW, Siekert RG, Lininger RE, et al: The bronchial arteries. An anatomic study of 150 cadavers. Surg Gynecol Obstet 86:395, 1948.
21. Feigelson HH, Ravin HA: Transverse myelitis following selective bronchial arteriography. Radiology 85:663, 1965.
22. Kardjiev V, Symeonov A, Chankov I: Etiology, pathogenesis, and prevention of spinal cord lesions in selective angiography of the bronchial and intercostal arteries. Radiology 112:81, 1974.
23. Parke WW, Michels NA: The nonbronchial systemic arteries of the lung. J Thorac Cardiovasc Surg 49:694, 1965.
24. Botenga ASJ: Selective Bronchial and Intercostal Arteriography. Leiden, Holland, HE Stenfert Kroese, 1970.
25. Rémy J, Beguery P, Froment T, et al: La vascularisation systémique du poumon: Technique d'exploration et anatomie radiologue appliquées au diagnostic topographique des hémoptysies. Ann Radiol (Paris) 18:47, 1975.
26. Bredin CP, Richardson PR, King TKC, et al: Treatment of massive hemoptysis by combined occlusion of pulmonary and bronchial arteries. Am Rev Resp Dis 117:969, 1978.
27. Greenfield AJ, Athanasoulis CA, Waltman AC, et al: Transcatheter embolization: Prevention of embolic reflux using balloon catheter. AJR 131:651, 1978.
28. Ellis FJ Jr, Grindlay JH, Edwards JE: The bronchial arteries. Experimental occlusion. Surgery 30:810, 1951.
29. Boushy SF, Helgason AH, North LB: Occlusion of the bronchial arteries by glass microspheres. Am Rev Resp Dis 103:249, 1971.
30. Hélénon CH, Chatel L, Bigot JM, Brocard H: Fistulae oesophago-bronchique gauche aprés embolisation bronchique. Nouv Presse Med 6:4209, 1977.

36

The Management of Massive Hemoptysis: Treatment by Bronchial Artery Embolization

P. C. Shetty, M.D.
Donald J. Magilligan, M.D.

Massive hemoptysis is defined as pulmonary hemorrhage of more than 600 ml within 24 hours. Most acute episodes of hemoptysis last less than 24 hours and gradually subside.[1, 2] However, when the hemoptysis is massive, it carries a mortality rate of 50% to 100%. It is generally agreed that surgery is the treatment of choice for patients with massive hemoptysis. In two different studies, an aggressive surgical approach limited mortality to 0.9% and 17%, respectively.[3, 4] However, with active massive hemoptysis at the time of surgery, the mortality in both series was 35%. An even greater therapeutic dilemma is presented by massive hemoptysis in patients having a specific contraindication to surgery. In actively bleeding patients with contraindications defined as postexpiratory volume of less than 40% of that predicted, occult site of hemorrhage, or bronchial carcinoma with involvement of the mediastinum or great vessels, mortalities have been reported at 69% and 71%.[4, 5] Transcatheter bronchial artery embolization for control of massive hemoptysis is employed in patients in whom surgery is contraindicated. This method is also used to control hemoptysis prior to surgery to decrease operative mortality.

PATIENT PREPARATION

If necessary, airway control is established by intubation. Only a small percentage of patients need endotracheal intubation. An alternative to the use of a double-lumen tube for control of hemorrhage is selective intubation of the normal bronchus with the help of a fiberoptic bronchoscope, or tamponade by endobronchial inflation of a balloon-tipped catheter.[5] Although bronchoscopy is routinely performed prior to angiography for bronchial artery embolization, bronchoscopy is not necessary in patients with established diagnosis and unilateral disease on the chest x-ray film.

Physical examination should be performed with special attention to neurologic and peripheral vascular status, especially of the lower extremities. The patient and appropriate family members should be informed of the details of the procedure, including related pain and discomfort and possible complications, with special emphasis on potential for injury to the spinal cord due to contrast material or embolization. An informed consent form is completed prior to premedication.

ANATOMY OF THE BRONCHIAL ARTERIES

There are three common forms of bronchial artery anatomy: (1) one bronchial artery on each side, with the right being an intercostal bronchial trunk (Fig. 36–1A); (2) one bronchial artery on the right and two on the left (Fig. 36–1B); and (3) a less common variation, two bronchial arteries arising on each side of the aorta (Fig. 36–1C). Most bronchial arteries arise along the ventral and lateral aspects of the thoracic aorta between the upper margin of the fifth and lower border of the sixth thoracic vertebrae.

Knowledge of the blood supply to the spinal cord is also necessary to avoid spinal cord injury, the most dreaded complication of this procedure. A single anterior spinal artery and the two posterior spinal arteries provide the dominant blood supply to the entire spinal cord. However, radiculomedullary branches "reinforce" the anterior and posterior spinal arteries at several levels. These radiculomedullary branches can arise at various levels from the ascending cervical, superior intercostal, posterior intercostal, subcostals, lumbar, iliolumbar, lateral and medial sacral, both vertebrals, paracervical, bronchial, phrenic, and renal arteries. The radiculomedullary branch, which may be seen to arise from any of these

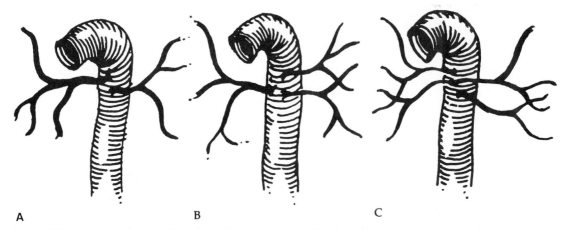

A   B   C

Figure 36–1. Common forms of bronchial artery anatomy. *A,* One bronchial artery on each side, with the right an intercostal bronchial trunk. *B,* One bronchial artery on the right and two on the left. *C,* Less commonly, two bronchial arteries may arise on each side.

arteries, has a typical hairpin appearance, as illustrated by the artery of Adamkiewicz (Fig. 36–2). The slender ascending branch is the radiculomedullary branch, while the descending undulating branch is the reinforced anterior spinal artery. The artery of Adamkiewicz is the largest known radiculomedullary artery, which in 75% of cases arises on the left side either from the ninth through twelfth intercostal arteries or from the left first and second lumbar arteries. In the mid-thoracic spinal cord region, the largest known radiculomedullary branch arises from the fifth thoracic intercostal artery, on either the right or the left side.

TECHNIQUE

Embolization is performed in a well-equipped angiographic suite by an angiographer with experience in interventional radiology (mainly embolization techniques). A scout film is obtained over the area of interest, which should provide good detail over the spine in order to identify the often small spinal artery. Appropriate filtration is used over the lung. A No. 5 or 6 French tapered catheter (Fig. 36–3) is introduced into the thoracic aorta through the common femoral artery by the Seldinger technique. We find that a Simmons I type of

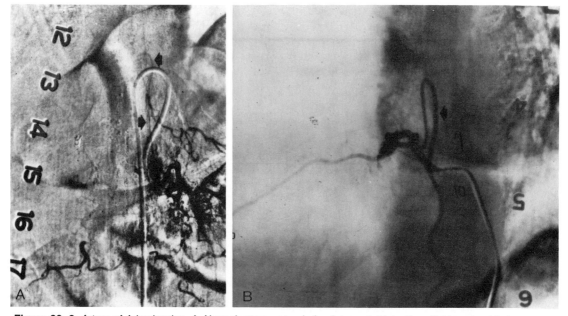

Figure 36–2. Artery of Adamkewicz. *A,* Normal artery seen during intercostal injection. *B,* Hypertrophied artery in a patient with an arteriovenous malformation (AVM) of the spinal cord.

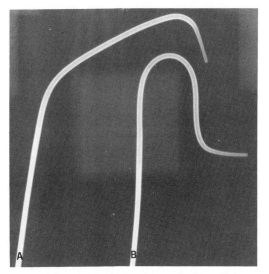

Figure 36–3. Two useful catheters for bronchial artery catheterization: spinal artery catheter (A); sidewinder I type curve with tapered tip (B).

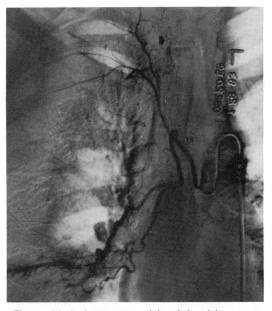

Figure 36–4. A common origin of the right supreme intercostal and right bronchial artery in a patient with right lower lobe neoplasm. A segment of the spinal artery is opacified (arrow). This artery was not embolized.

curve (Fig. 36–3B) in the tapered-tip catheter is easier to advance into the proximal bronchial artery; also, it is more stable during embolization. Meglumine iothalamate (Conray-60) is used as the contrast medium because it has been found to have minimal neurotoxic effects compared with other agents. A search is made to selectively enter the bronchial artery on the affected side. About 0.5 to 1 ml of contrast is injected to confirm the position of the catheter. Depending on the size of the bronchial artery, 3 to 6 ml of contrast is then injected, and serial films are obtained over the distribution of the bronchial artery. The films are carefully scrutinized to identify any blood supply to the spinal cord; this may require subtraction tech-

nique. A lateral film may also be necessary to identify the spinal artery. Use of digital subtraction technique, when available, with intra-arterial injection will reduce both the amount of contrast material and the time required for bronchial angiography.

If the spinal artery is opacified while injecting the bronchial artery or intercostal bronchial trunk, we consider this an absolute contraindication to embolization (Fig. 36–4). However, others feel this is only a relative contraindication. When there is a common origin of bronchial artery and intercostal artery, careful

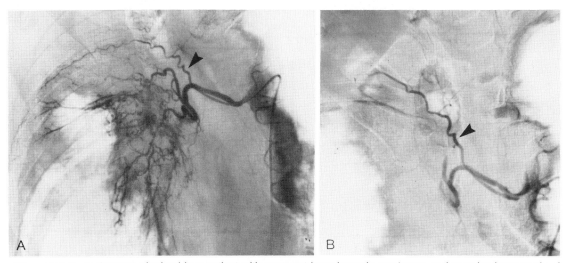

Figure 36–5. Angiograms obtained in a patient with recurrent bronchogenic carcinoma and massive hemoptysis. A, A common origin of the right fifth intercostal and right bronchial artery. B, The bronchial artery was successfully embolized, sparing the intercostal artery.

technique may allow selective catheterization of the bronchial artery, which is then embolized; the intercostal artery is thus preserved (Fig. 36–5).

Gelfoam is the most commonly used embolic material in the bronchial arteries.[6] Absolute alcohol and isobutyl-2-cyanoacrylate are alternatives, but we reserve these materials for patients with recurrent bleeding due to recanalization of the bronchial artery originally thrombosed by Gelfoam particles. Gelfoam particles, 1 to 4 mm in size, are soaked in dilute contrast and injected slowly through the catheter; injection is stopped when occlusion of the main branches of the bronchial artery is achieved.

When bronchial artery embolization is either completely or partially unsuccessful in arresting massive hemorrhage, the addition of balloon occlusion of the pulmonary artery may be life-saving. The capillary anastomosis normally present between bronchial and pulmonary arteries may be markedly increased in size in disease; in such cases, following bronchial arterial occlusion the enlarged anasto-motic network may allow pulmonary arterial flow in the diseased area. Therefore, temporary pulmonary artery occlusion by the occlusive balloon catheter should be considered if bronchial artery embolization fails to arrest bleeding in life-threatening hemoptysis.

ANGIOGRAPHIC FINDINGS

Angiographic findings in the bronchial artery are nonspecific. Commonly observed changes include hypervascularity (Fig. 36–6A); bronchial artery hypertrophy (Fig. 36–4); bronchial artery aneurysms (Fig. 36–7A); bronchopulmonary anastomosis (Fig. 36–7B); and neovascularity (Fig. 36–8). However, in some cases no definite abnormalities are seen (Fig. 36–9). Extravasation of contrast is seldom seen. In our series of 16 patients, bronchial artery–to–pulmonary artery shunting was seen only in chronic inflammatory processes. Angiographic evidence of neovascularity was seen in 50% of the known malignant neoplasms.

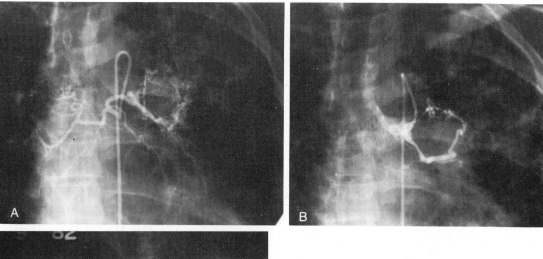

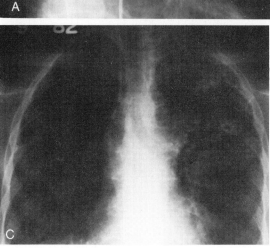

Figure 36–6. Angiograms obtained in a patient who presented with massive hemoptysis and unilateral left upper lobe abnormalities. *A*, The rare occurrence of a single bronchial trunk supplying the left and right lung, with hypervascularity over the left upper lobe. *B*, The branch to the left lung was selectively catheterized and embolized. *C*, The hemoptysis successfully arrested.

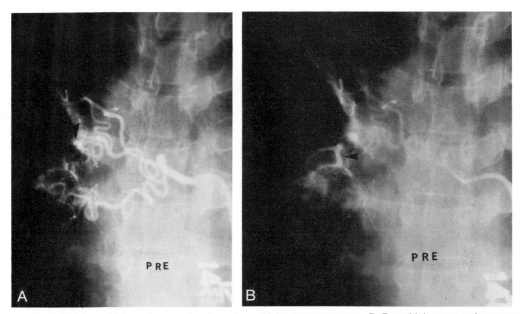

Figure 36–7. *A,* A bronchial angiogram showing a bronchial artery aneurysm. *B,* Bronchial artery–pulmonary artery shunting in a patient with active tuberculosis.

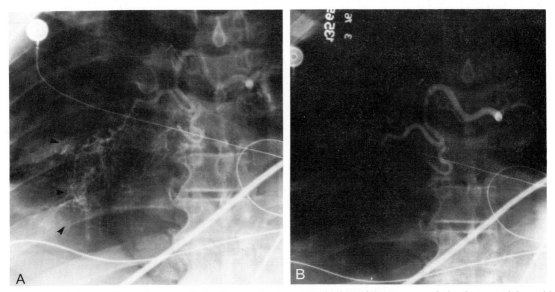

Figure 36–8. In a patient who presented with massive hemoptysis, bronchoscopy revealed a large endobronchial neoplasm. *A,* Selective right bronchial angiogram shows considerable neovascularity. *B,* After embolization of the major branches, hemoptysis ceased, and bronchoscopy and biopsy of the lesion were performed without complication.

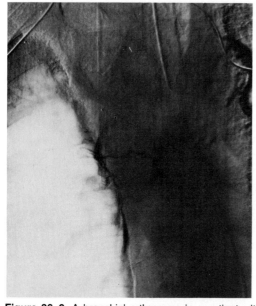

Figure 36–9. A bronchial arthrogram in a patient with recurrent squamous cell carcinoma after right upper lobectomy. Although this bronchial artery is small and without hypervascularity, the patient's hemoptysis ceased abruptly following embolization.

COMPLICATIONS

In addition to possible injury to the spinal cord and the complications related to femoral artery catheterization by the Seldinger technique, there are two additional possible complications related to bronchial artery angiography and embolization. One of these is transverse myelitis,[7] caused by the contrast medium used. Incidence and severity of the myelitis can be minimized by avoiding a flood aortogram, which seldom visualizes the bronchial arteries, and by using only small amounts of the less neurotoxic meglumine iothalamate.

The second possible complication is occlusion of the visceral or peripheral arterial branches following reflux into the aorta of material used for embolization. The risk can be minimized by injecting only small amounts of embolization material at a time, and by stopping injection when the major branches of the bronchial artery are occluded. If blood supply to the spinal cord is visualized while injecting the bronchial artery or, most commonly, the bronchointercostal trunk, emboli-

zation of such a bronchial artery should not be performed in order to avoid the risk of spinal cord injury (Fig. 36–5A). When there is a common bronchointercostal trunk without identifiable supply to the spinal cord, attempt must be made to embolize only the bronchial artery (Fig. 36–5B).

CONCLUSIONS

The success of transcatheter bronchial artery embolization in arresting hemoptysis is uniform in many series. In those patients who are hemorrhaging at the time of the procedure, the effect is immediate and dramatic. In a large series of actively bleeding patients, Rémy and colleagues successfully arrested hemorrhage in 41 of 49 cases.[8, 9]

Bronchial artery embolization for control of massive hemoptysis should be mainly reserved for patients who have contraindications to surgery. In patients who do not respond to medical management, this method may also be used prior to surgery to decrease the operative mortality.

References

1. Lindberg EJ: Emergency operation in patients with massive hemoptysis. Am Surg 30:158–159, 1964.
2. Pursel SE, Lindskog GE: Hemoptysis: a clinical evaluation of 105 patients examined consecutively on a thoracic surgical service. Am Rev Respir Dis 84:329–336, 1961.
3. Crocco JA, Rooney JJ, Frankishen DS, et al: Massive hemoptysis. Arch Intern Med 121:495–498, 1968.
4. Sehhat S, Oreize M, Moinedine K: Massive pulmonary hemorrhage: surgical approach as a choice of treatment. Ann Thoracic Surg 25:12–15, 1978.
5. Garzon AA, Govrin A: Surgical management of massive hemoptysis: a ten-year experience. Ann Surg 187:267–271, 1978.
6. Bookstein JJ, Moser KM, Kalafer ME, et al: The role of bronchial arteriography and therapeutic embolization in hemoptysis. Chest 72:658–661, 1977.
7. Feigelson HH, Ravin HA: Transverse myelitis following selective bronchial arteriography. Radiology 85:663–665, 1965.
8. Rémy J, Voisin C, Dupuis C, et al: Traitement des hémoptysies par embolisation de la circulation systémique. Ann Radiol 17:5–16, 1974.
9. Rémy J, Arnaud S, Fordor H, et al: Treatment of hemoptysis by embolization of bronchial arteries. Radiology 122:33–37, 1977.

XIII

The Use of Lasers for Tracheobronchial Lesions

*The world gains value from the extraordinary,
and duration from the average.*

—Paul Valéry (1871–1945)

In his quantum theory, Einstein (1917) established the theoretical basis *(stimulated emission)* of laser, but for almost 40 years laser remained in the realm of science fiction. A beam of energy intense enough to penetrate the hardest and most heat-resistant material, a beam that could be directed for short or long distances and focused with unerring accuracy was a dream in technology. But the dream was realized, as evidenced in this description by Schawlow (1981): "What instrument can shuck a bucket of oysters, correct typing errors, fuse atoms, lay a straight line for a garden bed, repair a detached retina, and drill holes in diamonds?" Each of us can add to this list because of the marvelous versatility provided by laser.

In the 1950's the physical properties of *maser* (Microwave Amplification by Stimulated Emission of Radiation) were described by several American and Russian scientists working independently (Schawlow, Townes, and Vasov), and Gordon and coworkers (1955) successfully demonstrated the application of maser.

The first laser (Light Amplification by Stimulated Emission of Radiation) beam in the visible light spectrum was developed in 1961 by Maiman, who excited a ruby rod by an intense pulse of light from a flash lamp. This report originated a new and fascinating era in technology.

Many substances—gas, liquid, or solid—can be used as the active medium in lasers. Each emits energy at a different and characteristic wavelength. In 1961, Javan and colleagues constructed the first gas laser, an electron-excited gaseous system, using a mixture of helium and neon. That same year a laser with energy in the near infrared spectrum was developed by Johnson using a neodymium-doped yttrium-aluminum-garnet rod (Nd:YAG). An argon laser in the blue-green portion of the spectrum was devised by Bennett and coworkers (1962), and the carbon dioxide laser with spectral energy in the infrared portion soon followed (Patel, McFarlane, and Faust, 1964).

By 1981 Goldman was able to list 13 different types of lasers used in medicine and biology, each with different physical characteristics and hence different applications.

The recognition that argon and Nd:YAG laser energy, unlike the CO_2 laser, could be transmitted through a flexible quartz fiber (Kiefhaber and colleagues, 1977; Toty and colleagues, 1981) increased the endoscopic application of laser to numerous organs and their pathology. Previously CO_2 laser coagulation of bleeding in experimentally induced gastric erosions in animals had been reported by Goodale and coworkers (1970). The use of a flexible fiberoptic delivery service for laser coagulation of bleeding in experimental gastric lesions in animals was described by Dwyer and associates (1975). Later that year, Frühmorgen and coworkers utilized the flexible laser for endoscopic gastrointestinal coagulation in humans.

Separate from the direct destruction of tissue or tumor by laser, another method of laser usage has developed. The observation that hematoporphyrin derivative preferentially localizes in malignant tumors (Figge, Weiland, and Manganiello, 1948) led to laser phototherapy of tumors, first in the urinary bladder

(Kelly and Snell, 1976) and subsequently in a wide variety of solid tumors of the skin and subcutaneous tissues (Dougherty and coworkers, 1978, 1979, 1981, 1982). When thus localized, the argon laser activates the photosensitive hematoporphyrin derivative, resulting in cytotoxicity for the malignant cell, presumably by singlet oxygen, although superoxide and the hydroxyl radical are also produced (Dougherty and Gomer, 1976; Weishaupt and coworkers, 1976; Buettner and Oberley, 1980). The application of this technique to lung carcinoma, chiefly in patients who are not candidates for other therapy, has been investigated at a number of centers, with encouraging results (Hayata and coworkers, 1982; Cortese and Kinsey, 1982). The possible use of photoradiation therapy for in situ carcinoma is exciting. Should hematoporphyrin derivative be used routinely in lung cancer patients undergoing surgery to detect other lesions of the tracheobronchial tree? Could hematoporphyrin derivative be used to check for tumor at resection margins? Are all lung cancers equally preferential in localizing hematoporphyrin derivative?

The definitive role of laser in thoracic surgery remains to be established. Its multiple uses and the applications that are currently being explored deserve watching and consideration by all thoracic surgeons. The following chapters describe how two institutions have found laser technology of benefit in a variety of thoracic problems.

The Use of Lasers for Tracheobronchial Lesions: Treatment of Obstructing Lesions by the Carbon Dioxide Laser

Richard B. McElvein, M.D.
George L. Zorn, Jr., M.D.

INDICATIONS FOR LASER THERAPY

Obstruction of the trachea and main-stem bronchi can be caused by a variety of benign and malignant diseases. Papillomas, granulation tissue, tracheal webs, and tracheal stenosis are all examples of such benign lesions. Primary malignant tumors of the trachea occur infrequently but primary pulmonary carcinoma is a relatively common cause of obstruction of the trachea and main-stem bronchi by direct involvement.

Prior to the introduction of lasers, these obstructing lesions were treated by other modalities, such as morcellation by biopsy forceps through a bronchoscope, electrocautery, cryotherapy, injection with sclerosing agents, injection with steroids, and dilatation. Each of these methods had its advantages and disadvantages, but in general they have been supplanted by the use of lasers.

SELECTION OF PATIENTS

The selection of patients who may benefit from CO_2 laser therapy should be based on the symptomatic presentation of respiratory tract obstruction in the trachea or main-stem bronchi demonstrated on chest x-ray films, conventional tomograms, endoscopy, or computed (axial) tomographic scans.

The ideal patient for CO_2 laser therapy is one who has symptomatic airway obstruction and, in the case of malignant disease, who has failed other therapy.[3] The lesion should protrude into the bronchial or tracheal lumen without obvious extension beyond the cartilage. The axial length of the endotracheal or endobronchial component should be less than 4 cm, and the lesion should be able to be visualized through a rigid bronchoscope. Ideally, there should be functioning lung tissue beyond the obstruction.

In practice, these ideal circumstances are infrequently encountered, but every effort using the methods described should be made to predetermine whether the treatment will be effective. In some cases in which it was impossible to predict the outcome, we nonetheless elected to use the laser and were pleasantly surprised at its ability to reopen an obstructed bronchus and provide symptomatic relief. Four patients, not included in our study, did not receive laser therapy because our evaluation indicated that therapy would be ineffective in opening the airway.

LASER CHARACTERISTICS

Laser is an acronym for *l*ight *a*mplification by *s*timulated *e*mission of *r*adiation. The concept was envisioned by Einstein about 1917; it remained for advances in mechanical, physical, electrical, and optical engineering to produce a functioning laser in the 1950s.

A wide variety of lasers is in use in both medicine and industry. The three lasers that are available for medical use are the carbon dioxide (CO_2), argon (Ar), and neodymium:yttrium aluminum garnet (Nd:YAG) lasers.[4]

The CO_2 laser, which is the instrument we used in our series, operates in the 10.6-μ range near the infrared spectrum. The beam can be passed in a straight line and reflected by means of mirrors; it is absorbed by water.

The Ar laser operates in the 0.5-μ range near the blue-green spectrum. Its beam can be passed through flexible fiberoptic bundles; it is absorbed in red tissues.

The Nd:YAG laser operates in the 1.06-μ range, which is near the infrared; the beam can be passed through flexible quartz fibers. Absorption is independent of tissue color.

Each of the lasers has a different absorption spectrum, power, and depth of penetration.

A laser beam can be visualized as a thermal beam that, when striking tissue, can be absorbed, reflected, scattered, or transmitted. The biologic effect of a laser is a function of the power of the laser, the duration of the impulse, the wavelength of the beam, and the power density developed by the lens system. The other elements of laser interaction with tissues are the physical properties of absorption, scatter, density, and thermal conductivity. A summation of these variables produces local tissue changes.

The production of a laser beam is based on the physical principle that molecules exist at a low energy level and can be stimulated by heat, light, or electricity to a higher energy level. This transient high energy level rapidly deteriorates to the low energy state with the release of photons. The photons are produced randomly, but in the case of the CO_2 laser, the photons strike a fully reflective mirror at one end and a partially reflective mirror at the other end, resulting in a laser beam (Fig. 37–1).

The CO_2 molecules are used to charge a cylinder that is activated by an electric current. The process is continuous as long as the electric current is applied and the cylinder is kept supplied with CO_2. The beam of coherent light contains a great deal of energy and can be transmitted by means of mirrors to the oper-

ating head of the bronchoscopic attachment, through which the beam can be directed at the obstructing lesion.

The CO_2 laser beam is absorbed in water and has a direct mechanical effect on tissues, with a resulting rise in temperature of the intracellular water to 100°C, which causes production of steam and disruption of cells. The rise in temperature also results in coagulation of proteins, which enhances destruction of the tissue.[5]

A CO_2 laser is hemostatic, and thus there is minimal bleeding with its use. Because of the sharp thermal drop-off from the edge of the beam to adjacent tissue, there is also minimal edema. The CO_2 laser beam has a shallow depth of penetration, 1 to 3 mm, and it will not penetrate the intact trachea or bronchi unless excessive power for prolonged periods of time is used. The laser treatment can be repeated without the risks typical of reoperation using other modalities, and there is no interference with other treatment for malignant lesions such as radiation therapy or chemotherapy administered either before or after the laser treatment. Because of the exquisite control possible with the laser beam as well as the sharp thermal drop-off, healing of the tissues is rapid. The shallow penetration allows the surgeon to remove only the involved tissues, thereby sparing underlying normal tissues.[6]

The disadvantages of a CO_2 laser include the necessity for direct vision of the lesion through a rigid bronchoscope. The shallow penetration of the CO_2 laser beam may require sequential application in order to achieve the desired result. General anesthesia is a necessity, but with the use of compressed air for ventilation administered through a Sanders ventilating bronchoscope, the risk of fire and hazard is minimal. The eyes of the patient and the personnel must be protected to avoid the possibility of concentration of stray laser beams in the eye, with subsequent retinal damage. Destruction of tissue results in particulate matter and smoke, but this is readily taken care of by the ventilating system. The instruments are expensive, but when they are shared with other surgeons, cost becomes an insignificant factor.[7]

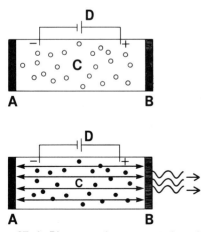

Figure 37–1. Diagrammatic representation of carbon dioxide laser. *A* = fully reflective mirror; *B* = partially reflective mirror; *C* = carbon dioxide molecules; *D* = electrical charge. *Top*, CO_2 molecules before activation; *bottom*, following activation by electrical current. (From McElvein RB: Laser endoscopy. Ann Thorac Surg 32:464, 1981.)

CLINICAL RESULTS

From May 28, 1979, to July 30, 1983, 89 patients received laser therapy for symptomatic respiratory tract obstruction at the University Hospitals, Birmingham, Alabama. These patients presented with perplexing clinical problems in a variety of forms that were treated or solved by the use of a carbon dioxide (CO_2) laser.[1,2]

Thirty-eight patients had benign lesions; 51 had malignant lesions. The youngest patient was 21 years of age, and the oldest was 72 years of age. There were 50 males and 39 females, who underwent from one to six therapeutic laser treatments of their obstructing lesion.

The results in the patients with benign lesions were uniformly good, except in certain patients with tracheal stenosis. Of our nine patients who received laser therapy for tracheal stenosis, five had a good result, but four required subsequent reconstruction. The stenosis in one of these patients remained refractory to therapy by any method. The poor results were related to disease causing specific pathologic changes in tracheal anatomy, as described in the following section.

The results in the patients with malignant disease were categorized into immediate and long-term results. Of the 51 patients, 46 had an immediate *good* result, defined as an improved airway at the completion of treatment, with partial or complete resolution of the clinical symptoms. An immediate poor result was defined as failure to improve the airway or death occurring shortly after treatment; five patients fit this category.

Long-term results in the patients with malignant lesions were judged according to an arbitrary survival period of 30 days following an initial (immediate) good response to treatment. Of these patients, 33 survived for at least 30 days and 18 for less than 30 days.

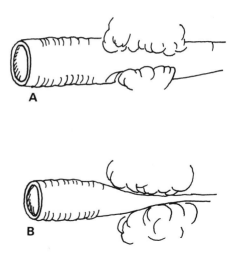

Figure 37–3. Bronchial lesions. *A,* Intrabronchial disease, amenable to laser treatment. *B,* Extrabronchial compression, not amenable to laser treatment.

CONCLUSIONS

Our experience with the CO_2 laser has led us to draw some general conclusions about the types of lesions most amenable to therapy and those not likely to respond favorably.

In patients with a tracheal stenosis or tracheal narrowing, if the lesion is composed of granulation tissue or a web with an intraluminal lesion, but with normal cartilaginous structures, then removal of the obstruction will result in an improved airway. However, if disease has caused disruption of the tracheal cartilages so that both the external and internal diameters of the trachea are narrowed, then removal of the obstructing lesion will result in destruction of a portion of the tracheal wall, with cicatrization and failure to relieve the obstruction on a permanent basis (Fig. 37–2).

We have also noted the problem of extrinsic compression of a main-stem bronchus by a tumor. By the same line of reasoning, if there is an intraluminal extension of the carcinoma into a main-stem bronchus, this lesion can be eradicated with the laser (Fig. 37–3). If, however, the tumor mass surrounds the bronchus and causes extrinsic compression and internal narrowing, then use of the laser will result in destruction of the bronchial wall with subsequent cicatrization and failure to improve the airway.

In summary, we have found a CO_2 laser attached to a rigid ventilating bronchoscope to be an effective tool for eradication of intraluminal tracheal and bronchial lesions, benign or malignant. Because of the advantages of minimal edema and bleeding, we have found

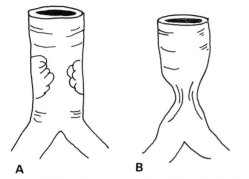

Figure 37–2. Tracheal lesions. *A,* Intraluminal disease, amenable to laser treatment. *B,* Stenosis, not amenable to laser treatment.

this to be superior to other methods. The treatment does not interfere with other therapy in the case of malignant disease, and we have found we have been able to provide an improved airway with a more comfortable existence for the patient so that additional therapy can be carried out.

References

1. McElvein RB: Laser endoscopy. Ann Thorac Surg 32:463–467, 1981.

2. McElvein RB, Zorn G: Treatment of malignant disease in trachea and main stem bronchi by carbon dioxide laser. J Thorac Cardiovasc Surg 86:858–862, 1983.

3. McDougall JC, Cortese DA: Neodymium-YAG laser therapy of malignant air obstruction. Mayo Clin Proc 58:35–39, 1983.

4. Minton JP, Ketcham AS: The laser, a unique oncolytic entity. Am J Surg 108:845–848, 1964.

5. Litwin MS, Glew DH: The biologic effects of laser radiation. JAMA 187:842–847, 1964.

6. McGuff PE, Deterling RA Jr, Gottlieb LS, et al: Surgical applications of laser. Ann Surg 160:765–777, 1964.

7. Strong MS, Vaughan CW, Polanyi T, Wallace R: Bronchoscopic carbon dioxide laser surgery. Ann Otol 83:769–776, 1974.

38

The Use of Lasers for Tracheobronchial Lesions: Utilization of Nd:YAG Lasers for Endobronchial Lesions

Michael Unger, M.D.
Grant V. S. Parr, M.D.
James Duckett, M.D.

Surgery by *laser* (*l*ight *a*mplification by *s*timulated *e*mission of *r*adiation) has become very much in vogue recently, and more and more specialties are finding applications for these new instruments. As with any new (and not so new) technique, controversies exist over the indications for and mode of utilization of the tool. The use of lasers for the treatment of endobronchial lesions is not exempt from these controversies.

TYPES OF LASERS: BIOPHYSICAL CHARACTERISTICS AND SPECIFIC USES

Whatever the specific therapeutic indications for the use of lasers, each type of laser produces different tissue reactions according to its specific biophysical characteristics.

Carbon Dioxide Laser

The carbon dioxide (CO_2) laser was the first to be used for the treatment of endobronchial lesions.[1] However, the mid-infrared wavelength (10,600 nm) beam of this laser cannot be safely transmitted through currently available fiberoptic bundles; moreover, its use requires cumbersome, articulated arms equipped with reflecting mirrors that must be manipulated through a specially coupled rigid bronchoscope. These drawbacks limit its utility in endoscopic procedures. On the other hand, the specific wavelength also determines the degree of biological response to the beam. In this spectrum the coefficient of absorption in water is very high, thus limiting penetration in depth. As a result, the CO_2 laser can be considered as an excellent cutter or "scalpel" in situations necessitating high precision and where the traditional instrument cannot be used safely.

Nd:YAG Laser

In contrast to that of the CO_2 laser, the beam of the Nd:YAG (neodymium:yttrium aluminum garnet) laser, with its near-infrared wavelength of 1060 nm, can be safely transmitted through fiberoptic light guides and has a much lower coefficient of absorption but a higher coefficient of scattering in the tissues.[2] This permits its use as an excellent in-depth coagulator and as a "hemostat" with a potential capacity to vaporize the tissues.

Argon Laser

The third type of laser with endobronchial application is the Argon (Ar) laser, with its beam in the visible spectrum and a wavelength in a range of 488 to 514 nm. This blue-green spectrum has a specific characteristic of high absorption by hemoglobin and thus is potentially useful for coagulation. Unfortunately, its penetration in nonpigmented tissue is shallow and not comparable to that of the Nd:YAG laser beam. The Ar laser also has been used as a pump laser for the rhodamine B dye for the early detection of carcinoma in situ and for its therapy.[3] This technique is based on utilization of various hematoporphyrin derivatives (HpD) or, more recently, dihematoporphyrin ether (DHE). These substances are photosensitizers producing stimulated singlet oxygen, which is cytotoxic.[4]

ENDOBRONCHIAL INDICATIONS FOR LASER THERAPY

The most common cause of a major endobronchial obstruction is a carcinoma. A less common cause of obstruction is benign tracheal strictures due to prolonged intubation or other traumas. Finally, various benign tumors may occasionally cause obstruction. We consider all these types of obstructions to be indications for laser therapy.

TECHNICAL CONSIDERATIONS

In our series of 175 patients and 446 procedures, we used the Nd:YAG laser (MediLas 2-MBB). The laser beam is transmitted via a fiberoptic light guide of 2.2-mm diameter. Since the Nd:YAG laser beam is in the invisible spectrum (1060 nm), precise aiming is facilitated by transmission through the same fibers of another low-power laser, the HeNe (helium–neon) laser, with a beam in the visible red spectrum (630-nm wavelength).

In contrast to the procedure reported by Dumon[5] and Toty[6] and their coworkers, who use the rigid scope, most of our procedures were done with the flexible fiberoptic bronchoscope (Olympus 1-TR) under topical anesthesia only (Table 38–1).[7] In cases where rapid and significant mechanical debulking was to be done, the rigid (Storz) bronchoscope was used after prior in-depth coagulation with the Nd:YAG laser; in these cases, general anesthesia was employed. One of the initial problems associated with the use of the rigid scope was the necessity for periods of hypoventilation during the procedure. This was overcome, however, with adaptation of the ventilatory technique utilizing the Sanders injector.[8, 9]

Table 38–1. Frequency of Use of Flexible Fiberoptic and Rigid Bronchoscopes in Nd:YAG Laser Therapy[a]

Instrument	No. of Patients	No. of Sessions
Flexible fiberoptic bronchoscope	142	407
Rigid bronchoscope	33	39
Total	175	446

[a]From Unger M, Atkinson GW: Nd:YAG laser applications in pulmonary and endobronchial lesions. In Joffe SN (ed): Neodymium-YAG Laser in Medicine and Surgery. New York, Elsevier, 1983, pp. 71–82.

Table 38–2. Histologic Diagnosis in 175 Patients Undergoing Laser Therapy for Endobronchial Lesions

Endobronchial Lesion	No. of Patients
Malignant	
Primary lung malignancies	
Epidermoid	94
Undifferentiated or mixed type	13
Adenocarcinoma	9
Adenoid cystic carcinoma	1
Hemangiopericytoma	1
Lymphoepithelioma	1
Carcinoid tumor	3
Metastatic cancer to the lung	
Renal cell carcinoma	8
GI tract carcinoma	5
Thyroid cancer	4
Breast cancer	3
Larynx cancer	2
Endometrial cancer	2
Melanoma	2
Hodgkin's lymphoma	2
Lymphosarcoma	1
Sarcoma	1
Benign	
Tracheobronchial granuloma or stenosis	19
Lipoma	1
Hamartoma	1
Sarcoidosis	1
Foreign body	1

CLINICAL FINDINGS

Diagnosis at Referral

Of our 175 patients, 147 had endobronchial or endotracheal malignant tumors no longer amenable to surgical procedures. Most of these patients were referred to us for "last resort" therapy by laser after all other applicable therapeutic modalities had been exhausted. In 94 of the 147 patients, the histologic diagnosis was consistent with epidermoid carcinoma, creating the major histologic group. Other primary lung neoplasms treated were 13 undifferentiated and 9 adenocarcinomas. Unusual primary lesions included three carcinoid tumors, one adenoid cystic carcinoma, one lymphoepithelioma, and one hemangiopericytoma. Metastatic lesions to the tracheobronchial tree were treated in 30 patients and included renal cell carcinoma, gastrointestinal tract carcinomas, and cancers of the thyroid, breast, larynx, and endometrium as well as melanomas, Hodgkin's lymphomas, lymphosarcomas, and sarcomas.

Benign tumors in our series included tracheobronchial granulomas or fibrotic stenosis, sarcoidosis, lymphoma, hamartoma, and foreign body (Table 38–2).

Location of Tumor

From the anatomic standpoint, a large majority of the tumors in our patients were localized to the trachea, the carina, and the major right and left bronchi. More peripheral lesions were treated by laser only in cases of severe respiratory impairment, intractable hemoptysis, or post-obstructive pneumonia with possible abscess refractory to other therapy.

RESULTS

In our 86 patients in whom laser therapy resulted in an excellent response, there was complete re-establishment of the obstructed airway lumen, with corresponding significant clinical improvement. For example, in one patient in whom total endobronchial obstruction with atelectasis was caused by a recurrent epidermoid carcinoma after right upper lobectomy (Fig. 38–1A), treatment with the Nd:YAG laser produced marked clinical improvement following reopening of the right main-stem bronchus and reaeration of the remaining right lower lobe (Fig. 38–1B). Laser therapy was also successful in the patient with endobronchial carcinoid tumor, a young man who had adamantly refused any other definitive surgical procedure.

As our numbers indicate (446 laser sessions in 175 patients), some of the patients necessi- tated more than one therapeutic laser session, and several among them had additional laser treatments at intervals of several months. For example, one of our patients was a 78-year-old man with squamous cell carcinoma causing severe obstruction of the trachea, the carina, and the left main-stem bronchus. The obstruction was successfully relieved following four sessions of laser therapy. The patient returned 4½ months later for another series of three sessions because of recurrence of the tumor; once more he left the hospital with significant reduction of the obstructing mass. He was not seen for an additional 2½ months, at which time two additional sessions of Nd:YAG therapy were given with only a fair response; however, he was still able to return to his family in stable condition.

In another group of 50 patients, laser therapy re-established the lumen only partially, but with complete hemostasis and some measurable clinical improvement. However, one patient with tracheal stenosis, a 14-year-old girl, eventually required tracheoplasty for relief of her symptoms. In a third group of 15 patients, in spite of complete hemostasis and debulking, the lumen could not be re-established. In these cases, there was generally complete obstruction of a major bronchi.

Less than optimal results reflect in large part our cautious approach to lesions in anatomic proximity to major pulmonary vessels, particularly in the area of the left main and left

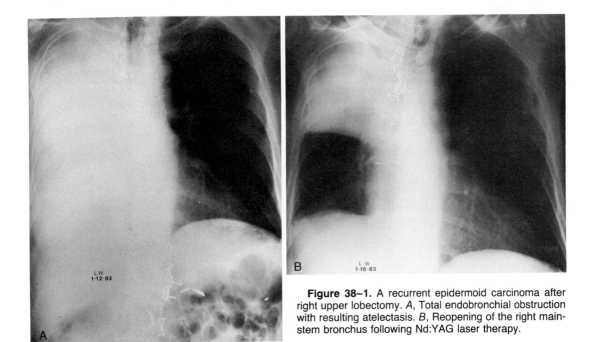

Figure 38–1. A recurrent epidermoid carcinoma after right upper lobectomy. *A,* Total endobronchial obstruction with resulting atelectasis. *B,* Reopening of the right main-stem bronchus following Nd:YAG laser therapy.

upper lobe bronchi. Moreover, in some cases the risk of significant distortion of normal pulmonary anatomy as a result of atelectasis and mediastinal shifts dictated a decision against completion of therapy. One of our patients was a 70-year-old man who was referred to us with hemoptysis and complete atelectasis of the left lung due to left mainstem obstruction by a squamous cell carcinoma. One laser therapy session was attempted with poor results. The bleeding was stopped, but the bronchial lumen could not be restored. However, at the same time, a left pulmonary angiogram showed significant vascular involvement by the tumor with very poor perfusion in this area. On this basis, we decided not to proceed with further laser therapy since it could not be justified on the physiologic basis.

COMPLICATIONS

In the experience of most clinicians utilizing the laser technique in endobronchial therapy, the most frequent complication cited was bleeding.[10] We seem to be more fortunate in this aspect and recorded only one episode of perioperative hemorrhage, with blood loss of about 100 ml. We attribute this low rate in part to the cautious technique of careful coagulation prior to ablation and vaporization; however, there was one episode of delayed catastrophic hemoptysis occurring 6 days after initial treatment. Autopsy revealed that as part of the tumor involvement and destruction, the pulmonary artery had come to lie in the bronchial wall. Incidental laser beam pulses had produced necrosis of the wall of the pulmonary artery, which eventually resulted in the delayed rupture and the fatal hemoptysis.

Another delayed death was not directly related to the laser treatment but rather was due to an unusual terminal alveolar block as a result of extrusion of necrotic tumor material after extensive laser therapy. In our series there was also one case of infection, despite successful reopening of the right upper lobe bronchus, related to post-obstructive abscess, which then spread to the lower lobes. Although we are aware of documented episodes of endobronchial combustion of the fiberoptic bronchoscope,[11] we did not encounter this potentially very serious complication in our experience in spite of the fact that most of our procedures were done with this instrument.

However, the possibility of this complication may influence the choice of the rigid over the flexible fiberoptic bronchoscope because the rigid metallic bronchoscope will not burn!

CONCLUSION

The classical surgical tools, the scalpel and the hemostat, have a new variation in the form of lasers. It should be understood that this new modality is not a replacement for the well-proved older techniques, but that lasers can be used successfully in conjunction with traditional instruments after careful study of the biophysical interaction characteristic of each laser type. In certain circumstances, however, such as in endobronchial obstruction in a patient unable to undergo a more traditional surgical procedure, utilization of lasers can achieve remarkable results. The curative techniques, employing dye lasers, deserve further study; however, the palliative aspect of removal of the obstruction with the help of the Nd:YAG laser is now well established. The overall statistics of cancer mortality for the time being most probably will not be affected; however, in certain cancer patients, laser therapy can provide much improved comfort and some prolongation of a useful life.

References

1. LaForet EG, Berger RL, Vaughan CW: Carcinoma obstructing the trachea. Treatment by laser resection. N Engl J Med 294:941, 1976.
2. Halldorsson T, Rother W, Langerholc FF Jr: Theoretical and experimental investigations prove Nd:YAG laser treatment to be safe. Proceedings of the International Medical Laser Symposium, Detroit, 1979.
3. Cortese DE, Kinsey JH: Endoscopic management of lung cancer with hematoporphyrium derivative phototherapy. Mayo Clin Proc 55:543–547, 1982.
4. Dogherty TJ, Kufman JH, Goldfarb A, et al: Photoradiation therapy for the treatment of malignant tumors. Cancer Res 38:2628–2635, 1978.
5. Dumon TF, Reboud E, Garbe L, et al: Treatment of tracheobronchial lesion by laser photoresection. Chest 81:278–284, 1982.
6. Toty L, Personne C, Colchen A, Vourc'h G: Bronchoscopic management of tracheal lesions using the Nd:YAG laser. Thorax 36:175–178, 1981.
7. Unger M, Atkinson GW: Nd:YAG laser applications in pulmonary and endobronchial lesions. In Joffe SN (ed): Neodymium-YAG Laser in Medicine and Surgery. New York, Elsevier, 1983, pp. 71–82.
8. Duckett JE, McDonnell TJ, Unger M, Parr GVS: General anaesthesia for Nd:YAG laser resection of obstructing endobrachial tumours using the rigid bronchoscope. Can Anes Soc J 32:67–72, 1985.

9. Parr GVS, Unger M, Trout R, Atkinson GW: One hundred neodymium-YAG laser ablations of obstructing tracheal neoplasms. Ann Thor Surg 38:374–381, 1984.

10. Dumon JF, Bourcereau J, Meric B, Aucomte F: Report of 1000 YAG laser endobronchial resections. In Joffe SN (ed): Neodymium-YAG Laser in Medicine and Surgery. New York, Elsevier, 1983, pp. 59–70.

11. Casey KR, Fairfax WF, Smith SJ, Dixon JA: Intratracheal fire ignited by the Nd:YAG laser during treatment of tracheal stenosis. Chest 84:295–296, 1983.

Section References

References for Section I: The Management of Zenker's Diverticulum

Bevan AD: Pulsion diverticulum of the esophagus: Cure by the Sippy-Bevan operation. Surg Clin N Am 1:449, 1917.

Girard C: Du traitement des diverticules de l'oesophage. Cong Franc Chir 392, 1896.

Goldmann EE: Die zweizeitige Operation von Pulsionsdivertikeln der Speiseröhre. Beitr klin Chir 61:741, 1909.

Hill W: Pharyngeal pouch treated by diverticulo-pexy. Proc Roy Soc Med, Sect Laryngol 11:60, 1918.

Jackson C: Oesophagoscopic observations, p. 2. In Jackson C and Shallow TA: Diverticula of the oesophagus, pulsion, traction, malignant and congenital. Ann Surg 83:1, 1926.

Jackson C: Peroral Endoscopy and Laryngeal Surgery. St. Louis, Mo., 1915.

Ludlow A: A case of obstructed deglutition, from a preternatural dilatation of, and bag formed in, the pharynx; in a letter from Mr. Ludlow, surgeon, at Bristol, to Dr. William Hunter. Read Aug. 27, 1764. Med Obs Inq 3:85, 1767.

Mosher HP: Webs and pouches of the oesophagus, their diagnosis and treatment. Surg Gynecol Obstet 25:175, 1917.

Nicoladoni K: Ein Beitrag zur operativen Behandlung der Oesophagusdivertikel. Wien Med Wchnschr 27:605; 654, 1877.

Niehans: Described by Girard (1896), p. 400.

Schmid HH: Vorschlag eines einfachen Operationsverfahrens zur Behandlung des Oesophagusdivertikels. Wien klin Wchnschr 25:487, 1912.

Wheeler WI: Pharyngocele and dilatation of pharynx, with existing diverticulum at lower portion of pharynx lying posterior to the esophagus, cured by pharyngotomy, being the first case of the kind recorded. Dublin J Med Sci 32:349, 1886.

Zenker FA, von Ziemssen H: Krankheiten des Oesophagus. 49–87. In Handbuch der Speciellen Pathologie und Therapie. Leipzig, F. C. W. Vogel, Vol. 7, 1877.

References for Section II: The Surgical Management of Recurrent or Persistent Pneumothorax

Bigger IA: Cited in Tyson MD, and Crandall WB: The surgical treatment of recurrent idiopathic spontaneous pneumothorax. J Thorac Surg 10:566, 1941.

Dominy DE, Campbell DC Jr: Surgically correctable acquired cystic disease of the lung as seen in flying personnel. Dis Chest 43:240, 1963.

Forlanini C: A contribuzione della terapia chirurgica della tizi, ablazione del polmone? pneumotorace artificiale? Gaz. d. Osp. Milano 3:537, 585, 601, 609, 617, 625, 641, 657, 665, 689, 705, 1882.

Hewson W: The operation of the paracentesis thoracis proposed for air in the chest; with some remarks on the emphysema, and on wounds of the lungs in general; by William Hewson, reader of anatomy. Communicated by Dr. Hunter. Read June 15, 1767. Med Obs Inq III, 372, 1767.

Itard JE: Sur le pneumo-thoraz on les congestions gazeuses qui se forment dans la poitrine. Dissertation, Paris, 1803.

Laennec RTH: De l'Auscultation Médiate. Paris, J. A. Brosson et J. S. Chaudé, 2 vols., 1819.

Lockwood: Discussion, on p. 438 in Watson EE, Robertson C: Recurrent spontaneous pneumothorax. Report of three cases. Arch Surg 16:431, 1928.

Martin EW: A case of pneumothorax shown by the roentgen rays. Lancet 2:846, 1901.

Miller WS: Human pleura pulmonalis, its relation to blebs and bullae of emphysema. AJR 15:399, 1926.

Spengler L: Zur Chirurgie des Pneumothorax. Beitr klin Chir 49:68, 1906.

Tyson MD, Crandall WB: The surgical treatment of recurrent idiopathic spontaneous pneumothorax. J Thorac Surg 10:566, 1941.

References for Section III: Malignant Pleural Mesothelioma

Cooke WE: Fibrosis of the lungs due to the inhalation of asbestos dust. Br Med J 2:147, 1924.

Cooke WE: Pulmonary asbestosis. Br Med J 2:1024, 1927.

Klemperer P, Rabin CB: Primary neoplasms of the pleura. Arch Pathol 11:385, 1931.

Law R, Gregor A, Hodson ME, et al: Malignant mesothelioma of the pleura: A study of 52 treated and 64 untreated patients. Thorax 39:255, 1984.

Mallory TB, Castleman B, Parris EE: Case records of the Massachusetts General Hospital. N Engl J Med 236:407, 1947.

Murray HM: Report Dept. Comm. on Compensation for Industrial Diseases. London, H.M.S.O., 34:3495, 1907.

Wagner JC: Experimental production of mesothelial tumours of the pleura by implantation of dusts in laboratory animals. Nature 196:180, 1962.

Wagner JC, Sleggs CA, Marchand P: Diffuse pleural mesothelioma and asbestos exposure in the North Western Cape Province. Br J Industr Med 17:260, 1960.

Weiss A: Pleurakrebs bei Lungenasbestose, in vivo morphologisch gesichert. Medizinische 3:93, 1953.

Willis RA, Willis AT: Principles of Pathology and Bacteriology. London, Butterworths, 1972, p. 532.

Woolley PG: A primary carcinomatoid tumor (mesothelioma) of the adrenals, with sarcomatous metastases. Trans Assoc Am Physicians 17:627, 1902.

References for Section IV: Needle Biopsy for the Diagnosis of Intrathoracic Lesions

Craver LF, Binkley JS: Aspiration biopsy of tumors of the lung. J Thorac Surg 8:436, 1938–39.

Forkner CE: Material from lymph nodes of man. I. Method to obtain material by puncture of lymph nodes for study with supravital and fixed stains. Arch Int Med 40:532, 1927.

Greig EDW, Gray ACH: Note on the lymphatic glands in sleeping sickness. Lancet 1:1570, 1904; Br Med J 1:1252, 1904.

Guthrie CG: Gland puncture as a diagnostic measure. Johns Hopkins Hosp Bull 32:266, 1921.

Kato H, Ono J, Niizuma M, et al: Transbronchofiberscopic aspiration biopsy using a special catheter. Jap J Thorac Dis 16:774, 1978; see also Kato H, Konaka C, Ono J, Takahashi M, Hayata Y: Cytology of the Lung. Techniques and Interpretation. Tokyo, Igaku-Shoin, 1983.

Leyden: Ueber infectiöse Pneumonie. VII. Verhandlungen des Vereins für innere Medicin. Deutsche Med Wchnschr 9:52, 1883.

Martin HE, Ellis EB: Biopsy by needle puncture and aspiration. Ann Surg 92:169, 1930.

Ménétrier P: Cancer primitif du poumon. Bull Soc Anat (Paris) 11:643, 1886.

Sappington SW, Favorite GO: Lung puncture in lobar pneumonia. Am J Med Soc 191:225, 1936.

Swierenga J, Versteegh RM: Trans-bronchiale punctiebiopsie. Ned Tijdschr Geneeskunde 100:2364, 1956.

Versteegh RM, Swierenga J: Bronchoscopic evaluation of the operability of pulmonary carcinoma. Acta Oto-Laryngol 56:603, 1963.

Ward GR: Bedside Hematology, p. 129. Philadelphia, WB Saunders Co., 1914.

White WC, Pröscher F: Spirochetes in acute lymphatic leukemia and in chronic benign lymphomatosis (Hodgkin's disease). JAMA 49:1115, 1907.

White WC, Proescher F: Experimental lymphatic spirillosis in guinea-pigs. JAMA 49:1988, 1907.

References for Section V: Thoracoscopy

Bloomberg AE: Thoracoscopy in perspective. Surg Gynecol Obstet 147:433, 1978.

Bozzini P: Der Lichtleiter oder Beschreibung einer einfachen Vorrichtung und ihrer Anwendung zur Erleuchtung innerer Höhlen und Zwischenräume des lebended animalischen Körpers. Weimar, 1807.

Brandt HJ, Loddenkemper R, Mai J: Atlas der diagnostichen Thorakoskopie. New York, Georg Thieme, 1983.

Brück: Das Uretroscop und das Stomatoscop zur Durchleuchtung der Blase und der Zahne und ihrer Nachbartheile durch Galvanisches Gluhlicht. Breslau, 1867.

Desormeaux AJ: De l'endoscope et de ses applications des affections de l'urethre et de la vessie. Paris, J.-B. Baillière et Fils, 1865.

Desormeaux AJ: Bull Acad Med, 1853; Quoted in Desormeaux, 1865.

Fisher J: Instruments for illuminating dark cavities. Phil J Med Phys Sciences 14:409, 1827.

Jacobeus HC: Endopleurale Operationen unter der Leitung des Thorakoskops. Beitr Klin Tuberk 1–35, 1916.

Jacobeus HC: The practical importance of thoracoscopy in surgery of the chest. Surg Gynecol Obstet 34:289, 1922.

Jacobeus HC: Ueber die Möglichkeit die Zystoskopie bei Untersuchung seröser Höhlungen anzuwenden. Muench Med Wchnschr 4:2090, 1910.

Kelling: Cited by Unverricht: Die Thorakoskopie und Laparoskopie. Klin Wchnschr 2:502, 1923.

Leiter J: Protokoll der Sitsung vom 29, Jäanner 1886. Anz. k.k. Gesselschaft der Aertze in Wein, 11 Feb. 1886, p. 36.

Newman D: On malpositions of the kidney. Glasgow Med J II:81, 1883, p. 132.

Nitze M: Eine neue Beobachtungs- und Untersuchungsmethode für Harnröhre, Harnblase und Rectum. Wien med Wchnschr 5:649; 713; 806; 779, 1879.

Nitze M: Lehrbuch der Kystoskopie. Ihre Technik und Klinische Bedeutung. Von Bergmann, Wiesbaden, 1889.

Ségalas: Cited by Fisher, 1827, p. 409: "On the 11th of December, 1826, M. Segalas exhibited to the Royal Academy of Sciences of France, an instrument for illuminating the urethra and bladder, which he calls the Speculum urethro-cystique."

Unverricht: Die Thorakoskopie und Laparoscopie. Klin Wchnschr 2:502, 1923.

References for Section VI: The Use of Radionuclide Scans in Lung Cancer

Anger HO: Scintillation camera. Rev Sci Instrumen 21:27, 1958.

Baumann E: Über das normale Vorkommen von Jod in Thierkörper. Ztschr physiol Chem 21:319, 1895–1896.

Blumgart HL, Yens OC: Studies on the velocity of blood flow. I. The method utilized. J Clin Invest 4:1, 1927.

Blumgart HL, Weiss S: Studies on the velocity of blood flow. II. The velocity of blood flow in normal resting individuals, and a critique of the method used. J Clin Invest 4:15, 1927.

Blumgart HL, Weiss S: Studies on the velocity of blood flow. III. The velocity of blood flow and its relation to other aspects of the circulation in patients with rheumatic and syphilitic heart disease. J Clin Invest 4:149, 1927.

Blumgart HL, Weiss S: Studies on the velocity of blood flow. IV. The velocity of blood flow and its relation to other aspects of the circulation in patients with arteriosclerosis and in patients with arterial hypertension. J Clin Invest 4:173, 1927.

Blumgart HL, Weiss S: Studies on the velocity of blood flow. V. The physiological and the pathologic significance of the velocity of blood flow. J Clin Invest 199, 1927.

Blumgart HL, Weiss S: Studies on the velocity of blood flow. VI. The method of collecting the active deposit of radium and its preparation for intravenous injection. J Clin Invest 4:389, 1927.

Blumgart HL, Weiss S: Studies on the velocity of blood flow. VII. The pulmonary circulation time in normal resting individuals. J Clin Invest 4:399, 1927.

Blumgart HL, Weiss S: Studies on the velocity of blood flow. VIII. The velocity of blood flow and its relation to other aspects of the circulation in patients with pulmonary emphysema. J Clin Invest 4:555, 1927.

Curie P, Curie MS: Sur une substance nouvelle radioactive contenue dans la pechblende. Compt Rend Acad Sci 127:173, 1898.

Hertz S, Roberts A, Evans RD: Radioactive iodine as an indicator in the study of thyroid physiology. Proc Soc Exp Biol Med 38:510, 1938.

Hevesy G: Absorption and translocation of lead by plants. Biochem J 17:439, 1923.

Lawrence J: Described in Myers WG, Wagner HN Jr: How it began. In Wagner HN Jr (Ed): Nuclear Medicine. New York, H. P. Publishing Co., 1975, p. 8.

Science: Availability of radioactive isotopes. Announcement from headquarters. Manhattan Project, Washington, D.C. Science: 103:697, 1946.

Seidlin, Marinelli, and Oshry: Described in Myers WG, Wagner HN Jr: How it began. In Wagner HN Jr (Ed): Nuclear Medicine. New York, H. P. Publishing Co., 1975, p. 9.

References for Section VII: Mediastinoscopy in Lung Cancer

Bricker EM, Modlin J: Role of pelvic evisceration in surgery. Surgery 30:76, 1951.

Carlens E: A method for inspection and tissue biopsy in the superior mediastinum. Dis Chest 36:343, 1959.

Daniels AC: A method of biopsy useful in diagnosing certain intrathoracic diseases. Dis Chest 16:360, 1949.

Eiselsberg: Discussion in Marschik (1919).

Haagensen CD: Diseases of the Breast. Philadelphia, W. B. Saunders Co., 1956, p. 660.

Harken DE, Black H, Clauss R, Farrand RE: A simple cervicomediastinal exploration for tissue diagnosis of intrathoracic disease. N Engl J Med 251:1041, 1954.

Heidenhain L: Ueber einen Fall von Mediastinitis suppurativa postica nebst Bemerkungen über die Wege, ins hintere Mediastinum einzudringen. Arch klin Chir 59:199, 1899.

Marschik H: Die Mediastinostomie. Wien klin Chir 32:103, 1919.

Marschik H: Zur Behandlung der Halsschüsse. Wien klin Chir 29:805, 1916.

Marschik H: Zur Geschichte der Mediastinostomie. Wien klin Chir 53:360, 1940.

Mihaljevic C: Erfahrungen bei 500 lateralen Mediastinoskopien. Ztschr Tuberk 128:34, 1968.

Milton H: Mediastinal surgery. Lancet 1:872, 1897.

Rasumowski: Described by von Hacker: Zur operativen Behandlung der perioesophagealen und mediastinalen Phlegmone nebst Bemerkungen zur Technik der collaren und dorsalen Mediastinostomie. Arch klin Chir 64:478, 1901.

Specht, G: Erweiterte Mediastinoskopie. Thoraxchir 13:401, 1965.

Storey CF, Reynolds BM: Biopsy techniques in the diagnosis of intrathoracic lesions. Dis Chest 23:357, 1953.

Steele JD, Marable SA: Cervical mediastinotomy for biopsy. J Thorac Surg 37:621, 1959.

Weber W: Hiloskopie—eine Methode in der thorakalen Differentialdiagnostick. Prax Pneumol 22:79, 1968.

References for Section VIII: The Extent of Resection for Localized Lung Cancer

Aeby C: Der Bronchialbaum de Säugetiere und des Menschen. Leipzig, 1880.

Archibald E: The technic of total unilateral pneumonectomy. Ann Surg 100:796, 1934.

Belcher JR: Thirty years of surgery for carcinoma of the bronchus. Thorax 38:428, 1983.

Block: Experimentelles zur Lungenresection. Deutsche Med Wchnschr 7:634, 1881.

Bowman AK: The Life and Teaching of Sir William Macewen; A Chapter in the History of Surgery. London, 1942.

Brewer LA, III: The first pneumonectomy. Historical notes. J Thorac Cardiovasc Surg 88:810, 1984, p. 820.

Churchill ED, Belsey R: Segmental pneumonectomy in bronchiectasis. The lingula segment of the left upper lobe. Ann Surg 109:481, 1939.

Ewart W: The bronchi and pulmonary blood vessels: their anatomy and nomenclature; with a criticism of Professor Aeby's views on the bronchial tree of mammalia and of man. London, Baillière, Tindall, & Cox, 1889, p. 65.

Gluck T: Experimenteller Beitrag zur Frage der Lungenexstirpation. Berlin klin Wschr 18:645, 1881.

Graham EA, Singer JJ: Successful removal of an entire lung for carcinoma of the bronchus. JAMA 101:1371, 1933.

Kramer R, Glass A: Bronchoscopic localization of lung abscess. Ann Otol Rhinol Laryngol 41:1210, 1932.

Macewen W: The Cavendish lecture on some points in the surgery of the lung. Br Med J 2:1, 1906.

Murphy JB: Surgery of the lung. JAMA 31:151; 31:208; 31:281; 31:341, 1898.

Nissen R: Exstirpation eines ganzen Lungenflügels. Zentralbl Chir 58:3003, 1931.

Ochsner A, DeBakey M: Primary pulmonary malignancy. Treatment by total pneumonectomy. Analysis of 79 collected cases and presentation of 7 personal cases. Surg Gynecol Obstet 68:435, 1939, p. 446.

Paget S: The Surgery of the Chest. Bristol, John Wright & Co., 1896, p. 458.

Rienhoff WF Jr: Pneumonectomy. A preliminary report of the operative technique in two successful cases. Bull Johns Hopkins Hosp 53:390, 1933.

Rienhoff WF Jr: The present status of the surgical treatment of primary carcinoma of the lung. JAMA 126:1123, 1944, p. 1128.

References for Section IX: New Anesthetic Techniques for Intrathoracic Operations

Lunkenheimer PP, Rafflenbeul W, Keller H, et al: Application of transtracheal pressure oscillations as modification of "diffusion respiration." Br J Anesth 44:627, 1972.

Öberg PA, Sjöstrand U: Studies of blood pressure regulation. Common carotid artery clamping in studies of carotid sinus baroreceptor control of the systemic blood pressure. Acta Physiol Scand 75:276, 1969.

Slutsky AS, Brown R, Lehr J, Rossing T, Drazen JM: High-frequency ventilation: A promising new approach to mechanical ventilation. Med Instrum 15:229, 1981.

Sykes MK: Editorial. High frequency ventilation. Thorax 40:161, 1985.

Tuffier et Hallion: Opérations intrathoraquies avec respiration artificielle par insufflation. Compt Rend Soc Biol 48:951, 1896.

Tuffier et Hallion: Etude expérimentale sur la chirurgie du poumon. Sur les effets circulatoires de la respiration artificielle par insufflation et de l'insufflation maintenue du poumon. Compt Rend Soc Biol 48:1047, 1896.

References for Section X: Management of Postoperative Thoracotomy Pain

Adams RC, Lundy JS, Seldon TH: Continuous caudal anesthesia or analgesia. A consideration of the technic, various uses and some possible dangers. JAMA 122:152, 1943.

Bier A: Versuche über Cocainisirung des Rückenmarkes. Deutsche Zent Chir 51:361, 1899.

Braun H: Ueber neue örtliche Anaesthetica. (Stovain, Alypin, Novocain). Deutsche Med Wchnschr 31:1667, 1905.

Cathelin F: Une nouvelle voie d'injection rachidienne. Méthode des injections épidurales par le procédé du canal sacré. Applications a l'homme. Compt Rend Soc 53:452, 1901.

Corning JL: Spinal anesthesia and local medication of the cord. NY Med J 42:483, 1885.

Dean HP: Discussion on the relative value of inhalation and injection methods of inducing anesthesia. Br Med J 2:869, 1907.

Dogliotti AM: A new method of block anesthesia. Segmental peridural spinal anesthesia. Am J Surg 20:107, 1933.

Dogliotti AM: Eine neue Methode der regionären Anästhesie: Die peridurale segmentäre Anästhesie. Zent Chir 50:3141, 1931.

Einhorn A: See Braun, 1905, p. 1669.

Freud S: Über Coca. Zent Ges Ther 2:289, 1884.

Halsted WS: Practical comments on the use and abuse of cocaine. NY Med J 42:294, 1885. (See also Hall RJ: Hydrochlorate of cocaine. NY Med J 40:643, 1884.)

Heile B: Der epidurale Raum. Arch klin Chir 101:845, 1913.

Irving FR: An improvement in catheter technic for continuous caudal anesthesia. JAMA 122:1181, 1943.

Koller K: Uber die Verwendung des Cocain zur Anasthesirung am Auge. Wien Med Blatter 7:1352, 1884.

Läwen A: Uber Extraduralanästhesie fur chirurgische Operationen. Ztschr Chir 1081, 1911.

Lemmon WT: A method for continuous spinal anesthesia. Ann Surg 111:141, 1940.

Love JG: Continuous subarachnoid drainage for meningitis by means of a ureteral catheter. JAMA 104:1595, 1935.

Manalan SA: Caudal block anesthesia in obstetrics. J Ind State Med Assoc 35:564, 1942.

Moréno T: In De Jong RH: Local Anesthetics, 2nd ed. Springfield, Charles C Thomas, 1977, p. 4.

(Niemann A): Ueber eine organische Base in der Coca. Justus Liebig's Ann Chem Pharm 114:216, 1860.

Pagés F: Anestesia metamerica. Rev Sanid Mil Madr 11:351, 385, 1921.

Sicard A: Les injections medicamenteuses extra-durales par vois sacro-coccygienne. Compt Rend Soc Biol 53:396, 1901.

Tuffier: Analgésie chirurgicale par l'injection sous arachnoïdienne lombaire de cocaïne. Compt Rend Soc Biol 51:882, 1899.

Tuffier: Analgésie cocaïnique par voie extradurale. Compt Rend Soc Biol 53:490, 1901.

Tuohy EB: Continuous spinal anesthesia: A new method utilizing a ureteral catheter. Surg Clin N Am 25:834, 1945.

References for Section XI: Muscle Flaps and Thoracic Problems

Abrashanoff: Plastiche Methode der Schlieszung vom Fistelgängen welche von inneren Organen kommen. Zentrbl Chir 38:186, 1911.

Antony M: Case of extensive Caries of the fifth and sixth Ribs, and disorganization of the greater part of the right lobe of Lungs, with a description of the operation for the same, &c. Phil J Med Phys Sciences 6:108, 1823.

'B.L.': Editorial reprinted from Phil Med Museum 2:343, 1806, citing the Bombay Courier for April 4, 1795. See further description in McDowell F: The Source Book of Plastic Surgery. Baltimore, The Williams & Wilkins Company, 1977, pp. 65–88.

Eggers C: The treatment of bronchial fistulae. Ann Surg 72:345, 1920.

Halsted AE, Thurston HF: The treatment of bronchial fistulas. Report of a case. JAMA 88:689, 1927.

Kanavel AB: Plastic procedures for the obliteration of cavities with non-collapsible walls. Surg Gynecol Obstet 32:453, 1921.

Kiricuta J: Use of the Omentum in Plastic Surgery. Oxford, Pergamon Press, 1980.

Pool EH, Garlock JH: A treatment of persistent bronchial fistula. Ann Surg 90:213, 1929.

Richérand LC: Histoire d'une résection des côtes et de la plèvre. Lue à l'Académie Royale des Sciences de l'Institut de France, le Lundi 27 Avril 1818, Paris. Paris, Caille et Ravier, 1818.

Taliacotii (Tagliacozzi), G: De Curtorum Chirurgia per insitionem. Venetiis, Apud Gasparem Bindonum iuniorem, MDXCVII.

Wangensteen OH: The pedicled muscle flap in the closure of persistent bronchopleural fistula. J Thorac Surg 5:27, 1935–36.

References for Section XII: The Management of Massive Hemoptysis

Alexander J: The Surgery of Pulmonary Tuberculosis. Philadelphia, Lea & Febiger, 1925.

Calmette A: Tubercle Bacillus Infection and Tuberculosis in Man and Animal. Tr by W. Soper and G. H. Smith. Baltimore, Williams & Wilkins, 1923, p. 191.

Cudkowicz L: The blood supply of the lung in pulmonary tuberculosis. Thorax 7:270, 1952.

Ehrenhaft JL, Taber RE: Management of massive hemoptysis, not due to pulmonary tuberculosis or neoplasm. J Thorac Surg 30:275, 1955.

Eloesser L: Observations on sources of pulmonary hemorrhage and attempts at its control. J Thorac Surg 7:671, 1938.

Fearn SW: Aneurism of the pulmonary artery. Lancet 1:679, 1841.

Gerstl B, Weidman WH, Newman AV: Pulmonary aspergillosis: Report of two cases. Ann Int Med 28:662, 1942.

Jewkes J, Kay PH, Paneth M, Citron KM: Pulmonary aspergilloma: Analysis of prognosis in relation to haemoptysis and survey of treatment. Thorax 38:572, 1983.

Liebow AA, Hales MR, Lindskog GE: Enlargement of the bronchial arteries, and their anastomoses with the pulmonary arteries in bronchiectasis. Am J Pathol 25:211, 1949.

Pitkin CE: Repeated severe hemoptysis necessitating pneumonectomy. Ann Otol Rhinol Laryngol 50:914, 1941.

Rafferty P, Biggs B, Crompton GK, Grant IWB: What happens to patients with pulmonary aspergilloma? Analysis of 23 cases. Thorax 38:579, 1983.

Rasmussen V: On hoemoptysis, especially when fatal, in its anatomical and clinical aspects. Edinburgh Med J 14:385; 486, 1868.

Ross CA: Emergency pulmonary resection for massive hemoptysis in tuberculosis. J Thorac Surg 26:435, 1953.

Ryan TC, Lineberry WT Jr: Pneumonectomy for pulmonary hemorrhage in tuberculosis. Am Rev Tbc 61:426, 1950.

Wood DA, Miller M: The role of the dual pulmonary circulation in various pathologic conditions of the lungs. J Thorac Surg 7:649, 1938.

Yesner R, Hurwitz A: A report of a case of localized bronchopulmonary aspergillosis successfully treated by surgery. J Thorac Surg 20:310, 1950.

References for Section XIII: The Use of Lasers for Tracheobronchial Lesions

Bennett WR Jr, Faust WL, McFarlane RA, Patel CKN: Dissociative excitation transfer and optical maser action oscillation in Ne-O_2 and Ar-O_2 rf discharges. Phys Review Letters 8:470, 1962.

Buettner GR, Oberley LW: The apparent production of superoxide and hydroxyl radicals by hematoporphyrin and light as seen by spin-trapping. FEBS Lett 121:161, 1980.

Cortese DA, Kinsey JH: Endoscopic management of lung cancer with hematoporphyrin derivative phototherapy. Mayo Clin Proc 57:543, 1982.

Dougherty TJ: Photoradiation therapy for cutaneous and subcutaneous malignancies. J Invest Dermatol 77:122, 1981.

Dougherty TJ, Gomer CJ, Weishaupt KR: Energetics and efficiency of photoinactivation of murine tumor cells containing hematoporphyrin. Cancer Res 36:2330, 1976.

Dougherty TJ, Kaufman JE, Goldfarb A, Weishaupt KR, Boyle D, Mittleman A: Photoradiation therapy for the treatment of malignant tumors. Cancer Res 38:2628, 1978.

Dougherty TJ, Lawrence G, Kaufman JH, et al: Photoradiation in the treatment of recurrent breast carcinoma. J Natl Cancer Inst 62:231, 1979.

Dougherty TJ, Weishaupt KR, Boyle DG: Photosensitizers. In DeVita VT Jr, Hellman S, Rosenberg SA (eds): Cancer: Principles and Practice of Oncology. Philadelphia, J. B. Lippincott Company, 1982, pp. 1836–1844.

Dwyer RM, Yellin AA, Bass M, Cherlow J: Laser-induced hemostasis in the canine stomach. JAMA 231:486, 1975.

Einstein A: Zur Quantentheorie der Strahlung. Phys. Z. 18:121–128, 1917.

Figge FHJ, Weiland GS, Manganiello LOJ: Cancer detection and therapy. Affinity of neoplastic, embryonic, and traumatized tissues for porphyrins and metalloporphyrins. Proc Soc Exp Biol Med 68:640–641, 1948.

Frühmorgen P, Bodem F, Reidenbach HD et al.: Endoscopic laser coagulation of bleeding gastrointestinal lesions with report of first therapeutic application in man. Gastrointest Endosc 23:73, 1976.

Goldman L (ed): The Biomedical Laser: Technology and Clinical Applications. New York, Springer-Verlag, 1981, p. 4.

Goodale RL, Okada A, Gonzales R, et al: Rapid endoscopic control of bleeding gastric erosions by laser radiation. Arch Surg 101:211, 1970.

Gordon JP, Zeigler HJ, Townes CH: The maser: New type of microwave amplifier, frequency standard, and spectrometer. Physiol Rev 99:1264, 1955.

Hayata Y, Kato H, Konaka C, et al: Hematoporphyrin derivative and laser photoradiation in the treatment of lung cancer. Chest 81:269, 1982.

Javan A, Bennett WR Jr, Herriott DR: Population inversion and continuous optical maser oscillation in a gas discharge containing a He-Ne mixture. Phys Rev Letters 6:106, 1961.

Kelly JF, Snell ME: Hematoporphyrin derivative: A possible aid in the diagnosis and therapy of carcinoma of the bladder. J Urol 115:150, 1976.

Kiefhaber P, Nath G, Moritz K: Endoscopic control of massive gastrointestinal hemorrhage by irradiation with a high-power neodymium-YAG laser. Prog Surg 15:140, 1977.

Maiman TH: Stimulated optical radiation in ruby. Nature 187:493, 1960.

Patel CKN, McFarlane RA, Faust WL: Selective excitation through vibrational energy transfer and optical maser action in N_2-CO_2. Phys Rev 13:617, 1964.

Schawlow AL: Quoted in Goldman, 1981, p. 4.

Toty L, Personne C, Colchen A, Vourc'h, G: Bronchoscopic management of tracheal lesions using the neodymium yttrium aluminum garnet laser. Thorax 36:175, 1981.

Weishaupt KR, Gomer CJ, Dougherty TJ: Identification of singlet oxygen as the cytotoxic agent in photoinactivation of a murine tumor. Cancer Res 2326, 1976.

INDEX

Page numbers in *italics* indicate illustrations. Page numbers followed by t indicate tables.